"I am delighted to welcome this important and wide-ranging book on offender rehabilitation in many different Asian countries. It should be of great interest to criminologists, psychologists, social scientists, and criminal justice policy-makers and practitioners throughout the world."

David P. Farrington, *Emeritus Professor of Psychological Criminology, Cambridge University*

"Chu and Daffern have assembled a marvelous collection of chapters that describe the efforts and challenges of developing and implementing rehabilitation across a diversity of Asian countries. This book will certainly become a fixture on the bookshelves of researchers and practitioners in Asia. For Western readers, however, do not be misled by the title. This book offers valuable lessons for rehabilitation programming in non-Asian jurisdictions."

James Bonta, *Ph.D., Author,* The Psychology of Criminal Conduct

"The book, *Approaches to Offender Rehabilitation in Asian Jurisdictions*, constitutes a laudable effort to draw attention to the field of forensic mental health. This edited volume – edited by Chi Meng Chu and Michael Daffern, two internationally recognized experts – represents a significant step in the study of offender assessment, management, and rehabilitation in the Asia continent. This book brings together scholars and practitioners from different Asian countries and adds to the literature on offender rehabilitation in several ways including better understanding how offender rehabilitation is strategized and delivered in different countries. It is an invaluable reference for scholars, field practitioners, policymakers, and graduate students interested in this field of study. Highly recommended!"

Heng Choon (Oliver) Chan, *Ph.D., Associate Professor of Criminology, Department of Social Policy, Sociology, and Criminology, University of Birmingham, Birmingham, United Kingdom*

T0372257

APPROACHES TO OFFENDER REHABILITATION IN ASIAN JURISDICTIONS

This book aims to understand how Asian jurisdictions conceptualise rehabilitation within both the correctional and forensic mental health sectors.

Little has been written about rehabilitation practices for people in criminal justice and forensic mental health services in Asia. Although there is some recognition of the need to develop and/or adjust rehabilitation practices for non-white/non-western peoples in Western jurisdictions, the extent to which Western-derived practices have been considered, adjusted, or adopted in Asian countries is not well known. This book includes contributions from an international team who explore the ways in which history, culture, religion, and resources impact how rehabilitation is conceptualised and offered in multiple Asian countries. It aims to provide an understanding of the relative merits of contemporary Western practices across different Asian countries and consider how these practices have been adopted and adapted within correctional and forensic mental health sectors.

This book is essential for administrators who are developing rehabilitation strategies and for practitioners working with people who have a history of offending behaviour.

Chi Meng Chu is Senior Principal Clinical and Forensic Psychologist, as well as Director of Translational Social Research Division and Strategic Planning Office at the National Council of Social Service in Singapore. He is also an adjunct associate professor at the Department of Psychology, National University of Singapore.

Michael Daffern is a clinical psychologist who has worked in prisons and in general and forensic mental health services. He is Professor of Clinical Forensic Psychology and Director of the Centre for Forensic Behavioural Science, Swinburne University of Technology, Australia.

International Perspectives on Forensic Mental Health

A Routledge Book Series
Edited by Patricia Zapf
Palo Alto University

The goal of this series is to improve the quality of health care services in forensic and correctional settings by providing a forum for discussing issues and disseminating resources related to policy, administration, clinical practice, and research. The series addresses topics such as mental health law; the organization and administration of forensic and/or correctional services for persons with mental disorders; the development, implementation and evaluation of treatment programs and interventions for individuals in civil and criminal justice settings; the assessment and management of violence risk, including risk for sexual violence and family violence; and staff selection, training, and development in forensic and/or correctional systems.

Published Titles

Diversity and Marginalisation in Forensic Mental Health Care
Edited by Jack Tomlin and Birgit Vollm

Safeguarding the Quality of Forensic Assessment in Sentencing: A Review Across Western Nations
Edited by Michiel van der Wolf

Globalization, Displacement, and Psychiatry: Global Histories of Trauma
Edited by Sanaullah Khan and Elliott Schwebach

Approaches to Offender Rehabilitation in Asian Jurisdictions
Chi Meng Chu and Michael Daffern

APPROACHES TO OFFENDER REHABILITATION IN ASIAN JURISDICTIONS

Edited by Chi Meng Chu and Michael Daffern

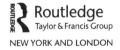

Routledge
Taylor & Francis Group

NEW YORK AND LONDON

Designed cover image: zennie © Getty Images

First published 2024
by Routledge
605 Third Avenue, New York, NY 10158

and by Routledge
4 Park Square, Milton Park, Abingdon, Oxon, OX14 4RN

Routledge is an imprint of the Taylor & Francis Group, an informa business

© 2024 selection and editorial matter, Chi Meng Chu and Michael Daffern; individual chapters, the contributors

The right of Chi Meng Chu and Michael Daffern to be identified as the authors of the editorial material, and of the authors for their individual chapters, has been asserted in accordance with sections 77 and 78 of the Copyright, Designs and Patents Act 1988.

ISBN: 978-1-032-42035-6 (hbk)
ISBN: 978-1-032-41867-4 (pbk)
ISBN: 978-1-003-36091-9 (ebk)

DOI: 10.4324/9781003360919

Typeset in Sabon
by MPS Limited, Dehradun

MD: For Lenore
CMC: For Adele and Eloise

CONTENTS

CONTRIBUTORS

Angelo de Alwis is a Consultant Forensic Psychiatrist with the Gold Coast Mental Health Service. He has previously worked as a consultant psychiatrist with Forensicare, Victoria, Australia and with the Forensic Mental Health Service in Sri Lanka. He has a special interest in the mental health and legal interface and in the history of psychiatry.

Brandon Burgess (he/him) is a clinical psychology student at the University of Manitoba, Canada. He has a Masters in Applied Forensic Psychology from Saint Mary's University in Halifax, Nova Scotia. His current research interests broadly involve improving forensic mental health service delivery for diverse or underserved populations.

Victor Cheng (Ph.D.) is a distinguished Senior Specialist at the Ministry of Justice Taiwan (R.O.C), with an extensive background in planning. An Adjunct Professor at Taiwan Police College, and a Visiting Scholar to renowned institutions like the University of Cambridge, Max Planck Institute, Zhejiang University, and Peking University. His extensive contributions shape the realms of criminal psychology, criminology and criminal justice across multiple nations.

Chi Meng Chu holds concurrent appointments at the National Council of Social Service as the Director (Translational Social Research Division), Director (Strategic Planning Office), and Senior Principal Clinical and Forensic Psychologist. He is also the Director (Special Projects) at the

Ministry of Social and Family Development, and an Adjunct Associate Professor at the Department of Psychology, National University of Singapore.

Wing Hong Chui is Professor and Head at the Department of Applied Social Sciences at The Hong Kong Polytechnic University. Prior to this, he was a youth social worker who worked with at risk youth and juvenile offenders. He has continued to seek to build a better world through his varied contributions at work.

Michael Daffern is a clinical psychologist who has worked in prisons and in general and forensic mental health services. He is Professor of Clinical Forensic Psychology and Director of the Centre for Forensic Behavioural Science, Swinburne University of Technology.

Andrew Forrester is Professor of Forensic Psychiatry at Cardiff University, and Consultant Forensic Psychiatrist with Oxleas NHS Foundation Trust. He has worked as a psychiatrist in prisons and criminal justice settings for over 25 years. His research focuses on mental health conditions in places of detention, mainly amongst marginalised groups.

Guru S. Gowda is an Assistant Professor in the Department of Psychiatry at the National Institute of Mental Health and Neuro Sciences (NIMHANS), Bengaluru, India. He is an early-career psychiatrist interested in diverse areas such as forensic psychiatry, ethics, social psychiatry, neuropsychiatry, and the mental health of special populations, particularly homeless individuals with mental illness.

Md. Amir Hussain is a Consultant Clinical Psychologist of Bangladesh who has worked in the mental health arena for over 14 years. He has several publications in national and international journals on drugs and marginalized populations issues. He has worked in the Bangladesh prison system from 2016 to 2022 and has developed a manual and conducted training in all 68 prisons in Bangladesh.

Yongmyeng Keum is the director of the Research Institute for Prisons and a university lecturer. He worked as a correctional officer for 30 years and researched prison design and Korean correctional policy. He is currently engaged in correctional studies, such as correctional practice, prison design, and prison history.

Al Aditya Khan (Dr.) is a consultant forensic psychiatrist in NHS, UK. He currently works in a medium secure psychiatric hospital. He is the associate clinical director for Kent Prisons and has worked in forensic psychiatry for over 17 years. His research interests include mental health and rehabilitation within prison and secure services.

Seung C. Lee (Ph.D.) is a research advisor for Public Safety Canada (Corrections Research Unit). He has researched and published articles on the validity of risk assessment instruments for violent and sexual offenses, as well as their application to different ethnic minority groups (e.g., Hispanic, Black, Indigenous, and Asian).

Jianhong Liu is a Distinguished Professor in the Faculty of Law at the University of Macau. He earned his Ph.D. from the State University of New York at Albany in 1993 and is the winner of the 2016 "Freda Adler Distinguished Scholar Award" and the 2018 "Gerhard O.W. Mueller Award" for Distinguished Contributions to International Criminal Justice. He is the Founding and Honorary President of the Asian Criminological Society.

Susitha Mendis (Dr.) is a consultant forensic psychiatrist from Sri Lanka. He was previously attached to the National Hospital Kandy and set up the new forensic psychiatric service. He works as an expert witness for criminal and civil cases and deals with victims and witnesses of crimes and mentally ill offenders. His interests include forensic phenomenology, forensic ethics, correctional psychiatry and deception. He dedicates his time to mental health law reforms, the development of forensic services and postgraduate training.

Pratima Murthy (Dr.) is a Senior Professor of Psychiatry and Director at the National Institute of Mental Health and Neuro Sciences (NIMHANS), Bengaluru, India. She has a keen interest in forensic psychiatry, substance use disorders and the history of psychiatry. She has served as a consultant to various international agencies, such as the United Nations Office on Drugs and Crime, the International Labour Organization, and the World Health Organization.

Carmelia Nathen is Chief Probation Officer and Director of the Probation and Community Rehabilitation Service in the Ministry of Social and Family Development in Singapore. Her involvement with statutory services spans over 25 years. As the former Director of Child Protective

Service, she supported a fundamental review of the child protection system and helped shape key policies. She continues to draw on her experiences to advance policies and practices in offender rehabilitation.

Alicia Nijdam-Jones (Dr., she/her) is a Registered Psychologist and Assistant Professor in the Department of Psychology at the University of Manitoba in Canada. She specialises in violence risk assessment, malingering assessment, community-based participatory research, and the use of forensic assessment measures with linguistically, ethnically, and culturally diverse samples.

Kala Ruby is Senior Assistant Director at the Probation and Community Rehabilitation Service in the Ministry of Social and Family Development in Singapore. She has over 10 years of experience in offender management programme development, research and training. She has contributed to multiple research studies to advance evidence-based work and continues to be involved in the development of data-driven policies and practices in the rehabilitation of probationers.

Howard Ryland (Dr.) is a clinical academic psychiatrist based in Oxford, UK. He completed his training in forensic psychiatry in 2017 and his DPhil (PhD) in Psychiatry from the University of Oxford in 2021. He has a strong interest in international mental health services and criminal justice systems. He was previously the President of the European Federation of Psychiatric Trainees.

Apichat Saengsin is a psychiatrist who has worked in general and forensic mental health services as well as prisons. Currently, he works at Galya Rajanagarindra Institute of Forensic Psychiatry, Bangkok, Thailand.

Weerapong Sanmontree is a mental health physician who has worked in general and forensic mental health services as well as prisons. Currently, he works at Galya Rajanagarindra Institute of Forensic Psychiatry, Bangkok, Thailand.

Jaydip Sarkar is a consultant forensic psychiatrist at Forensicare, Melbourne, Australia. He practises court room psychiatry in many jurisdictions. He was involved in a landmark case in Singapore that led to a legal precedence in a death penalty case. His co-edited book won the British Medical Association's "Best Medical Book in Psychiatry" award for "Clinical Topics in Personality Disorder".

Melvinder Singh is Deputy Director of Psychological Services and Policy Planning in the Psychological and Correctional Rehabilitation Division of Singapore Prison Service (SPS). Melvinder is a clinical psychologist by training and has been with the Public Service for over 20 years. He has served in a variety of positions in the areas of forensic psychology, research, programme evaluation and data science. He currently oversees the work of forensic psychologists and shapes the development and use of the risk assessment framework in SPS.

Zora A. Sukabdi (Dr.) is a forensic psychologist. One of her patents includes a 3D-Model of Motivation-Ideology-Capability Terrorism Risk Assessments and Rehabilitation. Zora works as a senior lecturer at the School of Strategic and Global Studies University of Indonesia and Executive Office Member of Indonesian Forensic Psychology Association (APSIFOR).

Masaru Takahashi is an associate professor of Ochanomizu University, Japan. Dr. Takahashi received his Ph.D. in Counselling Science from University of Tsukuba. His research interests focus on corrections, particularly offender recidivism risk assessment, risk communication, evaluation of psychological interventions for offenders, and addictive behaviours among correctional inmates.

Armon Tamatea (*Rongowhakāta; Te Aitanga-a-Māhaki*) (PhD., PGDipPsych (Clin) is a clinical psychologist who served as a senior advisor for the Department of Corrections (New Zealand) before being appointed to the University of Waikato. His research interests include institutional violence, psychopathy, New Zealand gang communities, and exploring culturally informed approaches to offender management.

Bhavika Vajawat (Dr.) is a Senior Resident in Forensic Psychiatry at the National Institute of Mental Health and Neurosciences (NIMHANS), Bangalore, India. She is an early career psychiatrist interested in forensic psychiatry, ethics, cultural psychiatry, and special populations like prisoners, children, women, and the elderly.

Yixuan Wang is a member of the Asian Society of Criminology and the Macau Society of Criminology. She is a currently a PhD student in the Faculty of Law at the University of Macau. Her research interests include criminal procedure, juvenile delinquency and criminal justice.

Kim J. Wheeler is the author of fifteen books of several different genres, an award-winning photographer and poet. Born in London, he became a self-taught photographer, poet, writer, and editor. He is a life coach at charity organisations for youth rehabilitation in Indonesia.

Aaron H. L. Wong is a part-time Research Assistant in the Department of Social and Behavioural Sciences at City University of Hong Kong. He holds an MPhil in Criminology from University of Cambridge and an LLM in Criminal Law and Criminal Justice from the University of Edinburgh.

Frank Wong is a Research Assistant in the Department of Social and Behavioural Sciences at City University of Hong Kong. He holds an LLB and a PCLL from the City University of Hong Kong.

Jeongsook Yoon (Ph.D.) is the Director of the Research Division for Crime Analysis and Survey at the Korean Institute of Criminology and Justice. Her primary research focuses on analysing the criminal and psychological characteristics of various types of crime, including violent and sexual crimes, and intimate partner violence.

ACKNOWLEDGEMENTS

We would like to thank Maree Stanford for assistance with proofreading and formatting.

INTRODUCTION

1

INTRODUCTION

Chi Meng Chu and Michael Daffern

Introduction

There are approximately 11 million people imprisoned around the world (Walsmley, 2018). Most will be released, and many will successfully reintegrate. What helps one person desist from crime and reconnect with their community may not work for another and what works in one country may not work for others. The way in which criminal justice and forensic mental health systems prioritise and seek to reform and reintegrate people who have broken the law varies around the world. We suspect these variations exist due to differences in history, culture, laws, politics and resources. Our focus in this book is on rehabilitation[1] practices in Asia. Many countries in Asia are ancient and there is considerable diversity in culture, religion, resources and history. As countries around the world reshaped their criminal justice systems during the 18th and 19th centuries, establishing prisons and laying a foundation for modern parole systems, many Asian countries were under colonial rule. Laws were imported, sentencing practices were founded to maintain order and control for economic advantage, and attitudes towards reformation and offender care and management were established.

In recent years, various assessment methods and approaches to rehabilitation that originated in the West have been questioned, based on whether they appropriately consider the values, morals and traditions of individuals from different demographic backgrounds. Questions have also been raised as to whether Western models should be imported into countries that are very different from the ones in which they originated.

DOI: 10.4324/9781003360919-2

It is also increasingly clear that other therapeutic modalities and preferences for working with people who have offended exist. The need for openness to explore various ways of helping people change and a comparative analyses of various interventions and rehabilitative approaches is burgeoning. Given increasing globalisation that has resulted in more culturally-diverse nations, it is important to consider how history, culture, religion and resources might impact on how people might work towards rehabilitation and reintegration. Such information can help practitioners and policy makers to create new services and adapt their own practices to better meet the needs of the communities they serve.

Context: Asia

Asia is the largest of the world's continents, with countries spread across its northernmost tip on the Arctic Ocean to its easternmost tip, the Pacific Ocean, the Indian Ocean to the south and Europe to the West. Some parts of Asia are densely populated and populous, including China and India, whereas other areas are sparse. There is variation in the wealth of different Asian countries, with several countries amongst the richest in the world, whereas some are the poorest. The resources that are available to criminal justice and forensic mental health services vary; accordingly, access to resources to support rehabilitation also varies.

Asia is the birthplace of several of the world's major religions, including Islam, Hinduism and Buddhism, and there is a diversity of religions practiced. Hinduism is the main religion in India and Islam is the dominant religion in Bangladesh, Indonesia, Malaysia and Pakistan. Indeed, there are more people of Islamic faith living in Indonesia than in any other country of the world. Buddhism is widely practiced in Thailand, South Korea, Singapore, Taiwan, Japan, Thailand, Sri Lanka and China. Christianity, Confucianism, Jainism, Judaism, Shinto, Sikhism and Taoism are also commonly practiced. Some religions incorporate all aspects of personal and social life and therefore have an influence on politics. Alarid and Wang (2001) note for instance that Buddhist groups are politically active in Sri Lanka, Burma, Thailand, Cambodia and Japan, much like Christianity and Islam impact politics in multiple other countries around the world. Religion therefore plays an important role in determining how crime is understood in Asia; specifically, how people who break the law should be regarded, and what reformative activity should look like in Asian correctional and forensic mental health services. As noted below, and discussed in several chapters, religious services and guidance are a part of many Asian countries' rehabilitation programmes. For example, although rehabilitation of people convicted of terrorism offences is not this book's priority, it is evident that deradicalisation programmes for people of Islamic faith often emphasise religious discussions and instruction, often led by clerics (e.g., Bjørgo & Carlsson, 2008).

The histories of Asian countries vary widely. Many countries were colonised during the period when prisons were being established around the world, and some countries remained under colonial rule until after World War II. European nations, including Spain, Holland, Portugal, the United Kingdom and France, colonised various Asian countries from the 16th to the 20th century. The impacts of colonisation on ideology, political structures and social systems are profound. Legal systems and criminal justice practices are a product of these different histories, with colonial rulers typically importing and imposing laws and criminal justice systems from their home countries. Much like the history of forced migration of offenders to countries like the United States and Australia, many people who offended in colonised countries were transported to other parts of Asia, both as a punishment and also to develop the economies of other colonies. Yang (2003) notes the influence of British colonisation of India and Ceylon and the use of transportation of offenders to other colonies, an act of banishment that served to punish and deter others, as well as providing free labour to enhance economic development in the growing British empire. In ancient Asian cultures, banishment and exile were common communal responses to crime (Horigan, 1996). Yang (2003) also notes the particular cultural significance of banishment in India, which encouraged its use by English colonial forces: "it was believed to have the added virtue of being a transgressive punishment, that is, it transgressed indigenous notions about the religious and cultural dangers of crossing the *kala pani* or the 'black waters'" (p. 186; a reference to travelling over surrounding seas). Consequently, transportation for life was regarded as more severe than a lifetime of incarceration, hence it was considered to have considerable deterrent impacts.

Zhong and Zhang (2021) highlighted the different histories that have contributed to the development of diverse criminal justice systems in Asia. For example, Japan learned mainly from the German and French systems during the 1868 Meiji Restoration, whereas China, Vietnam and North Korea are socialist states that have been greatly influenced by the Soviet Union. India, Hong Kong and Malaysia adopted models from the United Kingdom as they were previously British colonies. Furthermore, some Western countries provide aid to Asian countries for the development of criminal justice systems and this has influenced the type of rehabilitation programmes that exist across Asian countries.

Sentencing practices also differ throughout Asia. Several countries (e.g., China, Vietnam, Indonesia, Singapore, Bangladesh, Taiwan, Sri Lanka and Malaysia) maintain the death penalty (as at the time this book was written). This penalty is often the result of conviction for very serious crimes (e.g., murder), but drug offences in some countries also attract the death penalty. By contrast, some similar crimes in other Asian jurisdictions may seem to be intertwined with that country's political institutions such that judicial systems may be more tolerant of such offences (Zhong & Zhang, 2021). Take the case of Myanmar, where the government reportedly benefitted from the drug trade (Cornell & Swanstrom, 2006). Zhong and Zhang also noted the influence of gender hierarchies and gender-related subcultures that might mean family violence (specifically violence towards female intimates) is difficult to control through criminal justice institutions and practices.

Rates of incarceration vary widely in Asia, from relatively high rates in Thailand (411 people in prison per 100,000 of the national population) to 36 people per 100,000 of the national population in Japan. There are also differences in the proportion of women in custody, from 19.7% of the prisoner population in Hong Kong (China) to 1.6% of the prisoner population in Pakistan (World Prison Brief, 2021). This may suggest differences in criminal behaviour amongst men and women in Asian countries but also different criminal justice responses.

The Nelson Mandela and Bangkok Rules, United Nations Principles and Common Rehabilitation Principles and Frameworks

The United Nations Standard Minimum Rules for the Treatment of Prisoners (i.e., Nelson Mandela Rules, 2015) Rule 4 states that the purpose of imprisonment is to protect society from crime and to reduce recidivism. Signatories are encouraged to embrace policies and procedures that not only ensure the secure, safe and humane custody of prisoners but also reform, to aid reintegration, autonomy and desistance from crime. Precisely what each jurisdiction should do to reform incarcerated individuals is not dictated, but Rule 92 states:

> ... appropriate means shall be used, including religious care in the countries where this is possible, education, vocational guidance and training, social casework, employment counselling, physical development and strengthening of moral character, in accordance with the individual needs of each prisoner, taking account of his or her social and criminal history, physical and mental capacities and aptitudes, personal temperament, the length of his or her sentence and prospects after release.

How this rule manifests and the specific practices that are used in different jurisdictions around the world are neither mandated nor clear. The United Nations Office on Drugs and Crime's *Introductory Handbook on the Prevention of Recidivism and the Social Reintegration of Offenders* (2012) elaborates on the Mandela Rules, but notes the complexity of rehabilitation practices, suggesting these vary according to existing laws, available resources and the receptiveness of the population to rehabilitation practices. Relatedly, criminal justice systems often overlook the needs of justice-involved women and girls. Adopted in 2010 by the United Nations General Assembly, the United Nations Rules for the Treatment of Female Prisoners and Non-Custodial Measures for Women Offenders (i.e., the "Bangkok Rules") are important to protecting the rights of women who have offended and those who are in custody or incarcerated. In addition, these rules are important for looking into the different needs and situations of incarcerated women. The Bangkok Rules were initiated by the Government of Thailand, with Her Royal Highness Princess Bajrakitiyabha of Thailand having contributed crucially to their development.

Forensic mental health services and prisons also need to be mindful of the United Nations Principles for the protection of persons with mental illness and the improvement of mental health care, adopted by the United Nations General Assembly (resolution 46/1190) in 1991. These principles, in particular, principle 20, which refers to "criminal offenders" with mental illness, note that all other principles for care (Principle 1) and treatment (especially Principle 11) are relevant. Nevertheless, as seen in the various chapters in this book, forensic mental health services vary widely across Asian jurisdictions.

Overarching rehabilitation frameworks such as the Risk-Need-Responsivity model (RNR; Andrews & Bonta, 2010) and Good Lives Model (GLM; Ward & Brown, 2004), are suggested as potentially beneficial for offender rehabilitation by the United Nations Office on Drugs and Crime (2015). Originating from Canada in the 1990s, the Risk-Need-Responsivity model has been widely embraced in many Western jurisdictions. The mechanism for change that is indicated by the RNR model pertains to the modification of criminogenic needs, and there is broad acceptance of the importance of common ("Central Eight") criminogenic needs across jurisdictions worldwide. These criminogenic needs are typically the focus of rehabilitation efforts in criminal justice systems that embrace the RNR model.

Developed in New Zealand in the early 2000s, the GLM is a strength-based rehabilitation framework that is responsive to the interests, abilities and aspirations of people who have offended. It posits that all individuals have aspirations and needs and that individuals will need to acquire the skills and knowledge that are required to succeed in the world. Criminal behaviour results when individuals lack the internal and external resources necessary to satisfy their needs using pro-social means. Practitioners will have to work with people who have offended to develop intervention plans that will help the person acquire the capabilities to achieve outcomes that are personally meaningful to them.

Notwithstanding the widespread adoption of the RNR and GLM models in many Western jurisdictions, there is a dearth of literature examining their applicability, use and impact in Asia. There are reports of training and treatment efforts in Hong Kong, Japan, Singapore and South Korea (amongst other jurisdictions; e.g., Chu & Zeng, 2017; Chua et al., 2014; Hong Kong Psychological Society, 2021; Ministry of Justice, Japan, 2021; Yoon et al., 2021) that allude to the use of RNR and GLM principles, but there is little written on their implementation, adaptation and/or effectiveness in Asia. This is an important point because the cross-cultural and cross-jurisdictional applications of these models may pose implementation, and subsequently, efficacy challenges.

Relatedly, Pusch and Holtfreter (2017) observed that risk assessment measures and intervention programmes have primarily been developed in Western jurisdictions, and routinely used to assess risk and to intervene with people from different ethnicities, cultures and countries. Unfortunately, this practice is ubiquitous despite the limited knowledge about the cross-cultural transferability of these instruments and methods (Shepherd & Lewis-Fernandez, 2016). In particular, Schmidt et al. (2020) noted there is limited research on the psychometric properties of risk assessment instruments across different cultural groups – an absence of "separate test norms for culturally diverse populations, and a lack of attention to issues of diversity" (p. 2).

Schmidt et al. (2020) also argued that dynamic risk factors "vary across cultures with respect to their prevalence and their ability to predict reoffending" (p. 4). These authors have subsequently highlighted how many (purported) dynamic risk factors fail to identify crime-related problems amongst people in non-European and North American contexts; positing that dynamic risk factors are normative and influenced by legal judgements, as well as social and ethical values. The lack of cultural equivalence in these dynamic risk factors may lead to problems with the accuracy of risk assessment and formulations, development and placement in suitable interventions (Schmidt et al., 2021). Similarly, Friedman (1990) suggested that the values that are reflected within dynamic risk factors could be unstable across time and cultures. These could collectively explain why the adoption and effectiveness of intervention efforts may vary across jurisdictions. According to Schmidt et al. (2020) the cross-cultural transferability of dynamic risk factors, as delineated by the General Personality and Cognitive Social Learning model of crime (Andrews & Bonta, 2010), has not been adequately supported and therefore, it cannot be assumed that these are an appropriate basis for rehabilitation efforts.

To facilitate an understanding of how sociocultural context can affect individual agency, Strauss-Hughes et al.'s (2019) Cultural-Ecological Predictive Agency Model (CEPAM) "focuses on the interaction between persons and contexts while considering the historical process through which this came to be" (p. 9). Specifically, these historical processes include education, employment and leisure opportunities that may differ across cultures and affect the prevalence of crime. CEPAM highlights two pathways that could influence individual agency. First, inequitably structured context, in which individual action occurs, can lead to increased likelihood of indigenous contact with criminal justice systems. Second, intergenerational discrimination and deprivation within an individual's developmental context can lead to an increased likelihood of individuals forming general mental models of themselves and others, further contributing to offending behaviours in some situations. In translating this understanding, Strauss-Hughes et al. (2022) posited that a possible approach to rehabilitation practice is to incorporate different cultural values, principles, as well as norms of knowledge and practice. In particular, this would require embracing Western scientific and indigenous epistemologies in a meaningful and ethical way – without the need for separate practice frameworks for culture.

The Importance of Culture and Religion in Asian Criminal Justice Approaches

Cultures and communities specify which attitudes and behaviours are to be considered normal, and consequently, which behaviours are regarded as criminal (Bhugra et al., 2010; Lahlah et al., 2013). For example, how individuals express anger varies across different cultures (Matsumoto et al., 2010), and this could lead to differences in the manifestation and acceptance of violence. Hence, interventions for such behaviours may also differ across countries and cultures. Understanding the historical, cultural and religious factors that contribute to "criminal" behaviours is crucial to understanding criminal justice response to crime, which are also, invariably, influenced by the availability of resources and sociopolitical considerations at the point in time. Although priority is often given to rehabilitation in Western societies, this may not often be the case in non-Western jurisdictions, where punishment, deterrence and protection of the public may be prioritised.

Convened during an era of "Nothing works" and before the advent of RNR and GLM, the First Asian and Pacific Conference of Correctional Administrators in 1980 is one of the first known (to the best of our knowledge) attempts to bring together leaders in the correctional field within Asia; and its proceedings give an indication of relative preferences (rehabilitation versus punishment) and practices at the time. In the Opening Address of this conference, His Honour, the Chief Justice of Hong Kong, Sir Denys Roberts, highlighted the principle objective for correctional administrators should be rehabilitation, but that punishment and deterrence were also key considerations. Differences in criminal justice responses and rehabilitation philosophies across Asian jurisdictions in the 1980s were evident in these proceedings. For example, representations from Indonesia noted a transition from the colonial *Sistem Kepenjaraan* (which promoted harsh punishment that was believed to lead to deterrence and repentance) to *Sistem Pemasyarakatan*, which focused on the resocialisation of people in prison by assisting them to acquire skills to facilitate a healthy reintegration. The latter emphasised the notion that it is not enough for the criminal justice system to focus on community protection, that protection should also be accorded to people who are convicted. Similarly, Malaysia and Philippines prioritised education and skills acquisition to help people in prison to reintegrate, whereas Thailand reported a more punitive regime that advocated punishment as a form of retribution.

The following brief introduction to cultural, and religious factors introduces readers to some of the important factors that are elaborated in this book and hints at the ways that these might influence rehabilitation practices, putting into context the preferences and practices described in the following country-specific chapters.

Cultural Factors

Scholars and practitioners working in the field of offender rehabilitation have long acknowledged that cultural differences should be carefully noted and adequately addressed when considering intervention approaches. Laungani's (2004) study of Asian approaches to psychological interventions highlighted some critical differences between Asian and Western cultures, which can be explained through four key dimensions: (1) individualism–communalism, (2) cognitivism–emotionalism, (3) free will–determinism and (4) materialism–spiritualism. In addition, Naeem et al. (2019) posited that Asians tended to orient towards the community, be more receptive toward spiritual explanations, and also more accepting of a deterministic view of life - further highlighting the importance of religion in Asia. Gender may also influence participation in psychotherapy in some cultures; for example, Shaikh and Hatcher (2005) found that women from some cultures are less likely to attend therapy because they might require permission from a man and needed to be brought by men to the clinic. As such, it is not unexpected that explanatory models of mental health problems and criminal behaviour may vary across cultures and jurisdictions, leading to very different responses to crime.

Criminology and studies of social control have been explored in Asia with Zhong and Zhang (2021) drawing attention to the Asian paradigm. They noted:

> Asian societies [centre] on attachment, [honour], harmony, and the holistic cognitive mode, while Western countries [emphasise] independence, materialistic success, individual rights, and the analytical cognitive mode. Western social control of crime thus adopts a conflict-based approach with a focus on individualistic retribution and punishment. The Western control mode requires complex and mature formal justice and legal systems to ensure legal rights and fairness are guaranteed. In contrast, the Asian paradigm is solution-oriented, aiming to resolve all conflicts through working communities. That is, communities, offenders, and victims in Asia will work together to achieve justice. Such a paradigm is rooted in the collective social [organisations] and lifestyles of Asian people, as well as the less developed formal control systems in most Asian societies. (p. 5)

The potential for differences across cultures is noted within the United Nations Office on Drugs and Crime's (2012) Introductory Handbook on the Prevention of Recidivism and the Social Reintegration of Offenders. This handbook suggests that culture should be considered when designing programmes, although notes: "The challenge, of course, continues to lie in the difficulty of translating the abstract model upon which the framework is based into specific interventions adapted to different groups of offenders" (p. 23). Cognitive behavioural and social learning methods are advocated but the extent to which these modalities are emphasised in correctional and forensic mental health settings within Asia is unclear.

Religious Factors

The Nelson Mandela Rules highlight the fact that religious instruction may be an important feature of rehabilitation programming in some countries. Reporting on the work of Christian chaplains and Buddhist prison volunteers in Hong Kong, Chui and Cheng (2013) noted that chaplains "want inmates to learn include humility, respect, patience, and gratitude, all of which are intrinsically religious and come from biblical teachings. The chaplains explained that they explore the potentials or values that inmates possess and encourage them to develop these, and that they teach them how they could contribute to society" (p. 162). Similarly, they observed that "the Buddhist volunteers believe that religion is crucial to the rehabilitation of offenders. However, the emphasis is placed on making peace with oneself and more importantly, understanding the consequences of wrongful actions. This goes back to the Buddhist teaching of karma" (p. 162).

Reading this description, one may wonder how countries where a large proportion of the population identifies as Buddhist, such as Thailand, can also maintain the death penalty, particularly when observers (e.g., Horigan, 1996) note that a more compassionate response, including rehabilitation should be favoured, using "the path to enlightenment, which would enable even the most dangerous convicted killer to find his or her Buddha-nature" (p. 237; Horigan, 1996, as cited in Alarid and Wang, 2001). According to Alarid and Wang, the notion of *Karma*, the law of cause and effect, is central to Buddhist notions of morality, and even if somebody's actions bring benefit to oneself it cannot be considered good if it results in harm to another person. According to the five precepts of Buddha's teachings, people must not take a life (including to all living creatures), take what has not been given, engage in sexual misconduct, use "intoxicants" and engage in "false speech". Alarid and Wang posit that the death penalty is inconsistent with the precept concerning taking life, as it is in Christian countries where it violates one of the Ten Commandments but the maintenance of societal order may be preferred over adherence to this precept, particularly since Asian societies tend to emphasise a collectivistic orientation, valuing social harmony and self-restraint above individual needs and preferences.

The Focus and Orientation of This Book

This book seeks to describe contemporary rehabilitation practices in correctional and forensic mental health services across Asia. Little is known about rehabilitation practices in these countries. By encouraging local authors to describe preferences and practices we seek to understand and explicate the ways in which history, culture and religion may operate and create influence. We also hope to create a forum for these authors to collaborate and learn from each other, and for Westerners to learn more about Asian approaches. One of the key reasons for bringing together contributors is to determine whether Western-centric models (including RNR and GLM) are relevant cross-culturally and across different socio-political as well as legal contexts in Asia. Specifically, in which ways they have been used, modified, and are helpful. Another aim of this book is to consider the relative emphasis on rehabilitation within criminal justice settings in Asia. Rehabilitation, punishment, deterrence and the protection of the public are general principles that underpin sentencing practices around the world, hence their relative importance throughout Asia is of interest.

We do not claim to be experts in the cultures or rehabilitation practices in the Asian jurisdictions featured in this book; instead, we relied on local experts to present their knowledge, experiences and opinions. Our list of countries and contributors is not exhaustive, but we have included a selection of jurisdictions across Asia that will showcase the diversity in philosophy and practice. In the end, we secured chapters from Singapore, Japan, Hong Kong, South Korea, Indonesia, Thailand, Sri Lanka, India, Bangladesh, Taiwan, Macao and China. We had no avenues in North Korea; and despite having contacts from Malaysia, Pakistan and Philippines, we could not secure a commitment. Our perspective is that much of what has been written about rehabilitation practices in Asia may be known within each country; there are however few descriptions of practices in many of the countries featured in this book that have been published in Western-oriented, criminal justice and forensic mental health journals and books. We are hopeful that this book will provide a good starting point to improve our understanding of offender rehabilitation and forensic treatment work across Asia.

In addition to the abovementioned chapters, we also invited Dr. Armon Tamatea to provide a chapter to help situate rehabilitation within a broader ecological framework. Furthermore, we invited Dr. Alicia Nijdam-Jones and Mr. Brandon Burgess to close this book by commenting on how criminal justice and forensic mental health services might better conceptualise rehabilitation, when taking into account history, ethnicity, cultural needs and differences.

Final Thoughts

The observations from the First Asian and Pacific Conference of Correctional Administrators in 1980 occurred within the midst of the "Nothing works" era, well before the enunciation of the RNR principles and the development of contemporary rehabilitation-focused correctional and forensic mental health practices and models of care. An emphasis on rehabilitation clearly existed but did so within a vacuum of empirically derived principles. Research into offender rehabilitation has exploded in recent decades, yet little is known about practices in Asia.

Rehabilitation for criminal justice and forensic mental health system involved people occurs within a sociopolitical and cultural ecology but little has been written about how the ecology might impact rehabilitation. Greater awareness of the ecological framework has surrounded health interventions. According to Grzywacz and Fuqua (2000), the ecological perspective highlights the importance of the interaction between the person and their socio-physical environment. They argue that intervention programmes need to consider salient features of the person's sociopolitical and cultural context before intervening to improve health outcomes. Although their emphasis is on health outcomes, their general points are pertinent to the rehabilitation and reintegration of people who have offended. Ecological models encourage a comprehensive and focused approach to consideration of historical, cultural and environmental determinants of behaviour that can be sometimes ignored by clinicians.

A word on language used throughout this book. In recent years, our field has evidenced a preference for the use of person-centered language, avoiding terms like prisoner or offender that may be perceived as either stigmatising or labelling (Winder et al., 2021). We acknowledge the importance of this and we have encouraged authors to use person-first language in relation to justice-involved people. Our own preference has been to use terms like "people in prison", rather than "prisoner", "inmate", "convict" or "felon" to emphasise a more humanising and healing approach (although we note that reference to "offender" rehabilitation in the title of the book is inconsistent and a better title may have been "Approaches to the Rehabilitation of People Who Have Offended in Asian Jurisdictions"). Whilst we have encouraged authors to use person-first language, we respect the choices of authors and their personal preferences.

We have asked all authors to consider rehabilitation within correctional (adult and youth) and forensic mental health systems, but this was a tall order given constraints on word count and the breadth and complexity of these services. Authors have tended to emphasise either correctional or forensic mental health services practices, mostly because of familiarity, whilst also trying to show their particular jurisdiction's approach to rehabilitation more generally. We are cognisant that the authors bring practical and authentic experiences within relevant services in their jurisdictions. It is difficult to be an expert in every aspect of criminal justice and forensic mental health service provision for adults and youth, for men and women, even within one's own jurisdiction. Necessarily, there are some gaps in each chapter.

Finally, the chapters in this book elucidate contemporary practices and we can see how religion, history, culture, politics and resources have shaped rehabilitation practices. As you work through the chapters in this book your will note that, several jurisdictions are unfamiliar with the RNR framework and/or GLM, but Taiwan, Hong Kong, Japan, South Korea and Singapore are exceptions. These jurisdictions have been influenced by Western rehabilitation models yet they have modified, to varying degrees, Western practices to suit their local contexts. In some jurisdictions, historical, cultural and political contexts have significantly influenced the development of rehabilitation practices, whereby Western notions of offender rehabilitation have not found their way into common practice (see chapters on China and Macao). Some jurisdictions' rehabilitation practices are relatively less mature, and resources may be scant. Hence, religious instructions and interventions are common, in addition to employment-related training (see chapters on Bangladesh, India, Sri Lanka and Thailand). The impacts of colonialisation are apparent in several countries and colonial-era laws facilitating punitive responses to "control" law-breakers, which replaced more traditional and local responses to crime, are now being reconsidered (see chapter on Indonesia).

Although this book is not an exhaustive description of rehabilitation practices in Asian jurisdictions, this collection may be valuable for policy makers and practitioners to reflect on the experiences of their colleagues and neighbours in Asia. We also hope that by writing this book we might help people working in Western jurisdictions to appreciate the notion that different yet effective intervention strategies exist in non-Western jurisdictions. We also hope to shine a light on some jurisdictions in Asia and encourage the sharing of experiences and knowledge to help these systems develop further. Some may inevitably embrace Western frameworks, yet contextualise them to suit their own sociopolitical and cultural contexts. Equally important is the observation about how Western jurisdictions are now trying to adjust practices to ensure they are culturally sensitive and helpful. Through this endeavour, we hope to encourage respect for local cultural factors and priorities as international knowledge and experiences are considered.

Note

1 We have not sought to dictate the use of *rehabilitation* and *reform*, and these are used interchangeably in this chapter as both are used by authors of chapters in this book.

References

Alarid, L. F., & Wang, H. M. (2001). Mercy and punishment: Buddhism and the death penalty. *Social Justice, 28*, 231–252.

Andrews, D. A., & Bonta, J. (2010). *The psychology of criminal conduct* (5th ed.). New Providence, NJ: LexisNexis Matthew Bender.

Bhugra, D., Popelyuk, D., & McMullen, I. (2010). Paraphilias across cultures: Contexts and controversies. *Journal of Sex Research, 47*, 242–256.

Bjørgo, T., & Carlsson, Y. (2008). Early intervention with violent and racist youth groups. *Norwegian Institute of International Affairs, Working Paper No. 677*, p. 38.

Chu, C. M., & Zeng, G. (2017). The assessment and treatment of youth offenders in Singapore: The implementation of the risk, needs, and responsivity framework. In H. C. O. Chan & S. Ho (Eds.), *The psycho-criminological perspective of criminal justice in Asia*, pp. 200–218. London, UK: Routledge.

Chua, J. R., Chu, C. M., Yim, G., Chong, D., & Teoh, J. (2014). Implementation of the Risk-Need-Responsivity framework across the juvenile justice agencies in Singapore. *Psychiatry, Psychology and the Law, 21*, 877–889.

Chui, W. H., & Cheng, K. K. (2013). Self-perceived role and function of Christian prison chaplains and Buddhist volunteers in Hong Kong prisons. *International Journal of Offender Therapy and Comparative Criminology, 57*, 154–168.

Cornell, S., & Swanstrom, N. (2006). The Eurasian drug trade. A challenge to regional security. *Problems of Post-Communism, 53*(4), 10–28.

Friedman, L. M. (1990). *The republic of choice: Law, authority, and culture.* Cambridge, MA: Harvard University Press.

Grzywacz, G., & Fuqua, J. (2000). The social ecology of health: Leverage points and linkages. *Behavioral Medicine, 26*, 101–115.

Hong Kong Psychological Society. (2021). *Loving our work within the legal and law enforcement framework.* https://www.hkps.org.hk/zh-hant/conferences_and_events/detail/8/

Horigan, D. P. (1996). Of compassion and capital punishment: A Buddhist perspective on the death penalty. *American Journal of Jurisprudence, 41*, 271–288.

Lahlah, E., Van der Knaap, L. M., Bogaerts, S., & Lens K. M. E. (2013). Making men out of boys? Ethnic differences in juvenile violent offending and the role of gender role orientations. *Journal of Cross-Cultural Psychology, 44*, 1321–1338.

Laungani, P. (2004). *Asian perspectives in counselling and psychotherapy.* New York: Brunner-Routledge.

Matsumoto, D., Yoo, S. H., & Chung, J. (2010). The expression of anger across cultures. In M. Potegal, G. Stemmler, & C. Spielberger (Eds.), *International handbook of anger*, pp. 125–137. New York, NY: Springer.

Ministry of Justice, Japan. (2021). *Offender rehabilitation of Japan.* https://www.moj.go.jp/content/001345371.pdf

Naeem, F., Phiri P., Rathod, S., & Ayub, M. (2019). Cultural adaptation of cognitive-behavioural therapy. *BJPsych Advances, 25*, 387–395.

Pusch, N., & Holtfreter, K. (2017). Gender and risk assessment in juvenile offenders. *Criminal Justice and Behavior*, 45, 56–81. http://dx.doi.org/10.1177/0093854817721720

Schmidt, S., Heffernan, R., & Ward, T. (2020). Why we cannot explain cross-cultural differences in risk assessment. *Aggression and Violent Behavior*, 50, 101346.

Schmidt, S., Heffernan, R., & Ward, T. (2021). The cultural-agency model of criminal behavior. *Aggression & Violent Behavior*, 58, 101554.

Shaikh, B. T., & Hatcher, J. (2005). Health seeking behaviour and health service utilization in Pakistan: challenging the policy makers. *Journal of Public Health*, 27, 49–54.

Shepherd, S. M., & Lewis-Fernandez, R. (2016). Forensic risk assessment and cultural diversity: Contemporary challenges and future directions. *Psychology, Public Policy, and Law*, 22, 427–438. https://doi.org/10.1037/law0000102

Strauss-Hughes, A., Heffernan, R., & Ward, T. (2019) A cultural–ecological perspective on agency and offending behaviour. *Psychiatry, Psychology and Law*, 26(6), 938–958.

Strauss-Hughes, A., Ward, T., & Neha, T. (2022). Considering practice frameworks for culturally diverse populations in the correctional domain. *Aggression and Violent Behavior*, 63, 101673.

The United Nations Office on Drugs and Crime. (2012). *Introductory Handbook on the Prevention of Recidivism and the Social Reintegration of Offenders*. United Nations, New York, December 2012. https://www.unodc.org/documents/justice-and-prison-reform/crimeprevention/Introductory_Handbook_on_the_Prevention_of_Recidivism_and_the_Social_Reintegration_of_Offenders.pdf

The United Nations Office on Drugs and Crime. (2015). *The United Nations Standard Minimum Rules for the Treatment of Prisoners (the Nelson Mandela Rules)*. https://www.unodc.org/documents/justice-and-prison-reform/Nelson_Mandela_Rules-E-ebook.pdf

Walsmley, R. (2018). *World prison population list* (12th ed). https://www.prisonstudies.org/sites/default/files/resources/downloads/wppl_12.pdf

Ward, T., & Brown, M. (2004). The good lives model and conceptual issues in offender rehabilitation. *Psychology, Crime, and Law*, 10, 243–257.

Winder, B., Scott, S., Underwood, M., & Blagden, N. (2021). *Recommended terminology concerning people with a criminal conviction*. COPE Practice Brief 01/21. NTU Psychology, Nottingham Trent University.

World Prison Brief. (2021). Downloaded from https://www.prisonstudies.org/

Yang, A. A. (2003). Indian convict workers in Southeast Asia in the late eighteenth and early nineteenth centuries. *Journal of World History*, 14(2), 179–208.

Yoon, J., Marshall, W. L., Simas-Knight, J., & Lee, S. (2021). *Treating sexual offenders I: Development of K-MIDSA and sex offender treatment manuals (I)*. https://www.kicj.re.kr/board.es?mid=a20201000000&bid=0029&list_no=12600&act=view.

Zhong, H., & Zhang, S. Y. (2021). Social control of crime in Asia. In *Oxford Research Encyclopedia of Criminology and Criminal Justice*. Oxford University Press. 10.1093/acrefore/9780190264079.013.623.

2

CROSS-CULTURAL RESPONSIVENESS AND CROSS-NATIONAL APPROACHES IN OFFENDER REHABILITATION

Research and Practice Considerations

Armon J. Tamatea

Introduction

Two meaningful and significant forces that influence and shape the conduct and values of individuals, communities and societies are the *law* and *culture*. According to Rosen (2006), the law is integral to culture as the culture is to law – both are a society's means of expressing a sense of order. The basic function of the law is to govern individual and societal behaviour, establish standards of conduct, and protect individual rights and property through the provision of a set of rules and regulations. The law provides a framework for maintaining order and stability in society by defining and regulating behaviour and setting consequences for violations, in order to deter wrongful conduct. By contrast, culture shapes human behaviour by providing a collective sense of meaning and purpose through shared traditions, beliefs, values and customs. However, collisions between culture and the law can raise issues in the forensic arena. Consider the following: In July 2016, Qandeel Baloch, a 26-year-old Pakistani social media star and model who gained notoriety for her provocative posts on social media, was murdered (*qatl-i-amd*[1]) by her brother, Muhammad Waseem. Waseem confessed to the killing, stating that he was angry with Qandeel. In 2019, Waseem was sentenced to life in prison for Qandeel's murder but was acquitted three years later (Saifi et al., 2022).

This case raises important issues for mental health practitioners whose role may include the provision of advice to the court by making sense of behaviour, especially where culture is a factor. In this case, a critical issue is to *understand the context of the behaviour*. Waseem confessed to

DOI: 10.4324/9781003360919-3

the killing, stating that he murdered Qandeel in the name of honour because she had brought stigma and shame to the family through her social media posts (State v. Muhammad Waseem, 2019). D'Lima et al. (2020) described the form of patriarchy that exists in India and Pakistan as providing an enabling environment for honour killings in these two countries, creating a system in which men maintain control over women throughout their lives.

A second issue is to determine whether the defendant's behaviour was *consistent with cultural norms*. *Karo-Kari* is a form of premeditated killing which has origins in rural and tribal areas of Pakistan. These homicides are primarily committed by men against women who are thought to have brought dishonour to their family – usually by participating in illicit pre-marital or extra-marital relations. In order to restore this honour, a male family member must kill the female in question (Patel & Gadit, 2008). Although illegal, socio-cultural factors (e.g., traditional patriarchal interpretations of Islam) and gender role expectations (e.g., valorisation of female chastity, women as property) have given legitimacy to *karo-kari* within some tribal communities. The case of State v. Muhammad Waseem (2019) highlighted the issue of honour killings in Pakistan and the challenges that women face in a patriarchal society where their actions and choices are often tightly controlled by family members and societal norms.

A third issue is to formulate the case and make the situation *intelligible* for a just decision to be determined and administered. This is made even more complex when considering the legal context at the time when the *Pakistan Penal Code (Act XLV of 1860)* allowed a murder victim's family to pardon a convicted killer.[2] While Islam allows compassion for the offender and encourages a pardon to be given to the culprit, with pardon and compassion comes the duty to recompense the family (Ismail, 2012). D'Lima et al. (2020) note that the limited understanding of local context, combined with scarce data on honour killings, has contributed to the continued hidden nature of this form of violence across Pakistan. As this example illustrates, the relationship between psychology and the law is a complex one.

The aim of this chapter is to explore key practice issues and provide some departure points for correctional and forensic mental health practitioners in relation to the following questions:

- What preparations can mental health practitioners make when anticipating working with cultural diversity in psycho-legal settings?
- What steps can be taken to incorporate cultural information into forensic assessments?

However, it is *not* the aim of this chapter to provide an overview of this context, but to canvass the psycho-legal landscape where the interface between mental health practice, the law, and culture-specific issues converge, and to introduce some of the practice issues that are relevant for mental health practitioners who work routinely with culturally diverse clients in a psycho-legal environment. Further, given the scope of this book and space limitations, there is no focus on one specific nation or culture. As such, the comments presented here are somewhat generalised. Indeed, many of the issues raised in this chapter will likely apply across the criminal justice spectrum to include adults and youth as well as forensic mental health settings. Readers are invited to reflect on the issues raised and apply to their context as appropriate.

The Importance of Culturally Responsive Practices

It is recognised that in order to demonstrate adequate competence when working with culturally diverse clients, practitioners must draw upon a range of knowledges, each of which derives from contrasting epistemological bases and application. General features of this knowledge are displayed in Table 2.1. This table can best be seen as presenting a range of conceptual 'anchors' to consider the emphases of knowledge and application within the respective domains, but also recognising that different areas of knowledge do not easily relate to each other. Culture is complex! As such, a challenge for mental health practitioners is to become accustomed to recognising the limits of their knowledge and expertise, but also to develop practices to bridge these areas.

Asia: Conflicts and Tensions

As Ganapathy and Balachandran (2016) point out, 'Asia' is not a mere geopolitical entity that is distinct from the West, and delineating this notion of 'Asia' as an amorphous collective of peoples involves much theoretical, methodological, and ideological work. Indeed, Asia is an incredibly diverse continent with a rich tapestry of cultures, languages, religions, and ethnic groups. It is the world's largest and most populous continent, comprising more than 40 countries and home to over 4.4 billion people (United Nations Department of Economic and Social Affairs, 2022). One of the key features of Asia is its diversity with regard to ethnic groups (e.g., Han Chinese, the Tamils of South India, the Ainu of Japan, and the various indigenous peoples of Southeast Asia), religions (e.g., Hinduism, Buddhism, Islam, Christianity), and languages (e.g., Mandarin Chinese, Hindi, Arabic and Malay).

TABLE 2.1 Comparisons of Clinical, Scientific, Legal and Cultural Knowledges*

	Clinical	Experimental	Legal	Cultural
Context	Health and wellbeing	Individual/group differences and similarities	Formalised social contracts	Heritage
Codified as	Intrapsychic or behavioural principles	Natural laws	Legislation	Cultural norms
'Problems'	Psychopathology	Statistical deviation	Offending, crime	Transgressions, violations of rules/codes
Knowledge foundations	Empirical literature Problem-based Clinical practice	Theoretical psychology Concept-based Inductive reasoning	Case law Case-based Adversarial	Traditions and rites; Regional and tribal differences Cosmology, religious beliefs and practices The supernatural
Research/ Scholarship examples	Predictive validity of assessment tools Intervention effectiveness Trauma Epidemiology of relevant behaviours (e.g., violence)	Memory Perception Child development Group decision-making	Mental health law Criminal justice Legal trends (e.g., therapeutic jurisprudence)	Somato-psychological and socio-religious models of health and wellbeing Human rights, inequities in health and justice outcomes Cultural perceptions/norms of antisocial behaviour
Application	Risk assessment Rehabilitation Integrating science into practice	Consultation re: jury selection, litigation strategy Expert witness	Policy and legislative consultation	Culturally safe practices Assessment and rehabilitation practices

* Adapted from Brigham (1999), Haney (1980) and Tseng (1999) – with liberties.

Moreover, there are challenges and conflicts that have shaped Asia's history and continue to influence the region today. Although Western nations are not immune from political conflicts, relevant contexts across Asia include:

- *Colonialism and imperialism:* Many Asian countries were colonised or controlled by foreign powers (e.g., India, Vietnam, the Philippines, and Indonesia). The effects of colonisation are still evident in these countries today, including in economic disparities, social hierarchies, and political power structures.
- *Nationalism and independence movements:* The struggle for independence from colonial rule has been a major theme for many countries in Asia, especially in modern times. For instance, India achieved independence from British colonial rule in 1947 after decades of struggle. Vietnam, the Philippines, and Indonesia experienced significant independence movements.
- *Territorial disputes:* Many countries in Asia have ongoing territorial disputes with their neighbours (e.g., the South China Sea dispute involves China, Vietnam, and the Philippines, among other countries).
- *Ethnic and religious conflicts:* Many Asian countries have complex ethnic and religious dynamics that have led to political conflict and subjected people to violence and persecution (e.g., Myanmar), which have led to violence and social unrest.

Further, the universalist assumptions of science imply a ready-made applicability of explanations of crime across time and space. In the forensic context, psychological theories and practices are juxtaposed against legal, social and health frameworks which are driven by different imperatives and are themselves located within specific cultural frameworks. The notion of forensic psychology as a science and therefore somehow separated from cultural biases is flawed. Indeed, economically and politically, the Asian region is dynamic and diverse and provides varied examples of social transition from relative poverty to wealth, conflict to reconstruction, and comparative isolation to globalisation (Ganapathy & Broadhurst, 2008).

Forensic mental health and criminal justice practitioners must critically evaluate the values inherent in their practice – those practitioners who deny their own values and biases risk imposing them on clients. Some key orienting questions for each domain may include (from Tamatea & Waipara-Panapa, 2022):

1 *Clinical:* What are the psychological and ethical issues? What is the *function* of the person's behaviour? What dilemmas or *conflicts* does the case present?

2 *Experimental:* What can I *explain/predict* about a given individual's behaviour? What is known about other people who present with the same/similar known *risk* (health, recidivism) and *protective* (support, resilience) factors?

3 *Legal:* What *questions* do I need to address in a judicial context? What are the legal *obligations* and *constraints* of my practice?

4 *Cultural:* What do I understand about the person, their community, and their way of life/norms/beliefs? Can their behaviour be considered more *meaningfully*? Do they present exceptions or challenges to the above domains?

Risk Assessment: Establishing Dangerousness

Broadly construed, 'forensic' refers to (1) the application of scientific methods and techniques to the investigation of crime and (2) relating to courts of law. Mental health practitioners are routinely tasked with considering psychopathology and risk of dangerousness as it relates to offending and the law. In addition to being informed by theoretical frameworks, the relevant research literature, risk tools and assessment guidelines to evaluate the information gathered, practitioners also construct formulations and seek to address the referral question. Similarly, clinicians are required to evaluate the role (and legitimacy) of cultural norms, beliefs and practices.

In countries such as Canada, Australia and New Zealand, correctional and forensic mental health practitioners, particularly psychologists and psychiatrists, have had an increasingly central role in providing expert commentary on the prediction, nature and management of an individual's level of dangerousness in order to (1) assist the *court* to make scientifically informed judgements to advise sentencing; (2) assist *prisons and forensic mental health services* to allocate rehabilitation resources (e.g., programmes, psychological intervention); and, (3) assist community *probation and community forensic mental health* services to plan and support an individual's reintegration and resettlement while anticipating and managing any ongoing threats to community safety that an individual may pose.

Culturally Responsive Psychological Assessment

Affirming cultural legitimacy implies creating opportunities for dialogue and enhancing respectful and ethical practices. A number of schemes and

TABLE 2.2 Phases of Cultural Assessment (adapted from Ridley et al., 1998)

Phase	Function	Awareness/Skill of Psychologist
Identify cultural data	Recognise salient and significant demographic, clinical, and non-verbal information	Know *where* and *what* to look for
Interpret cultural data	Ascertain meaning of the information from the client's perspective/outlook	Know *how* to look
Incorporate cultural data	Ensure accurate, comprehensive assessment that reflects the client's context	Understand *why*

approaches have emerged to integrate cultural material into clinical assessment (Suzuki et al., 2001), diagnosis (Petrovich & Garcia, 2016), case formulation (Dana, 2005), and treatment (Hays & Iwamasa, 2006; Leach & Aten, 2010; Slattery, 2004; Sue & Sue, 2013). For simplicity, the cultural assessment process of Ridley et al. (1998) is displayed in Table 2.2 as a framework for practitioners to adapt to their own professional context to facilitate culturally informed assessments and rehabilitation practices.

As an example of this approach in practice, consider cases of violence towards women in heterosexual relationships in China. In a review of the domestic violence literature in China, Su et al. (2022) revealed that the classification of what are actually violent crimes as 'family affairs' reflects deep-rooted cultural influences in China, in particular traditional Confucian beliefs (Identification) in social harmony and the assumed social norms of not interfering with the affairs of other people. Disclosure of the violence may result in loss of face for both partners and the ensuing public humiliation and belittling of the female partner in front of others would undermine her social standing and his reputation. The embarrassment, shame or humiliation caused by the husband's abuse (and the wife's victimisation) would strain the relationship and damage their reputation in the eyes of others (Interpretation). The commission of this behaviour behind closed doors reduces the likelihood of interception and social condemnation, increasing the likelihood of future violence (Incorporation). A belief that such violence is viewed as a 'family affair' means that such behaviour is beyond the reach of the law and may obscure the extent and reality of the violence, thus serving to minimise the emotional impact of the behaviour for the perpetrator.[3]

Principles of Risk Assessment

Of most concern to the public are antisocial behaviours – especially those involving violence and/or harmful sexual behaviour. The ability to identify those at risk of these behaviours, and to prevent these behaviours, supports safer communities and judicious resource allocation for criminal justice organisations. Conroy and Murrie (2007) advocate a systematic procedure that includes defining the question and being clear about what is being asked; this is a critical starting point in any psychological assessment. This means that the assessor needs to be context-specific. That is, what kind of behaviour, over what time span, and relevant to what settings? Incidents such as 'dowry deaths' in India (i.e., immolation of women) are linked to cultural traditions and customs (Belur et al., 2014). However, the nature of the violence associated with these deaths can be unreliably reported as either homicides or suicides, and accounts can change, especially if there is pressure on the family to promote a specific narrative of the offending. The phenomenon of 'death brokering' is a similar practice which refers to activities of authorities to declare individual deaths as culturally appropriate (Timmermans, 2005). All of these factors would impact on how an incident is officially recorded (i.e., accident or crime) and what behaviours are tolerated within a society or community – all of which has implications for the quality of a risk assessment.

A second issue is that of the behaviour in the overall population. Base rates, the rate of a given behaviour (e.g., interpersonal violence) in a particular sub-population, have become increasingly important as a source of empirical data in the development of predictive tools and the framing of risk statements. However, and as noted above, base rate data are not always reliable. As Cooke and Michie (2002) commented, it is a dangerous error to assume that a risk assessment procedure developed in one country will function the same way in another. A good foundation for developing valid risk assessment tools is the ability to use local normative data. The literature[4] on risk assessment tools that have been validated in Asian countries is comparatively scarce and reflects differential adoption of Western practices and tools.

Cultural Issues with Risk Assessment

The measures that have been validated in Asian countries are typically factorial (e.g., HCR-203, LSI-R, PCL-R) which relies on a detached and disaggregated model of personhood (compared with holistic conceptualisations of people). These tools also reflect an imported knowledge and research traditions that do not necessarily mirror cultural views of people, behaviour or criminal justice realities in these countries. Furthermore not all studies in Asia testing the predictive validity of risk assessment tools developed in Western contexts report predictive validity outcomes although some report positive findings. For instance, the HCR-20[3] and RSVP have good inter-rater and concurrent validity in South Korean research (Sea & Bang, 2021; Sea & Hart, 2021). Measures like the Stable-2007 add incremental predictive value when combined with the Static-99R (Tsao & Chu, 2021), and tools such as the SVR-20 reveal predictive validity for general offending (and not sexual recidivism for which it was designed) (Tsao & Chu, 2021).

It should also be noted that validation studies tend to use ethnicity, rather than culture, as organising variables. Accordingly, psychologists are encouraged to be judicious in the use and interpretation of risk measures and the implication such measures have on personal liberties. As per Ridley et al. (1998 – see Table 2.2), practitioners are also encouraged to seek cultural information to assist with interpretations of this information to develop more incorporated case formulations. For instance, an individual who rates on risk assessment items such as 'non-compliance' or 'negative attitudes to authorities' (or variations thereof) may also have collective national histories of negative interactions with police that in turn have informed anti-authoritarian attitudes (e.g., distrust) and behaviours (e.g., non-cooperation, 'resistance', or even compliance to avoid further aversive consequences). While the behaviours may indicate apparent risk on statistical grounds, the data in support of the item would necessitate a culturally informed approach.

Lastly, the method of conceptualising the causes of offending in Asian communities has some significant implications for the way in which risk is assessed in a context in which the over- or under-assessment of a particular need may result in the delivery of an inappropriate level of intervention, or result in an inaccurate risk classification.

In summary, a primary challenge facing any applied psychologist is to understand individuals in their context. Appreciating the perspective of peoples' cultural reality will often involve attempts to understand an alternative worldview that does not superimpose neatly, if at all, on Western notions of knowledge in general, or offending behaviour in particular. The risk assessment literature has been largely indifferent to the impact (or even notion) of *cultural* differences on how behaviour is perceived and formulated.

Offender Rehabilitation: Change in Coercive Contexts

A robust rehabilitation plan is informed by observing cultural processes that serve to ensure that treatment gains are relevant to the individual's context. Inferential errors due to overlooking culturally significant material (see Table 2.2) can result in poorly-informed assessments that, in turn, lead to inadequately designed interventions and poor outcomes. 'Errors', in this context, may result as a consequence of clinician bias that reflects a dismissive attitude towards the values, beliefs, socialisation practices, ways of knowing, or social role expectations of the person. Poor outcomes may equate to overestimating harm and criminality across a given group, overlooking potentially advantageous social supports, and undermining the individual's coping style by way of inducing (or reinforcing) passivity and avoidance in interactions with authorities. Additionally, 'resistant' behaviour towards the practitioner may emerge from a perception of coercion for individuals who are wary of discrimination and oppression, and who may feel that the information offered in the assessment may be misused to increase their experience of stigmatisation (Korbin, 2002; Patel & Lord, 2001). In this last section, emphasis is given to culturally responsive practices that promote the understanding of context and the realities of people who are culturally different from the psychologist.

Understand the Issues for the Person's Community

Practitioners are advised to learn about the communities from which their clients come. As noted earlier, clients from across Asia may well present with backgrounds that reflect dislocation, migration, diverse spiritual and religious beliefs, cultural conceptions of cause of offending behaviour, and trauma. Dislocation, for instance, means separation from place and community, and can incur loss of meaningful role identity, introduction of downward social mobility (e.g., unemployment), and the erosion of family structures and community sanctions and attitudes. Understanding a person's community requires an understanding of systems and rules (identifying – see Table 2.2) that inform their *role(s)* within a given community (e.g., in relation to elders, members of the opposite sex, children, etc.) and *codes of conduct* that signal behaviour that is reinforced or prohibited. Acquired knowledge of these norms can assist in placing the person's offending behaviour in cultural context. For instance, Ahn and Gilbert's (1992) study of sexualised behaviour in Asian-American homes reported that a significant proportion of Vietnamese, Korean, and Cambodian participants (mothers) considered it permissible for a grandfather to touch his 3-year-old grandson's genitals with pride – a behaviour that would attract disapproval and condemnation in Western countries. Ultimately, the challenge for the practitioner is to understand the meaning of specific behaviour (e.g., interpreting – see Table 2.1) under these conditions.

Some challenging issues in rehabilitation include language, attitudes to victims, and disclosure. Language can present an obvious barrier to not only effective communication, but also the fidelity of the assessment – especially if there are no equivalent offence-related terms in the person's language. For instance, Gahir and Garrett's (1999) study of rehabilitation in India revealed no word for 'rape' in Punjabi, despite the social recognition of the act. Furthermore, describing and discussing sexual offending behaviour can be confronting for some individuals whose culture holds a strong taboo against discussing sexual matters.

Develop Culturally Responsive Practices

Cultural problems can emerge when communication is poor and a lack of practitioner awareness or responsiveness to cultural issues is evident in the form of stereotyping (Patel & Lord, 2001) or unintended (or unconscious) cultural projections onto the perpetrator (i.e., 'cultural countertransference'; Stampley & Slaght, 2004). Bias amongst practitioners is often inadvertent, denied and typically beyond immediate awareness (Dana, 2005). Furthermore, the careless use of tools that require inference in order to interpret creates opportunities for the expression of bias that may promote negative stereotypes and caricatures that serve to dehumanise as well as over-pathologise the individual. Common ethnocultural biases can be (1) confirmatory (i.e., searching for information and evidence that supports a hypothesis while ignoring data that is inconsistent), (2) misattribution (e.g., the client may favour a sociocultural explanatory model, whereas a practitioner is likely to favour the personal characteristics of the person as due cause), and (3) judgement heuristics (i.e., quick decision rules that save time when approaching data, but also short-circuit our ability to engage in self-correction) (Smith, 2005; Sue & Sue, 2013). The following suggestions are made with a view towards promoting a practice environment that is culturally supportive and safe to raise awareness. They are also intended to de-bias unhelpful practitioner perceptions and behaviours, build capacity through knowledge generation, and encourage the development of skills:

- Identify and *address stereotypical beliefs* via professional supervision, self-evaluation, education, and reflective practice. Trying new ways of engagement and seeking feedback and support from individuals who have sufficient cultural capital and expertise to guide observations and considerations for engagement can facilitate effective interpersonal behaviours (Smith, 2005).
- Similarly, *address polarised understanding* of ethnic and cultural issues (Kelly, 2005). Learning to tolerate ambiguity is an important attribute

when working with individuals whose model of the world and how they interact with it may be distinct or somewhat at odds with the practitioner's own cultural outlook and values.

- Engage in *educational experiences* that are culturally informative and promote learning and experience with other ways of perceiving and knowing. This may mean looking beyond the agency into allied institutions with existing cultural capacity (e.g., mental health or child advocacy).
- If appropriate, seek the *involvement of others* in decision-making (e.g., community leader) to understand and enhance support structures in the offender's community.

Cultural responsiveness involves the development of specific and nuanced understanding of cultural expectations and boundaries. Critical in-session processes and skills to consider in enhancing effectiveness with culturally different offenders include:

- Developing *credibility and trust* (Comas-Díaz, 2012) can be a considerable challenge where there is distrust, hostility, or marginalisation (Rodriguez et al., 2007). Developing trust can take time, especially for peoples who place great value on relationships and connectedness.
- Explore *explanatory models of offending behaviour*. An individual's explanation of their offending behaviour may be discrepant from empirical notions of risk and file information. However, understanding the client's perspective can offer important insights into what they believe to be the causal factors (e.g., spiritual or socio-political factors), how controllable (and by extension, how treatable) they believe their offending behaviour to be, as well as who else should be involved in making decisions. By learning more about culturally different populations, practices and procedures can be developed that are appropriate to those peoples (Yessine & Bonta, 2009).
- Pay attention to *etiquette* – mundane behaviours can carry social significance and communicate respect across cultural spaces. Kapitanoff et al. (2000) identified a range of situations that practitioners can observe and consider in the course of assessment with clients from different cultures that include: (1) use of the native language with correct pronunciation, (2) knowledge of proper terms regarding traditional cultural beliefs, attitudes and practices, (3) knowledge of topics that may be considered inappropriate to discuss with strangers, (4) appropriate use or avoidance of eye contact or physical touch, (5) customs regarding the sharing of food, and (6) understanding the importance of spending time to get to know each other and create a trusting working alliance before assessment procedures begin.

In Closing

Revisiting the aims of this chapter, the reader is invited to reflect on: (1) what knowledge, awareness, and skill preparations need to be made when anticipating psychological work with culturally different clients in psycho-legal settings; (2) what steps need to be taken to incorporate cultural information into psychological assessments; and, (3) what factors, issues, concepts, processes, and relationships need to be contemplated when constructing culturally-informed reports for decision-making bodies. Working with clients and their cultural contexts requires time and effort and a sensitised way of working and understanding the person.

Notes

1 A person who, with the intention of causing death and/or bodily injury to a person, commits an act which is likely to cause death or with the knowledge that the act is of such imminent dangerousness that it must in all probability cause death, and causes the death of such person, is said to commit *qatl-e-amd* (Pakistan Penal Code 1860, s300).

2 The penalty of *Arsh* means that specific offences could be addressed by compensation to be paid to the victim or their (i.e., male) heirs.

3 This is not to say that such a dynamic is not applicable in Western countries. For instance, Nicolson (2019) identifies social activism as being a successful impetus for legal change and better support for women survivors of domestic violence. However, he points out that public discourse implicating perpetrators and survivors persists in Europe and North America, and that this may also exert a suppressive effect on reporting this behaviour.

4 Note: This literature is limited to peer-reviewed research that is published in the English language.

References

Ahn, H. N., & Gilbert, N. (1992). Cultural diversity and sexual abuse prevention. *Social Service Review, 66*(3), 410–427.

Belur, J., Tilley, N., Daruwalla, N., Kumar, M., Tiwari, V., & Osrin, D. (2014). The social construction of "dowry deaths." *Social Science & Medicine, 119*, 1–9.

Brigham, J. C. (1999). What is forensic psychology, anyway? *Law & Human Behavior, 23*, 273–298.

Comas-Díaz, L. (2012). *Multicultural Care: A clinician's guide to cultural competence*. Washington D.C.: American Psychological Association.

Conroy, M. A., & Murrie, D. C. (2007). *Forensic Assessment of Violence Risk*. Hoboken, NJ: Wiley.

Cooke, D. J., & Michie, C. (2002). Towards valid cross-cultural measures of risk. In R. R. Corrado, R. Roesch, S. D. Hart, & J. K. Gierowski (Eds.), *Multi-problem Youth: A foundation for comparative research on needs, interventions and outcomes* (pp. 241–250). Amsterdam, The Netherlands: IOS.

D'Lima, T., Solotaroff, J. L., & Pande, R. P. (2020). For the sake of family and tradition: Honour killings in India and Pakistan. *ANTYAJAA: Indian Journal of Women and Social Change*, *5*(1), 22–39.

Dana, R. H. (2005). *Multicultural Assessment: Principles, applications, and examples*. Mahwah, NJ: Erlbaum.

Gahir, M., & Garrett, T. (1999). Issues in the treatment of Asian sexual offenders. *Journal of Sexual Aggression*, *4*(2), 94–104.

Ganapathy, N., & Balachandran, L. (2016). Crime and punishment in Asia. *Journal of Contemporary Criminal Justice*, *32*(3), 196–204.

Ganapathy, N., & Broadhurst, R. (2008). Organized crime in Asia: A review of problems and progress. *Asian Criminology*, *3*, 1–12.

Haney, C. (1980). Psychology and legal change: On the limits of a factual jurisprudence. *Law & Human Behavior*, *4*, 147–199.

Hare, R. D. (2003). *Manual for the Revised Psychopathy Checklist* (2nd ed.). Toronto, Ontario, Canada: Multi-Health Systems.

Hays, P. A., & Iwamasa, G. Y. (Eds.). (2006). *Culturally Responsive Cognitive–Behavioral Therapy: Assessment, practice, and supervision*. Washington, DC: American Psychological Association.

Ismail, S. Z. (2012). The modern interpretation of the Diyat formula for the quantum of damages: The case of homicide and personal injuries. *Arab Law Quarterly*, *26*(3), 361–379.

Kapitanoff, S. H., Lutzker, J. R., & Bigelow, K. M. (2000). Cultural issues in the relation between child disabilities and child abuse. *Aggression & Violent Behavior*, *5*(3), 227–244.

Kelly, E. (2005). Review Essay: Sectarianism, Bigotry and Ethnicity–The Gulf in Understanding. *Scottish Affairs*, No. 50.

Korbin, J. E. (2002). Culture and child maltreatment: Cultural competence and beyond. *Child Abuse & Neglect*, *26*(6-7), 637–644.

Leach, M. M., & Aten, J. D. (Eds.). (2010). Counseling and psychotherapy. *Culture and the Therapeutic Process: A guide for mental health professionals*. New York, NY: Routledge.

Nicolson, P. (2019). *Domestic Violence and Psychology*. London: Routledge.

Patel, S., & Gadit, A. M. (2008). Karo-Kari: A form of honour killing in Pakistan. *Transcultural Psychiatry*, *45*(4), 683–694.

Patel, K., & Lord, A. (2001). Ethnic minority sex offenders' experiences of treatment. *Journal of Sexual Aggression*, *7*(1), 40–50.

Petrovich, A., & Garcia, B. (2016). *Strengthening the DSM: Incorporating resilience and cultural competence* (2nd ed.). New York, NY: Springer.

Prentky, R. A., Li, N.-C., Righthand, S., Schuler, A., Cavanaugh, D., & Lee, A. F. (2010). Assessing risk of sexually abusive behavior among youth in a child welfare sample. *Behavioral Sciences & the Law*, *28*(1), 24–45.

Ridley, C. R., Li, L. C., & Hill, C. L. (1998). Multicultural assessment: Re-examination, reconceptualization, and practical application. *Counseling Psychologist*, *26*, 827–910.

Rodriguez, M. M., McNeal, C. T., & Cauce, A. M. (2007). Counseling with the marginalised. In P. B. Pedersen, J. G. Draguns, W. J. Lonner, & J. E. Trimble

(Eds.), *Counseling across Cultures* (6th ed., pp. 223–238). Thousand Oaks, CA: Sage Publishing.

Rosen, L. (2006). *Law as Culture: An introduction.* Princeton, NJ: Princeton University Press.

Saifi, S., Syed, A., & Mogul, R. (2022, February 15). Court frees brother who confessed to killing social media star Qandeel Baloch. CNN. https://edition.cnn.com/2022/02/15/asia/pakistan-qandeel-baloch-brother-acquittal-intl-hnk/index.html

Sea, J., & Bang, S. (2021). The interrater reliability and concurrent validity of the HCR-20 version 3 in South Korea. *The Journal of Forensic Psychiatry & Psychology, 32*(6), 879–901.

Sea, J., & Hart, S. D. (2021). Interrater reliability and concurrent validity of the risk for sexual violence protocol for Korean sexual offenders: A field study. *International Journal of Offender Therapy and Comparative Criminology, 65*(13-14), 1423–1445.

Slattery, J. M. (2004). *Counseling Diverse Clients: Bringing context into therapy.* Belmont, CA: Cengage.

Smith, T. B. (2005). A contextual approach to assessment. In T. B. Smith (Ed.), *Practicing Multiculturalism: Affirming diversity in counseling and psychotherapy* (pp. 97–119). Boston, MA: Pearson.

Stampley, C., & Slaght, E. (2004). Cultural transference as a clinical obstacle. *Smith College Studies in Social Work, 74*(2), 333–347.

State v. Muhammad Waseem (2019), Pakistan Law Decisions 2019 District & Sessions Court, Multan, 298.

Su, Z., McDonnell, D., Cheshmehzangi, A., Ahmad, J., Chen, H., Šegalo, S., & Cai, Y. (2022). What "family affair?" Domestic violence awareness in China. *Frontiers in Public Health, 10,* 795841.

Sue, D. W., & Sue, D. (2013). *Counseling the Culturally Diverse: Theory and practice* (6th ed.). New York, NY: Wiley.

Suzuki, L., Ponterotto, J. G., & Meller, PJ. (2001). Multicultural assessment: Trends and directions revisited. In L. A. Suzuki, J. G. Ponterotto, & P. Meller (Eds.), *Handbook of Multicultural Assessment* (2nd ed., pp. 359–382). San Francisco, CA: Jossey-Bass.

Tamatea, A. J., & Waipara-Panapa, A. (2022). Māori, psychology, and the law: Challenges and opportunities for practitioners. In F. Seymour, S. Blackwell, & A. Tamatea (Eds.), *Psychology and the Law in Aotearoa New Zealand* (4th ed., pp. 11–41). Wellington, NZ: New Zealand Psychological Society.

Timmermans, S. (2005). Death brokering: Constructing culturally appropriate deaths. *Sociology of Health & Illness, 27*(7), 993e1013.

Tsao, I. T., & Chu, C. M. (2021). An exploratory study of recidivism risk assessment instruments for individuals convicted of sexual offenses in Singapore. *Sexual Abuse, 33*(2), 157–175.

Tseng, W. S. (1999). Culture and psychotherapy: Review and practical guidelines. *Transcultural Psychiatry, 36*(2), 131–179

United Nations Department of Economic and Social Affairs (Population Division). (2022). *World Population Prospects 2022: Summary of Results*. UN DESA/POP/2022/TR/NO. 3. https://www.un.org/development/desa/pd/sites/www.un.org.development.desa.pd/files/wpp2022_summary_of_results.pdf.

Yessine, A., & Bonta, J. (2009). The offending trajectories of youthful aboriginal offenders. *Revue Canadienne de Criminologie et de Justice Pénale*, *51*(4), 435–472.

Zhang, X. Y. (2017). Predicting reoffending using the structured assessment of violence risk in youth (SAVRY): A 5-year follow-up study of male juvenile offenders in Hunan Province, China. *PloS One*, *12*(1).

EAST ASIA

EAST ASIA

3

REFORM AND PUNISHMENT

An Overview of Correctional Rehabilitation in Mainland China

Yixuan Wang and Jianhong Liu

Introduction

Rehabilitation in China has a complicated and distinctive development, and to understand contemporary rehabilitation policies and practices it is important to examine how different political and social contexts have influenced rehabilitation during different stages of China's history. This chapter will show how punishment and rehabilitation have been moulded in China's development and how rehabilitation and punishment are intertwined.

In the following sections, the discussion takes a broader-than-usual view of rehabilitation to reflect contemporary China's perspective. In China, which is essentially an authoritarian state, the government has been granted tacit approval to intervene in the activities of citizens. In other words, apart from reforming criminal offenders, the government has legitimised early intervention before delinquent non-criminal behaviour develops into more serious criminal behaviour (Chen, 2004; Wu & Vander Beken, 2018). As such, this chapter covers responses to criminal offenders and those who have committed illegal (yet non-criminal) acts,[1] including various groups, such as those who are drug dependent and minors who have committed criminal acts but are under the age of criminal responsibility.

Moreover, an overview of rehabilitation will be given with reference to the individual and society. The former focuses on individual enhancement and positive change, while the latter is more concerned with the development of the individual at the societal level and the

DOI: 10.4324/9781003360919-5

consideration of public good. Viewed from this perspective, we will see that (in Chinese practice) more resources are devoted to reducing recidivism and controlling crime, but less attention is paid to correcting individual deficiencies and restoring their interests or rights (Li, 2022). This is due to the perception that individualised treatment (e.g., clinical psychological treatment and analysis of the causes of offending) is less efficacious.

A Brief Review of Historical Development of Rehabilitation in China

From the period of Confucianism to the founding of the People's Republic of China in 1949, the adoption of the socialist market economy in 1992 and on to the establishment of the "rule of law" today, the concepts and practice of rehabilitation have evolved. The idea of rehabilitation is rooted in traditional Chinese philosophy and political institutions. The rulers of the Xia, Shang, Zhou, and Qin dynasties (2029–206 BC) relied on severe penalties to maintain rule; cruel punishment existed for discipline and deterrence by dictators (Tao & Xiao, 2007). As Chinese civilisation progressed (Han dynasty onwards; ~202 BC) under the influence of Confucianism, Legalism, and Taoism, the disposal of offenders began to shift towards a correctional model in which punishment and rehabilitation co-existed. Along with the idea of punishment, these philosophical thoughts shaped the development of rehabilitation ideas in China.

The Early Phase of PRC Correction (1949–1977)

The founding of the People's Republic of China in 1949 was a significant turning point in China's history. Traditional perspectives on rehabilitation and politics produced mixed correctional policies. The war created numerous adversaries and labeled individuals as counter-revolutionary 'offenders,' contributing to a significant increase in prison populations (Jin, 1990). According to Mao Zedong's philosophy of reforming offenders through labour-guided reformation, prisons were rebuilt into labour reform farms and production/construction units were created for rehabilitation through labour (Li, 2019). In 1955, the Central Committee of the Communist Party of China proposed a new form of quasi-penal punishment, Re-education Through Labour (RETL, *laojiao*). As a non-criminal, compulsory rehabilitation measure, RETL was to be applied to those people who had not met the criteria for conviction but whose placement in society would increase unemployment. Labour was therefore used as a means of rehabilitation, which had the dual purpose of education and employment (Li, 2019; Wang, 2008). Accordingly, offenders participating in such labour processes learned vocational skills that would enable them to earn a living after release, develop good work habits and a self-sufficient mindset, and ultimately be transformed (State Council Information Office, 1992).

The Cultural Revolution occurred between 1966 and 1976, during which China's rehabilitation work severely regressed and the institutional structure was destroyed. Instead of being respected and rehabilitated, deviants who broke administrative laws or committed crimes were regarded as a hostile class and were subjected to severe punishment and persecution (Wang, 2009).

The Standardisation Phase (1978–2011)

At the end of the Cultural Revolution, the country's leadership, led by Deng Xiaoping, embarked on a comprehensive policy of reform and opening up, ushering in a second period of sweeping social change. With a rapidly growing market economy and modernisation, the by-products of reform and opening up – anomic behaviours – increased dramatically, and so did crime. To reestablish social order and to fight crime, a "strike hard" (crackdown on crime) campaign was launched. The campaign did not reach the ideal result, and after a slight decline, crime rose again (Li & Dai, 1991), leading to a new correctional system.

In 1994, the first Prison Law was adopted, which underlined the notion of combining punishment and rehabilitation for the purpose of rehabilitation (Jia, 2018). The introduction of this law means that the execution of sentences in China has taken on a corrective/rehabilitative character, which has created more humane and scientific rehabilitation (Yan, 2020). In addition, the RETL system was widely used for crime prevention and was extended to: those who had committed minor offences that did not warrant criminal punishment, those who were subject to compulsory drug rehabilitation, those who had repeatedly engaged in prostitution or solicitation, and those who were disobedient and disruptive to public order (Chu, 2007).

Several "strike hard" on offenders campaigns have led to overcrowding and underfunding in prisons (Wang, 2009). High expectations were placed on reform forces outside prisons; for example, learning from the Western community-based correctional programmes. Since 2003, pilots of community-based correction have been run in some areas. However, unlike in the West, Chinese community-based correction also has a collectivist characteristic. There is a tradition of clan and village autonomy in China since ancient times, and many problems can be solved within the collective. Therefore, along with correctional officers, community forces such as village committees and neighbourhood committees have become part of the rehabilitative team, which is also a practice of the "mass line" advocated by the Chinese Communist Party (Gao & Luo, 2006; Jiang et al., 2014).

The Law-based Phase (2012–present)

The reform and opening-up policy have brought a huge development dividend to China and also led to the maintenance of the regime being more dependent on legitimacy. After Xi Jinping assuming the office of the President of China, the rule of law became an important governing philosophy, which led to a series of legislative and legal revisions, and the correctional system was placed within a new legal framework. Firstly, the RETL system was criticised, because it infringes on citizens' freedom by imposing quasi-custodial sentences on people who had not committed a crime (Hung, 2002); secondly, RETL was at odds with China's Constitution and Law on Administrative Penalty, as these laws clearly state that all administrative punishments that restrict personal freedom should be prescribed by law[2] (Hung, 2002). The decision to abolish RETL was made in 2013.

Due to rapid economic development and dramatic changes in the social fabric, new social risk factors have developed, new types of crime (cybercrime, telecommunications fraud, etc.) have emerged and punitive and rehabilitative approaches seem to have failed. Consequently, the Chinese criminal justice system began to pay more attention to the concept of "risk". Through numerous amendments to criminal law, more risky behaviour has been recognised as a crime; judicial officers use the riskiness of a suspect to decide whether to make an arrest, and law enforcement officers can also assess the riskiness of an offender as a reference for sentence reduction or release[3] (Epstein & Wong, 1996; Lao, 2019). With this comes more criminal offenders. The number of criminal offenders tried in their first instance in Chinese courts increased from 1,173,406 in 2012 to 1,714,942 in 2021 (see Table 3.1). Combined with the reform of the Personnel Quota System, the criminal justice system is under unprecedented pressure – too many cases, not enough officers. In response,

TABLE 3.1 Summary Statistics of the Number of Criminal Offenders Tried by the Courts in the First Instance Source: National Bureau of Statistics, 2021

Year	2021	2020	2018	2016	2014	2012
Total number of criminal offenders (person)	1,714,942	1,526,811	1,428,772	1,219,569	1,183,784	1,173,406

Source: National Bureau of Statistics, 2021.

the Leniency System for Admitting Guilt and Accepting Punishment (*renzui renfa congkuan*), and criminal settlement (*xingshi hejie*) were promoted. Thanks to these mitigated criminal regimes, more offenders have access to avoid being sent to prison and instead accept community corrections. With this, community corrections were officially recognised in 2019 after more than a decade of piloting.

In an anomic social structure, minors are a source of risk and are threatened by it. Against the backdrop of several cases of vicious crimes against minors, school violence and sexual assault, the public demand for the protection of minors and the control of crime has received an official response. As stated in the Law on the Prevention of Juvenile Delinquency and the Law on the Protection of Minors (amended in 2020), deviant behaviours and offences committed by minors and the corresponding rehabilitation measures are more systematically regulated: (*a*) misbehaviours – supervision and education; (*b*) serious misbehaviours – special educational measures; and (*c*) criminal behaviours – special corrective educational measures[4] (Yuan, 2021). This means that the correctional work of minors is formally separated from procedures for adults and the correctional rehabilitation programme for minors in China has moved towards a more systematic and standardised process.

Diversity in Rehabilitation Practices

Progress in the rule of law has led to rehabilitation receiving more attention. This is not to say that punishment is being substituted, because in the view of the Chinese public, the two are not a dichotomy that forces a choice – punishment and rehabilitation co-exist in the practice of correction in China (Jiang et al., 2016). In the rehabilitation mechanism, different rehabilitation measures are implemented depending on the nature and the severity of behaviour and/or personal characteristics of the offender. The following section describes rehabilitation measures in prison and community settings and identifies aspects of the rehabilitation of minors and drug users.

Rehabilitation in Prison

Chinese philosophy is dominated by Confucianism, which emphasises that "anyone can be rehabilitated". This philosophy is expressed in prison, where rehabilitation relies on intensive supervision. The correction of inmates' is conducted through custodial, educational and/or labour, and psychological counselling.

Custodial rehabilitation involves the classification and management of inmates according to their sex, age, type of crime, sentence length, and other characteristics. The prisons are under the jurisdiction of the Ministry of Justice, which ensures that inmates of different sexes and ages are separated and supervised in different locations. Moreover, prisons adopt a quantitative management method based on a points system, which records and evaluates inmates' daily performance and activities. The points are used as an indicator for deciding the punishment and reduction of sentences for inmates. For example, a prison in Yunnan Province has implemented a dynamic points system of graded treatment, which assigns inmates to different levels of management based on their points and applies different rehabilitation methods accordingly. The points are adjusted periodically and the process is dynamic (Zhang, 2022). This mechanism can motivate inmates to reform themselves and reduce corruption in prisons.

The second means is educational rehabilitation, which consists of three courses: ideological, vocational, and cultural education. Ideological education aims to instil Marxist ideology and correct inmates' erroneous worldviews and values. Vocational education aims to teach inmates useful skills and knowledge that can help them find employment after release. The cultural education aims to improve inmates' literacy and general knowledge. The third means, labour rehabilitation, complements educational rehabilitation. According to Marxist ideology, inmates lack labour experience, which leads them to commit crimes. Therefore, labour is seen as an effective way to transform inmates into law-abiding, normal human beings by reforming their moral qualities and life skills (Liu & Chui, 2018). Inmates are required to follow a weekly schedule of "five days of work, one day of classroom education and one day of rest".

In recent years, a fourth means of psychological rehabilitation has become increasingly adopted, including psychological counselling, diagnostic evaluation and behavioural correction. This aims to address the mental health issues of inmates and help them cope with stress and trauma. For example, the staff at Foshan Prison will adjust the correctional rehabilitation according to inmates' mental condition and psychological testing. The prison also provides online and onsite psychological counselling for inmates by doctors and psychologists (Ji & Shen, 2014).

Rehabilitation in Community-based Correction

Compared with prison rehabilitation, community-based rehabilitation is less punitive and more rehabilitative, as it allows offenders with lower risk to receive open correction in the community, lessen their problems of living, studying and employment, and helping to reintegrate with the help of informal correctional forces (Wodahl & Garland, 2009). In China, community correction officers are assigned multiple rehabilitative responsibilities, including supervision and management, education and assistance, and psychological rehabilitation.

The responsibility of supervision and management involves monitoring the offenders' behaviour, enforcing restrictions, and encouragement to fulfil obligations. For example, offenders may need to report to the correctional officer before leaving their original residence, comply with prohibition,[5] and attend community service, addiction treatment or group study sessions (Wu, 2021).

The responsibility of education and assistance involves providing cultural education, including legal and general knowledge, as well as vocational education. To enhance offenders' sense of social responsibility, they are encouraged to participate in voluntary activities. Essential assistance is provided for offenders living in hardship. For example, some areas have set up halfway houses to offer temporary accommodation for those who have no home, no relatives and no means of subsistence (Rong & Liu, 2009).

The responsibility of psychological rehabilitation involves paying attention to the psychological condition of offenders and employing professionals to provide them with psychological correctional services as required by law. An example is given by an empirical evaluation in Yixing, Jiangsu Province, which showed that the 915 offenders assessed were significantly higher than the national average in the "psychopathic" item (an item of mental health measurement), meaning that offenders are more prone to mental illness than the general population and more in need of clinical psychological rehabilitation. This example shows how the risk of recidivism is assessed for offenders and how different assessment criteria are followed – "lenient, ordinary and strict" – to ensure that offenders with a higher risk of recidivism receive more resources for rehabilitation (Wang & Huang, 2012).

Rehabilitation of Deviant Minors

The correction and rehabilitation of juvenile delinquents in China follows the philosophy of education and rehabilitation, with education as the mainstay and punishment as a supplement. It explains how China uses non-criminal means to deal with minors who have deviated to the farthest extent possible, and how it avoids severe penalties for minors who are criminally liable by not applying the death penalty and by mitigating or reducing the penalty (Zhang et al., 2013). The placement and rehabilitation of the minors depend on whether they have committed an offence and are criminally liable. There are two types of rehabilitation for juvenile offenders: reformation in reformatories for juvenile delinquents (i.e., juvenile prisons), and community-based correction. Reformation in reformatories is of a penal nature, but it relies mainly on educational methods, with minors having access to educational resources similar to those in regular schools. Furthermore, labour is not a required form of rehabilitation for minors, because by law minors under 16 years are not required to work. Community-based correction is a more lenient form of correction, which does not deprive minors' of their liberty and growth environment, but requires them to report their activities to correctional officers regularly and to be supervised and helped by their guardians, teachers or community volunteers (Wu, 2022).

For deviant minors who have committed criminal acts but have not reached the age of criminal responsibility, older versions of the Criminal Law stipulate that they must accept compulsory "shelter and rehabilitation" (*shourong jiaoyang*) by the government. Shelter and rehabilitation is the resettlement of deviant minors in a fixed place for education and supervision, which separates them from the environment that caused their delinquent behaviour – guiding them to develop a correct outlook on life and values (Wang, 1992). By comparison, work-study schools were set up to accommodate minors who have committed serious deviant (non-criminal) behaviours, offering general compulsory education, off-campus hobby programs, technical courses, and psychological counselling (Yao & Sun, 2017). However, there are drawbacks to these two means of rehabilitation, including management chaos, unclear nature, and the risk of stigmatisation or cross-infection of vices. Therefore, Amendment (XI) to the Criminal Law abolished "shelter and rehabilitation" and replaced work-study schools with special schools, establishing a more systematic correctional rehabilitation programme for minors (Wu, 2021). The Prevention of Juvenile Delinquency Law requires government education departments to set up special schools in each region to receive juvenile delinquents, and to provide them with basic educational classes, targeted courses, and probationary activities.

Rehabilitation of People Addicted to Drug

In China, drug use is considered harmful so using drugs it prohibited; it is regarded as an administrative (rather than criminal) offence. Drug users are considered "sick" or "victims" of drugs, and the government is required to provide users with rehabilitation rather than punishment

(Tibke, 2017).There are four drug treatment models depending on how often the police find the person using drugs: voluntary drug rehabilitation, community-based drug rehabilitation (CDR), isolated compulsory drug rehabilitation (ICDR), and community-based recovery.

The law provides that those who voluntarily attend drug rehabilitation institutions will not be subject to administrative penalties. In other words, voluntary drug rehabilitation is a non-coercive and liberal treatment for drug addiction. However, owing to its voluntary character, the lack of adequate supervision and management, and the high cost of drug treatment, voluntary drug rehabilitation has been ineffective. The average cost of a course of rehabilitation at a voluntary drug rehabilitation centre in Guangdong, for example, is RMB13,400 (approximately USD1,990) per course of treatment, making it difficult to achieve rehabilitation using one course of treatment, and the high cost discourages many people (Zheng et al., 2011).

CDR is promoted as a people-centred approach, presupposing that people who are addicted are situated in the community. By maintaining the "individual-family-community" links, it avoids the isolation from society that comes with compulsory isolation facilities and integrates multiple resources to achieve the goals of rehabilitation and reintegrating (Zhao, 2015). Within 15 days of receiving a decision letter from the police on CDR, addicts need to register in their town or sub-district offices and officers will set up a CDR working team for them. This consists of full-time staff, community police, community doctors, volunteers and family members (Li, 2018). For example, based on practical experience, the Qingcun Judicial Office in Shanghai classifies and manages addicts according to a graded management model of "three levels and four stages", which divides them into high-risk, medium-risk and low-risk groups according to their risk of relapse, and imposes three types of rehabilitation measures – strict, medium and lenient, while the four stages of individual education are based on the duration of rehabilitation (Zhou & Yang, 2016).

After exhausting the above drug rehabilitation forms, if drug users still cannot overcome their addiction, the police can use ICDR. At ICDR centres, addicts receive professional medical and physical treatment as well as psychological correction. Additionally, because ICDR is similar to the coercive nature of prison, staff rely on labour and education to help facilitate rehabilitation. Adults have to work for pay within a fixed time and can attend educational activities such as anti-drug or psychological education and hobby classes (Liu & Hsiao, 2018). According to a survey by the Yunnan Provincial Drug Rehabilitation Administration, the reuse rate of drug addicts three years after completing their rehabilitation was

66.49% (Chen, 2021). These data show that ICDR as a last resort for recovery from drug addiction remains unsatisfactory for many people.

In practice, community-based recovery is a follow-up service to ICDR, which takes into account the fact that people in ICDR have a long history of drug use or are highly addicted, and need to rely on community workers to maintain supervision and rehabilitation for a period of time in order to prevent them from reverting to drugs after their return to society (Zhao, 2015). Community-based recovery is like CDR, in that community workers provide various services to drug abusers, including psychological treatment, employment guidance and assistance, and encouragement to reestablish confidence in their lives.

An Overview of Forensic-Psychological Rehabilitation

In China, psychological correction[6] is regularly mentioned, and most rehabilitation measures have a psychological correction component, consisting of basic psychological assessments and simple psychological counselling services. The widely applied risk needs responsivity (RNR) model and good lives models (GLM) may provide some ideas for forensic rehabilitation in China (Robertson et al., 2011). Although we can find a few studies on RNR, GLM (or similar programmes) in China, most of them are individual or small-scale, even immature, and no unified standard of measurement has been developed (Xiao & Yang, 2014). There is a need for both paradigms to be trialled and studied in China. Given the size of China's rehabilitation population, relying on precise risk identification and quickly taking treatment measures may achieve the two reform goals of personal improvement of offenders and prevention of recidivism. In the future, China needs to invest more in offender rehabilitation and bring in more people with the expertise to explore theories and techniques of rehabilitation appropriate for China.

Conclusion

In the context of China's increasing rule of law, the offender rehabilitation programme is moving towards a more regulated and legalised path. Although Chinese officials are still looking for various rehabilitation measures to weaken the punitive overtones of correction, criticism from all sides continues unabated. Many critics insist that the essence of rehabilitation in China is punishment, or even mind control, rather than rehabilitation (Dutton, 1992; Li, 2013; Wu, 1997). In the future, China needs to find a judicial and human rights-based path to face challenges and criticism. Instead of seeking to rehabilitate and punish offenders, as well as building a perfect correctional system with a grand narrative, perhaps preventing more people from entering prison is the right path to manage the increasing numbers of offenders.

Notes

1 In China, illegal acts include criminal acts, i.e., violations of criminal law; and, administrative offences, i.e., violations of administrative law but not criminal law.
2 According to the hierarchy of China's legal system, the highest level is the constitution, followed by laws, and then administrative regulations, local regulations, etc. The laws at the lower level may not contradict the laws at the higher level. As RETL is a coercive measure to restrict personal freedom, according to the legal hierarchy it should be regulated by the second level of laws, but in fact it is regulated by the third level of administrative regulations, so it violates the legal hierarchy.
3 Within penal enforcement agencies such as prisons, staff assess the behaviour of offenders based on a uniform point accumulation mechanism. These scores reflect the offenders' daily performance, with higher scores meaning that they are doing better on their sentence and are at a lower risk of reoffending.
4 Under the provisions of the Prevention of Juvenile Delinquency Act: Misbehaviours are unlawful transgressions such as smoking, drinking, truancy, truancy and gambling. Serious misbehaviours are acts committed by minors in violation of the provisions of criminal law, which are not criminally punishable because they are under the legal age of criminal responsibility, and acts that seriously endanger society. Criminal behaviours refer to acts committed in violation of the criminal law and for which the legal age of criminal responsibility has been reached and which require criminal punishment.
5 Under criminal law, the court may, at the time of sentencing, prohibit the offender from having access to certain people, places or occupations, depending on the circumstances of the offence and the need to prevent reoffending.
6 Psychological correction is the application of psychological principles and techniques by professionals to understand the psychological situation of offenders, to help them regulate their bad moods and prevent, improve and eliminate psychological problems.

References

Chen, X. (2004). Social and legal control in China: A comparative perspective. *International Journal of Offender Therapy and Comparative Criminology*, 48(5), 523–536.

Chen, X. (2021). Practice and reflections on deepening the basic model of national unified judicial administration for drug treatment – An empirical analysis based on the return survey of discharged detainees [深化全国统一司法行政戒毒工作基本模式的实践与思考——基于解戒人员回访调查的实证分析]. *Justice of China*, 02, 94–99.

Chu, H. (2007). The direction of the re-education through labour system [劳动教养制度走向]. *Crime and Rehabilitation Studies*, 9, 2–4.

Dutton, M. (1992). Disciplinary projects and carceral spread: Foucauldian theory and Chinese practice. *Economy and Society*, *21*(3), 276–294.

Epstein, E. J., & Wong, S. H.-Y. (1996). The concept of dangerousness in the People's Republic of China and its impact on the treatment of prisoners. *The British Journal of Criminology*, *36*, 472.

Gao, Q., & Luo, C. (2006). A preliminary study of the clan trial system in ancient Chinese society [中国古代社会宗族审判制度初探]. *Journal of Central China Normal University (Humanities and Social Sciences)*, *1*, 84–89.

Hung, V. M.Y. (2002). Improving human rights in China: Should re-education through labor be abolished? *Columbia Journal of Transnational Law*, *41*, 303–326.

Jia, L. (2018). Review and prospects of China's prison development in the past 40 years of reform and opening up [改革开放四十年中国监狱发展的回顾与展望]. *Journal of Henan Judicial Police Vocational College*, *16*(04), 14–21.

Jiang, S., Jin, X., Xiang, D., Goodlin-Fahncke, W., Yang, S., Xu, N., & Zhang, D. (2016). Punitive and rehabilitative orientations toward offenders among community correctional officers in China. *The Prison Journal*, *96*(6), 771–792.

Jiang, S., Xiang, D., Chen, Q., Huang, C., Yang, S., Zhang, D., & Zhao, A. (2014). Community corrections in China: Development and challenges. *The Prison Journal*, *94*(1), 75–96.

Ji, X., & Shen, M. (2014). *The Transformation of China's Rehabilitation of Criminals—Also on the Model of Criminal Rehabilitation in China* [中国改造罪犯模式之转型:兼论改造罪犯的中国模式]. Beijing: Publishing House of Local Records.

Jin, J. (1990). Building a socialist work reform criminology with Chinese characteristics [建设有中国特色的社会主义劳动改造罪犯学]. *Crime and Rehabilitation Studies*, *5*, 1–4+43.

Lao, D. (2019). Rethinking criminal law theory of risk [风险刑法理论的反思]. *Political Science and Law*, *11*, 30–43.

Li, E. (2013). The new drug détoxification system in China: A misused tool for drug rehabilitation. *East Asia Law Review*, *9*, 168.

Li, E. (2022). Rehabilitation in a risk society: 'The case of China'. In M. Vanstone & P. Priestley (Eds.), *The Palgrave Handbook of Global Rehabilitation in Criminal Justice* (pp. 89–106). Cham: Springer.

Li, Q., & Dai, Y. (1991). Labour reform work in China in the 1990s [九十年代的中国劳改工作]. *Crime and Rehabilitation Studies*, *1*, 46–48.

Li, Y. (2019). The successful development of 70 Years of rehabilitation of offenders in new Chinese prisons [新中国监狱70年改造罪犯的成功发展之路]. *Crime and Rehabilitation Studies*, *10*, 23–39.

Li, Z. (2018). Reflections on guidance and support for community-based drug treatment and rehabilitation by drug rehabilitation agencies of the administration of justice [司法行政戒毒机关指导支持社区戒毒、社区康复工作思考]. *Crime and Rehabilitation Studies*, *11*, 66–70.

Liu, L., & Chui, W. H. (2018). Rehabilitation policy for drug addicted offenders in China: Current trends, patterns, and practice implications. *Asia Pacific Journal of Social Work and Development*, *28*(3), 192–204.

Liu, L., & Hsiao, S. C. (2018). Chinese female drug users' experiences and attitudes with institutional drug treatment. *International Journal of Offender Therapy and Comparative Criminology*, 62(13), 4221–4235.

Robertson, P., Barnao, M., & Ward, T. (2011). Rehabilitation frameworks in forensic mental health. *Aggression and Violent Behavior*, 16(6), 472–484.

Rong, R., & Liu, Y. (2009). The Sunshine halfway house model in Chaoyang District, Beijing [北京市朝阳区积极探索阳光中途之家工作模式]. *Studies in Crime and Rehabilitation*, 6, 47–49.

State Council Information Office of the People's Republic of China (SCIO). (1992). *The State of Rehabilitation of Offenders in China*. Beijing: SCIO.

Tao, Y., & Xiao, Y. (2007). Ancient Chinese debates on the purpose of punishment and utilitarian and anti-utilitarian values [中国古代关于刑罚目的以及功利主义与反功利主义价值观的争论]. *Political Science and Law*, 3, 185–190.

Tibke, P. (2017). Drug dependence treatment in China: A policy analysis. *International Drug Policy Consortium Publication*, 2017, 1–16.

Wang, J., & Huang, P. (2012). Psychological correction: A remedy for community sentenced persons – The use and effectiveness of psychological correctional techniques in community correctional work [心理矫治:社区服刑人员矫正的一剂良药——心理矫治技术在社区矫正工作中的运用与成效]. *People's Mediation*, 1, 31–35.

Wang, M. (2009). A century of brilliance – A review of 60 years of prison work in New China - 1 [一个甲子的辉煌——新中国监狱工作60年的回顾 - 1]. *Crime and Rehabilitation Studies*, 9, 27–33.

Wang, S. (1992). The nature of juvenile reception and correction [少年收容教养的性质之我见]. *Tribune of Political Science and Law*, 3, 63–68.

Wang, Y. (2008). On China's re-education through labour system and its reform [试论我国的劳动教养制度及其改革]. *Qinghai Social Sciences*, 4, 175–177.

Wodahl, E. J., & Garland, B. (2009). The evolution of community corrections. *The Prison Journal*, 89(1 suppl), 81S–104S.

Wu, H. (1997). China's gulag: Suppressing dissent through the *laogai*. *Harvard International Review*, 20(1), 20–23.

Wu, J. (2021). The system and the way out: Dilemmas and reconfigurations of the specialized correctional education system [制度与出路：专门矫治教育制度困境与重构]. *Chongqing Social Sciences*, 8, 91–103.

Wu, W., & Vander Beken, T. (2018). Understanding criminal punishment and prisons in China. *The Prison Journal*, 98(6), 700–721.

Wu, Z. (2021). *Research on the Standardization of Community Corrections in China* [中国社区矫正规范化研究]. Beijing: Beijing Normal University Publishing Group.

Wu, Z. (2022). On the key issues and solutions for underage community corrections [论未成年社区矫正的关键问题与解决方法]. *Community Corrections Studies*, 1(01), 8–20.

Xiao, Y., & Yang, B. (2014). Theoretical foundations of evidence-based corrections – An interpretation of the RNR model [循证矫正的理论基础——RNR模型解读]. 犯罪与改造研究, 3, 14–18.

Yan, J. (2020). Reflections on the path to the realisation of the right to education for prison offenders [监狱罪犯受教育权实现路径的思考]. *China Prison Journal*, 35(04), 31–43.

Yao, J., & Sun, J. (2017). From 'work-study' to 'specialized' – The dilemma and way out of work-study education in China [从"工读"到"专门"——我国工读教育的困境与出路]. *Juvenile Delinquency Prevention Research*, 2, 46–56+12.

Yuan, N. (2021). On the legal construction of the three-tier prevention model for juvenile delinquency – A perspective on the amendment of the law on the prevention of juvenile delinquency [论未成年人犯罪三级预防模式的法律建构——以《预防未成年人犯罪法》的修订为视角]. *Juvenile Delinquency Prevention Research*, 2, 42–50.

Zhang, J. (2022). Practice and research on the management model of graded treatment of offenders in the new situation – Iterative upgrade of the dynamic point system of graded treatment [新形势下罪犯分级处遇管理模式的实践与研究——动态积分制分级处遇的迭代升级]. *China Prison Journal*, 37(05), 69–74.

Zhang, Y., Wang, D., & Li, X. (2013). Study on the application of non-custodial sentences for minor offenders [未成年罪犯非监禁刑适用问题研究]. *Juvenile Delinquency Prevention Research*, 4, 62–66+83.

Zhao, F. (2015). Exploration and practice of a social work model for community drug rehabilitation [社区戒毒社会工作模式的探索与实践]. *Social Work and Management*, 15(05), 5–13+87.

Zheng, Y., Wang, H., Luo, H., Wang, Y., & Yang, D. (2011). A comparative analysis of the advantages and disadvantages of two different models of voluntary drug treatment facilities [两种不同模式自愿戒毒机构的优势及弊端对比分析]. *Chinese Journal of Drug Abuse Prevention and Treatment*, 17(02), 107–110.

Zhou, C., & Yang, W. (2016). Some reflections on the education and correction of community drug addicts (rehabilitation) [(社区戒毒(康复)人员教育矫治工作的若干思考). *Crime and Rehabilitation Studies*, 10, 55–57.

4

OFFENDER REHABILITATION IN HONG KONG

Current Practice and Service Development

Aaron H. L. Wong, Frank Wong, and Wing Hong Chui

Introduction

Hong Kong is one of the safest cities in the world, with its overall crime rate per 100,000 population decreasing from 1,159 in 2000 to 961 in 2022 (Census and Statistics Department, 2011, Table 15.1; Hong Kong Police Force, 2023). Violent crimes are infrequent in Hong Kong. Only 13% of the reported crimes in 2022 were violent (Hong Kong Police Force, 2023), and the homicide rate, which is less susceptible to under-reporting (Broadhurst et al., 2017), is very low, the rate being 0.41 per 100,000 population in 2022 (Census and Statistics Department, 2023; Hong Kong Police Force, 2023). Robbery (6th out of 69 jurisdictions) and kidnapping (6th out of 79 jurisdictions) are also relatively uncommon when compared to other countries (United Nations Office on Drugs and Crime, 2022a, 2022b).

Consistent with the declining crime trend, the penal population in Hong Kong has also decreased by around 50% in the past decade (2011: 14,129; 2022: 7,209), while the total population has grown by about 4% (2011: 7,071,600; 2022: 7,346,100) (Census and Statistics Department, 2022, Table 1.1, 2023; Correctional Services Department [CSD], 2023a). Furthermore, over 90% of prisoners (2011: 11,576, 2021: 7,013) were sentenced to imprisonment of less than 3 years, reflecting that most prisoners did not commit the most serious crimes (Census and Statistics Department, 2022, Table 15.11).

Contributing to the low crime rate and penal population, the correctional services of Hong Kong play an important role in public protection

DOI: 10.4324/9781003360919-6

and crime prevention. The aim of these services is to lead prisoners towards law-abiding and constructive lives during imprisonment and after release (Correctional Services Department, 2022a). While China resumed its exercise of sovereignty over Hong Kong in 1997, Hong Kong retained its own criminal justice system, correctional services included, under the policy of "One Country, Two Systems". With Hong Kong simultaneously being a global city and "the gateway to China", how this unique context of "East meets West" (Adorjan & Chui, 2014a, p. 98) shapes its rehabilitation policy poses an interesting case study.

This chapter explores the rehabilitation strategies employed by correctional services in Hong Kong and how they successfully address the complex needs of prisoners. It is structured into four sections. The first section traces the history of rehabilitation policy in Hong Kong's correctional services. The second section explores current rehabilitation efforts in correctional institutions (including prisons, youth correctional institutions, drug addiction treatment facilities and psychiatric treatment facilities) and the community. The third section discusses how Western rehabilitation models are applied in Hong Kong and the final section examines the effectiveness of Hong Kong's rehabilitation efforts using official statistics and data. Limitations of the official data are highlighted.

Early Rehabilitation Policy in Hong Kong

Hong Kong's rehabilitation practices can be traced to 1853, when, under British colonial rule (Chan, 2017), rehabilitation was limited to religious support provided by visiting chaplains. Consistent with English practices, penal philosophy emphasised prisoners' opportunity for self-reflection. In the 1930s, industrial and reformatory schools were established to cater for young people's rehabilitative needs (Chan, 2017). In the 1960s, drug addiction treatment centres were established in response to the increase in opium and heroin addiction (Garner, 1976), whereas in the 1970s, a detention centre was established to provide wider sentencing options to deal with young offenders (Adorjan & Chui, 2014b).

The work of Hong Kong's correctional services continues to be guided by the "rehabilitative ideal" (i.e., punishment should serve a therapeutic function to bring positive changes to offenders) (Allen, 1959), even when such a concept was threatened in the West when the "nothing works" mantra became popular during the 1970s (Chui, 2022; Gray, 1999). The establishment of psychological services in correctional facilities in 1977 and the renaming of the Prisons Department as the Correctional Services Department in 1982 further reflect the growing institutional emphasis on rehabilitation (Chan, 2017; Hui & Lo, 2017).

Although the overall service model of the Correctional Services Department was built during British colonial rule, many practices that bear British roots were adapted to respond to local needs and changing environments. For example, arrangements were made for Buddhist volunteers to regularly visit correctional institutions and speak with prisoners (Chui & Cheng, 2013a) and rehabilitation centres for young offenders were established in 2002 to provide an additional sentencing option, beyond detention and training centres (Security Bureau, 1999). With the adaptation of Western theories to create localised assessment tools and treatment programmes, Hong Kong's rehabilitation practice has become increasingly localised, theory-informed, and evidence-based (Chan et al., 2017).

Offender Rehabilitation Efforts in Hong Kong

Rehabilitation Services in Prisons

Rehabilitation services delivered in prisons can be divided into: (1) psychological services, (2) welfare and counselling services, (3) education, (4) work and vocational training, and (5) employment support.

Psychological services

In Hong Kong's prisons, clinical psychologists assist offenders with settling into custody, enhancing their mental well-being, and bringing a positive change to their offending behaviour. Their work includes managing casework and providing individual counselling for offenders with psychological or complex emotional issues (Correctional Services Department, 2021a), as well as developing systematic assessment tools and psychological treatment programmes (Security Bureau, 2017a).

Further to adopting the Risk-Need-Responsivity (RNR) model, the Correctional Services Department developed the Risks and Needs Assessment and Management Protocol for Offenders in 2006. This is a systematic tool for assessing the custodial and reoffending risks and rehabilitative needs of offenders (Security Bureau, 2007). Under the Protocol, risk of reoffending is assessed according to the person's age, educational background, and past conviction and drug abuse history (Audit Commission, 2015). Rehabilitative needs are assessed in seven need domains: (1) family/marital, (2) employment, (3) community functioning, (4) associates, (5) personal/emotional, (6) criminal attitude, and (7) drug abuse. The Correctional Services Department offers corresponding programmes to match those needs, and aims to fulfil at least one rehabilitative need before discharge (Audit Commission, 2015). Localised violence and sexual offending risk assessment scales have also been developed (Chan et al., 2017).

A Sex Offenders' Evaluation and Treatment Unit was established in the 1990s, incorporating RNR and elements of the Good Lives Model (to sustain [offenders'] motivation for positive change) in its cognitive behavioural therapy (CBT) based treatment (Chan & Woo, 2017). In the 2000s, the Violence Prevention Programme was established. Comprising ten modules (e.g., cognitive restructuring, anger management, conflict resolution, and empathy training) the Violence Prevention Programme is designed to address violent offenders' criminogenic needs and prevent violent reoffending (Lee et al., 2017).

Female prisoners account for over 25% of the prison population, a ratio that is much higher than elsewhere in the world (6.9%) (Correctional Services Department, 2023a; Fair & Walmsley, 2022). To address females' unique risks and needs, the Correctional Services Department developed a separate assessment tool for females (Mak et al., 2017). Furthermore, a "Psychological Gymnasium" (Psy Gym) was established in 2011; the first facility in Asia aimed at addressing female offenders' specific needs (e.g., emotional and self-harm issues, victimisation and dysfunctional relationships) (Mak et al., 2018). The environment of the Psy Gym is specifically designed so that treatment can be conducted in a "cozy, cheerful, personalised, and generally less institutional atmosphere" (Mak et al., 2018, p. 1066). Combining both CBT and positive psychology, the Psy Gym programme has been empirically proven to reduce symptoms of depression, anxiety and stress as well as enhance hope and gratitude (Mak et al., 2018).

In 2018, the Correctional Services Department launched a "Life Gym" for male prisoners which serves as a "positive living" centre targeting male-specific needs and risks (GovHK, 2018). Both the Psy Gym and Life Gym programmes take several months to complete and aim to create a therapeutic community that encourages mutual support among participants and allows participants to implement newly learned psychological skills into practice in daily life (GovHK, 2018; Mak et al., 2017). The Correctional Services Department has designed other specialised treatment programmes such as the Offending Behaviour Programme for young offenders and the Drug Abuse Rehabilitation Programme for drug-dependent offenders in drug addiction treatment centres (2021a).

Welfare and counselling services

The Correctional Services Department provides welfare and counselling services for all prisoners, sometimes in collaboration with non-government organisations and volunteers. Prison officers assist prisoners with their personal issues and guide them in adapting to prison life. Prisoners can join educational tutorial classes and interest groups held by volunteers and non-government organisations (Correctional Services Department, 2023a). Chaplains and volunteers from religious organisations also offer religious services, which include visits, teaching, counselling, religious worship and recreational activities to all prisoners regardless of their religious belief or background (Correctional Services Department, 2020a).

Education

Difficulty in securing employment is a major obstacle faced by ex-prisoners in Hong Kong (Chui & Cheng, 2014). Most prisoners (excluding retirees) were either unemployed or non-skilled workers prior to custody (Society for Community Organization, 2019). As education is a path to employment in Hong Kong's competitive labour market (Chui & Cheng, 2013b, 2014) a key goal of the Correctional Services Department is to educate to help offenders "make a living, and eventually help them reintegrate into society" (Correctional Services Department, 2022a).

The Correctional Services Department offers half-day compulsory education courses conducted by qualified teachers to young offenders under 21. From 2014 to 2018, more than 2,500 young prisoners received education in correctional institutions (Correctional Services Department, 2019a). The Correctional Services Department also encourages prisoners to sit for public examinations, including the Hong Kong Diploma of Secondary Education Examination (Correctional Services Department, 2022b). The Correctional Services Department encourages adult prisoners to study for distance learning degrees offered by the Hong Kong Metropolitan University (Correctional Services Department, 2022b). Libraries and e-learning resource corners have been set up at various institutions to facilitate participation in distance learning courses, and multiple education funds are provided to cover academic expenses (The Hong Kong Government [GovHK], 2015). Between 2019 and 2021, 19 prisoners were awarded bachelor's degrees and one prisoner was awarded a master's degree (Correctional Services Department, 2022c).

Work and vocational training

To help prisoners acquire good working habits and reduce idleness, prisoners are required by law to work (Correctional Services Department, 2023b). In 2022, a daily average of 3,475 prisoners engaged in the production of various items, including garments, personal protective equipment, road signs, metalwork, etc. Modern technologies, such as 3D scanners and 3D printing equipment, have also been introduced in prison workshops to enhance working efficiency and facilitate prisoners' reintegration (Correctional Services Department, 2023b).

Similarly, the Correctional Services Department offers a wide range of vocational training courses to help prisoners gain accredited skills and cultivate good working habits (Correctional Services Department, 2022d). Over 40 vocational training programmes, covering building services, commercial practice, information technology are offered. In 2020–21, over 1,400 training places were offered, attracting over 900 prisoner enrolment (Correctional Services Department, 2021a). Prisoners may also participate in external examinations held by City and Guilds, the London Chamber of Commerce and Industry, and other vocational training bodies (Correctional Services Department, 2022b).

Employment support

For participants who have successfully completed certain vocational training courses, a voluntary employment follow-up service is offered (Correctional Services Department, 2023c). In addition, the Correctional Services Department also maintains a job-matching platform for all prisoners. Prisoners who are to be released within 3 months may file a job application, and the correctional institutions will facilitate job interviews, whether in person or over the telephone or the internet.

Correctional Institutions for Specific Groups of Offenders

To better address their rehabilitative needs, young offenders and offenders with drug dependence or mental health issues may be sentenced to special correctional institutions. The design of these institutions and their rehabilitation programmes are described below.

Correctional institutions for young offenders

The Correctional Services Department manages three types of custodial institutions for young offenders: a detention centre, training centres, and rehabilitation centres. The detention centre admits offenders aged between 14 and 24 (male only), and both the training centres and rehabilitation centres admit offenders aged between 14 and 20 (male and female). While the law prescribes the minimum and maximum detention time for each type of order, the actual length of the sentences is indeterminate. Correctional Services Department officers will periodically review the performance of young offenders, and better performance will expedite release (Security Bureau, 1998).

A detention centre order is designed to give a "short, sharp shock" to young offenders through physically demanding disciplinary training (Chui, 1999; Security Bureau, 1998). During the detention period, physical exercise, foot drills, shoe polishing and bed-making are part of the daily routine (Chui, 2005). Among the three types of youth institutions, the detention centre has the shortest detention periods: 1 to 6 months (for offenders aged 14 to 20 years) and 3 to 12 months (for offenders aged 21 to 24 years). Past data show that the average custodial times for the former and latter age groups are 4 months and 8 months, respectively (Correctional Services Department, 2010).

A training centre order involves a longer period of residency, ranging from 6 to 36 months (average is 18 months), with a focus on education and vocational training, and a longer post-release supervision period (Wong Chun Cheong v HKSAR, 2001). Compulsory half-day occupational training and half-day education classes are provided (Security Bureau, 1998). Extracurricular activities, such as scouting, hobby classes, and physical and recreational activities, are also provided to enhance young people's well-being and allow them to explore their interests. The training centre programme aims to develop young offenders' positive character and enhance their employability or academic results (Chan, 2017). The training centre programme's post-release supervision period is 3 years.

In the early 2000s, a new intermediate sentencing option for young offenders was made available: the rehabilitation centre order. A rehabilitation centre order is deemed suitable for offenders who are physically unfit to be sentenced to a detention centre and who have not committed a serious crime warranting a lengthier custodial time at a training centre. The detention period in a rehabilitation centre is between three and 9 months (Rehabilitation Centres Ordinance, 2001). Offenders serve 2 to 5 months in a rehabilitation centre, receiving disciplinary training, counselling services, social skills training, and basic work skills training (GovHK, 1999). Afterwards, they are transferred to a halfway house, where they may work or study as permitted during the daytime (Security Bureau, 2017b). Post-release statutory supervision lasts 12 months (Rehabilitation Centres Ordinance, 2001).

Drug addiction treatment centre

Drug addiction treatment centres provide compulsory treatment for drug-dependent offenders. Any person who has been convicted of "an offence punishable with imprisonment" and found "addicted to any dangerous drug" can be sentenced to a Drug Addiction Treatment Centre (Drug Addiction Treatment Centres Ordinance, 1968, secs 2 & 3). A Drug Addiction Treatment Centre order lasts between 2 and 12 months, depending on the progress of treatment, and there is a 1-year statutory post-release supervision period which includes regular drug tests to ensure supervisees remain free from drugs. Besides medication, the programme also offers outdoor physical work, such as gardening, to improve discipline and physical health (Correctional Services Department, 2010; Narcotics Division, Security Bureau, 2021a). Vocational training, a counselling service and employment support are also available (Narcotics Division, Security Bureau 2021b).

Psychiatric centre

A recent study estimated 7% of the total prison population in Hong Kong had a mental disorder (Siu et al., 2022). Operated as both a prison and a psychiatric treatment centre, Siu Lam Psychiatric Centre is the first and only correctional facility in Hong Kong designed for treating mentally ill offenders (Siu et al., 2022). From 2018 to 2022, approximately 200 people per year underwent assessment or treatment in the Siu Lam Psychiatric Centre (Correctional Services Department, 2023d). Siu Lam Psychiatric Centre provides psychiatric assessment and treatment for convicted and remanded offenders referred from other Correctional Services Department facilities and for offenders subject to a court hospital order (Siu & Lam, 2018). Occupational therapy, voluntary education, recreational activities, and sports classes are also provided (Correctional Services Department, 2002). Transfer to facilities outside Siu Lam Psychiatric Centre (e.g., Castle Peak Hospital) may be arranged for prisoners to receive necessary psychiatric treatment (Siu & Lam, 2018).

Rehabilitation in Community Settings

Hong Kong also actively promotes rehabilitation in community settings through (1) discretionary early-release schemes, (2) post-release supervision and support, and (3) community sentences.

Discretionary early-release schemes

To promote rehabilitation and early reintegration, prisoners may apply for early release through two schemes: the Release under Supervision Scheme and the Pre-release Employment Scheme (Security Bureau, 2021a). Applications are considered by the Release under Supervision Board, an independent advisory body that makes recommendations on the applications for and conditions of early release to the Chief Executive of Hong Kong (Security Bureau, 2021b).

Similarly, the Long-term Prison Sentences Review Board considers early release applications from those serving (1) a long-term sentence of over 10 years, (2) a determinate sentence when convicted under 21 years of age or (3) an indeterminate sentence. A prisoner may be granted early release (with post-release supervision requirements) under the Conditional Release Scheme or the Supervision After Release Scheme. The Board also has the power to recommend a shortened determinate sentence or a conversion from an indeterminate sentence to a fixed-term sentence (Security Bureau, 2021c).

Statutory post-release supervision administered by the Correctional Services Department is also applicable to (1) offenders who have served long-term imprisonment of over 6 years or who were convicted of specified serious offences and imprisoned for over 2 years, (2) offenders sentenced to a Drug Abuse Treatment Centre, and (3) young offenders sentenced to the three youth correctional institutions and prisons. A breach of the conditions imposed under statutory supervision may lead to reincarceration (Correctional Services Department, 2022e).

Post-release supervision and support

To facilitate prisoners' rehabilitation and reintegration, Correctional Services Department officers begin building rapport with supervisees and their families during the custody period in order to assist in the prisoners' career planning; they also provide guidance and support following the prisoners' discharge (Security Bureau, 2021d). Like offenders under probation, the usual conditions of post-release supervision include meeting with Correctional Services Department officers regularly, and an expectation of engagement in approved employment and residing at a specified address (Correctional Services Department, 2023a). Some additional conditions, such as a curfew, taking regular drug tests and attending counselling, may also be imposed. Correctional Services Department supervision officers also regularly visit the offender's workplace or home to ensure compliance with the supervision conditions (Correctional Services Department, 2023c).

Correctional Services Department officers may refer ex-prisoners to other government departments and non-government organisations for post-release support (GovHK, 2015), including social work support, hostel services, employment support, and short-term rental assistance (Social Welfare Department, 2022a). In recent years, multi-purpose family and rehabilitation service centres have been established to provide psychological and counselling services for ex-offenders (Correctional Services Department, 2023e). Following statutory supervision, a voluntary follow-up counselling programme is available for ex-supervisees in need under the Correctional Services Department's Continuing Care Project (Correctional Services Department, 2020a).

Community sentences

Community sentences are alternatives to imprisonment for (usually first- or second-time) offenders convicted of less serious offences (Chui, 2017). The two types of (noncustodial) community sentences available in Hong Kong are probation and community service orders; these involve close supervision and guidance by a probation officer from the Social Welfare Department. This department also provides welfare services to general ex-offenders and discharged prisoners (Social Welfare Department, 2022b).

Offenders under probation orders are placed under statutory supervision for 1 to 3 years (Probation of Offenders Ordinance, 1956). A standard probation order requires the offender to contact the probation officer regularly and inform them of any change of address (Chui, 2017). The court may impose additional conditions, such as "work and reside as directed", "abstain from dangerous drugs", "psychological treatment" and "curfew order" (Chui, 2004, p. 450).

A community service order requires offenders to perform unpaid work not exceeding 240 hours within 12 months under the supervision of a probation officer (Community Service Orders Ordinance, 1984). Like supervision under a probation order, probation officers meet offenders regularly to provide personal guidance (Social Welfare Department, 2022c), and conduct site visits to monitor offenders' performance.

With all probation officers being social workers, the provision of community sentences adopts a social work model to "advise, assist and befriend" offenders in the hope of transforming offenders into law-abiding citizens (Chui, 2022; Probation of Offenders Rules, 1958). Offenders' voluntary participation is a prerequisite for a community sentence (Probation of Offenders Ordinance, 1956), increasing the likelihood offenders participate in community programmes. Community sentences aim to bring positive changes in offenders' attitudes and behaviour, enhance their life coping skills and strengthen their family support (Social Welfare Department, 2022d). Probation officers will also assist offenders secure employment (Chui & Cheng, 2014).

The Role of Western Rehabilitation Models in Hong Kong's Practice

Correctional Services Department's Risks-Needs Assessment Protocol was developed in line with the Risk-Need-Responsivity (RNR) model to identify offenders with a higher risk of reoffending and their criminogenic needs. Corresponding treatment programmes are then provided (Chan et al., 2017). While elements of the GLM are incorporated into treatment programmes (Chan & Woo, 2017; Correctional Services Department, n.d.; Lee et al., 2017), GLM is not the guiding model. For offenders serving a community sentence, one-to-one counselling sessions are conducted by probation officers, focusing on personal, relationship and employment issues (Chui, 2016). Some ex-offenders under post-release supervision would also formulate a discharge plan with the help of supervision officers (Security Bureau, 2021d), but a "good lives plan" is not an explicit focus in these sessions. That said, staff do seek to promote "good lives" for offenders. For example, education and vocational training in correctional institutions assist offenders in terms of satisfying the primary goods of knowledge and excellence in work (see Ward et al., 2012). By assisting offenders in dealing with personal issues and seeking employment and introducing community resources to them during imprisonment, community sentences and post-release supervision, the primary goals of excellence in agency and community can also be advanced (Ward et al., 2012).

Therefore, Hong Kong's rehabilitation services have incorporated elements of both RNR and GLM models. There are also locally developed services and instruments that have emerged from these models/theories, as evidenced by the invention of Hong Kong's own risk assessment scales for sexual and violent offenders and the design of Psy Gym and Life Gym centres. Although authorities have not declared an official model that guides overall service delivery, it can be seen that, in line with both the RNR model and the GLM, "managing risk of reoffending" and "enhancing offender well-being" (Ward & Fortune, 2013, p. 34) have been the main foci in rehabilitation work in Hong Kong.

Effectiveness of Hong Kong's Rehabilitation Efforts

There are several official statistics that shed light on the success of Hong Kong's rehabilitation efforts. Firstly, the Correctional Services Department releases the recidivism rate of local ex-prisoners, in which recidivism is defined as readmission to a correctional institution within 2 years of discharge. In recent years, there has been a steady decrease from 36.5% (2004) to 23.3% (2020) in the official recidivism rate (Correctional Services Department, 2016, 2023f).

Secondly, Correctional Services Department releases the success rate of rehabilitation programmes with a post-release statutory supervision period. The success rate is defined as an absence of re-conviction within the supervision period (Audit Commission, 2015). In 2022, eight out of ten rehabilitation programmes had a success rate of over 95%. Only the Drug Abuse Treatment Centre programme and the Training Centre Programme had lower success rates (53.7% and 81.5%, respectively). The lower success rate of Drug Abuse Treatment Centre may be due to the additional "success" criterion of no relapse into drug abuse within the supervision period (Audit Commission, 2015).

Thirdly, the Social Welfare Department releases the successful completion rate of their supervision programmes. In 2021–22, 89% and 97%, respectively, of probation and community service orders were successfully served (Social Welfare Department, 2022e). The high success rate in completing community sentences adds support to the effectiveness of the social work approach and community-based rehabilitation programmes. Additionally, ex-offenders do not generally face significant difficulties in seeking employment. Correctional Services Department statistics from 2018 to 2022 show that over 80% of ex-offenders (who joined the follow-up service) secured employment within 6 months of being discharged (Correctional Services Department, 2023h).

Although the rehabilitation programmes of the Correctional Services Department and the Social Welfare Department appear to be successful in reducing recidivism, there are a few caveats. Firstly, the official recidivism rate calculates readmission within 2 years of discharge. Furthermore, due to the time between the offending behaviour and conviction, the time of readmission may fall outside the 2-year reporting period. Secondly, self-reported data indicate a higher recidivism rate (compared to the official rate). Chui and Chan (2012) found that around 30% of juvenile probationers self-reported reoffending within months and 38% of adult probationers self-reported having reoffended within 1 year (Chui, 2004). In another self-report study with a small sample size, four out of five interviewees admitted to reoffending after being released from youth correctional institutions (Chui, 1999). Thirdly, the low recidivism rates do not equate to successful and shame/stigma-free reintegration (Adorjan & Chui, 2012; Chui, 2005; Gray, 1999).

Conclusion

The rehabilitation approach in Hong Kong was greatly influenced by British practices when Hong Kong was under British rule. However, over the past decades, local adaptations have dominated, as evidenced by the establishment of rehabilitation centres and the design of localised risk-assessment tools and locally developed psychological treatment programmes. Western rehabilitation theories have played an important role in the development and provision of rehabilitation services. While a predominantly RNR-based assessment and treatment approach is adopted, the strengths-based GLM approach also features in some psychological treatment programmes. Furthermore, by providing education, work, and vocational training in correctional facilities, the Correctional Services Department aims both to address offenders' criminogenic needs and assist offenders in better reintegrating into society and living a good life. A social work approach drives supervision for those on community orders. Through counselling and supervision, it is believed that offenders can be rehabilitated in the community and become an asset to society (Chui, 2022).

Both the crime and recidivism rates in Hong Kong have significantly decreased over the past decades. Together with the high success rate of the rehabilitation programmes within institutions and in the community, these figures appear to support Hong Kong's rehabilitation programmes attempts to spark offenders' inner motivation to change and avoid reoffending (Correctional Services Department, 2022a).

Finally, the effectiveness of newer rehabilitation measures requires further evaluation. A "Change Lab", focussed on de-radicalising protesters convicted of offences related to the 2019 Hong Kong Anti-Extradition Bill protests, has recently been established (Correctional Services Department, 2022c). In recent years, the Correctional Services Department has also been developing the "smart prison" concept, in which one of the measures involves installing a "self-service kiosk" to enhance prisoners' self-management skills (Correctional Services Department, 2019b). Further research is needed to evaluate these new initiatives; for example, whether the increased use of technology will benefit offenders' rehabilitation, or, conversely, bring unintended harm to rehabilitation by reducing communication and undermining trust between prison staff and prisoners.

References

Adorjan, M., & Chui, W. H. (2012). Making sense of going straight: Personal accounts of male ex-prisoners in Hong Kong. *The British Journal of Criminology*, 52(3), 577–590. 10.1093/bjc/azr093

Adorjan, M., & Chui, W. H. (2014a). Aging out of crime: Resettlement challenges facing male ex-prisoners in Hong Kong. *The Prison Journal*, 94(1), 97–117. 10.1177/0032885513512095

Adorjan, M., & Chui, W. H. (2014b). *Responding to youth crime in Hong Kong: Penal elitism, legitimacy and citizenship.* Routledge. 10.4324/9780203067642

Allen, F. A. (1959). Criminal justice, legal values and the rehabilitative ideal. *The Journal of Criminal Law, Criminology, and Police Science, 50*(3), 226–232. JSTOR. 10.2307/1141037

Audit Commission. (2015). *Rehabilitation services provided by the Correctional Services Department.* https://www.aud.gov.hk/pdf_e/e64ch08.pdf

Broadhurst, R., Chan, C. Y., & Lee, K. W. (2017). Crime trends. In W. H. Chui & T. W. Lo (Eds.), *Understanding criminal justice in Hong Kong* (2nd ed., pp. 57–80). Routledge.

Census and Statistics Department. (2011). *Hong Kong annual digest of statistics: 2011 Edition.* https://www.statistics.gov.hk/pub/B10100032011AN11B0100.pdf

Census and Statistics Department. (2022). *Hong Kong annual digest of statistics: 2022 Edition.* https://www.censtatd.gov.hk/en/data/stat_report/product/B1010003/att/B10100032022AN22B0100.pdf

Census and Statistics Department. (2023, February 16). *Table 110-01001: Population by sex and age group.* Retrieved April 12, 2023, from https://www.censtatd.gov.hk/en/web_table.html?id=110-01001

Chan, C. C. L., Hui, S. H., Cheung, H. K., & Pau, B. K. Y. (2017). Development of psychological services in the Hong Kong Correctional Services Department. In H. C. (Oliver) Chan & S. M. Y. Ho (Eds.), *Psycho-criminological perspective of criminal justice in Asia* (pp. 114–125). Routledge.

Chan, K. P. J., & Woo, C. P. (2017). The development of psychological treatment programmes for incarcerated sex offenders in Hong Kong: From relapse prevention to a positive treatment approach. In H. C. (Oliver) Chan & S. M. Y. Ho (Eds.), *Psycho-criminological perspective of criminal justice in Asia* (pp. 160–183). Routledge.

Chan, S. (2017). Offender rehabilitation: The Hong Kong Correctional Services Department. In H. C. (Oliver) Chan & S. M. Y. Ho (Eds.), *Psycho-criminological perspective of criminal justice in Asia* (1st ed., pp. 89–113). Routledge.

Chui, W. H. (1999). Residential treatment programs for young offenders in Hong Kong: A report. *International Journal of Offender Therapy and Comparative Criminology, 43*(3), 308–321. 10.1177/0306624X99433005

Chui, W. H. (2004). Adult offenders on probation in Hong Kong: An exploratory study. *The British Journal of Social Work, 34*(3), 443–454. 10.1093/bjsw/bch047

Chui, W. H. (2005). Detention center in Hong Kong: A young offender's narrative. *Journal of Offender Rehabilitation, 41*(1), 67–84. 10.1300/J076v41n01_03

Chui, W. H. (2017). Probation and community service orders. In W. H. Chui & T. W. Lo (Eds.), *Understanding criminal justice in Hong Kong* (2nd ed., pp. 291–311). Routledge.

Chui, W. H. (2022). Approaches to rehabilitation in Hong Kong. In M. Vanstone & P. Priestley (Eds.), *The Palgrave handbook of global rehabilitation in criminal justice* (pp. 219–236). Springer International Publishing. 10.1007/978-3-031-14375-5_13

Chui, W. H., & Chan, H. C. O. (2012). Criminal recidivism among Hong Kong male juvenile probationers. *Journal of Child and Family Studies*, *21*(5), 857–868. 10.1007/s10826-011-9546-0

Chui, W. H., & Cheng, K. K. (2013a). Self-perceived role and function of Christian prison chaplains and Buddhist volunteers in Hong Kong prisons. *International Journal of Offender Therapy and Comparative Criminology*, *57*(2), 154–168. 10.1177/0306624X11432128

Chui, W. H., & Cheng, K. K. (2013b). The Mark of an ex-prisoner: Perceived discrimination and self-stigma of young men after prison in Hong Kong. *Deviant Behavior*, *34*(8), 671–684. 10.1080/01639625.2013.766532

Chui, W. H., & Cheng, K. K. (2014). Challenges facing young men returning from incarceration in Hong Kong. *The Howard Journal of Criminal Justice*, *53*(4), 411–427. 10.1111/hojo.12088

Correctional Services Department. (n.d.). *Violence prevention programme.* Retrieved April 12, 2023, from https://www.csd.gov.hk/psy_gym/InDesign/en/violence/violence.htm

Correctional Services Department. (2002). *Report of the special task group set up in relation to the death of inmate Mr. CHEUNG Chi-kin in Siu Lam Psychiatric Centre on 19 November 2001 (Annex A of LC paper no. CB(2)947/02-03(01)).* https://www.legco.gov.hk/yr02-03/english/panels/se/papers/se0123cb2-947-01-e.pdf

Correctional Services Department. (2010). *Hong Kong Correctional Services annual review 2009: operations and institutional management.* https://www.csd.gov.hk/annualreview/2009_long/west/chapter1/index.htm

Correctional Services Department. (2016, April 27). *LCQ9: Rehabilitation programmes for persons in custody and recidivism rate.* https://www.csd.gov.hk/english/news/news_pr/20160427.html

Correctional Services Department. (2019a). *Examination of estimates of expenditure 2019–20: Controlling officer's reply: Reply serial no. SB396.* https://www.csd.gov.hk/images/doc/news/news_st/eee1920/SB396e.pdf

Correctional Services Department. (2019b). *Examination of estimates of expenditure 2019–20: Controlling officer's reply: Reply serial no. SB188.* https://www.csd.gov.hk/images/doc/news/news_st/eee1920/SB188e.pdf

Correctional Services Department. (2020a, May 14). *Religious services.* https://www.csd.gov.hk/english/reh/reh_overview/reh_overview_religious/reh_over_rs.html

Correctional Services Department. (2021a, January 4). *Psychological services.* https://www.csd.gov.hk/english/reh/reh_overview/reh_overview_psy/reh_ps.html

Correctional Services Department. (2022a, December 30). *4 critical success factors towards a safer and more inclusive society.* https://www.csd.gov.hk/english/about/about_4factors/reh_over_4csf.html

Correctional Services Department. (2022b, December 30). *Education.* https://www.csd.gov.hk/english/reh/reh_overview/reh_overview_education/reh_edu.html

Correctional Services Department. (2022c). *Examination of estimates of expenditure 2022–23: Controlling officer's reply: Reply serial no. SB030.* https://www.csd.gov.hk/images/doc/news/news_st/eee2223/SB030e.pdf

Correctional Services Department. (2022d, December 20). *Vocational training unit*. https://www.csd.gov.hk/english/reh/reh_ivt/reh_ivt_vt/reh_vt.html

Correctional Services Department. (2022e, October 20). *Supervision services*. https://www.csd.gov.hk/english/reh/reh_overview/reh_overview_supervision/reh_ru_supn.html

Correctional Services Department. (2023a, February 13). *Admissions of persons in custody to correctional institutions*. https://www.csd.gov.hk/english/statistics/ins_mgt/napucci.html

Correctional Services Department. (2023b, March 24). *Industries units*. https://www.csd.gov.hk/english/reh/reh_ivt/reh_ind/reh_ind.html

Correctional Services Department. (2023c, January 5). *CSD Q&A corner*. https://www.csd.gov.hk/english/info/qa/qa.html

Correctional Services Department. (2023d, February 20). *Number of persons under CSD management*. https://www.csd.gov.hk/english/statistics/ins_mgt/npuc.html

Correctional Services Department. (2023e, April 11). *CSD multi-purpose family and rehabilitation service centres*. https://www.csd.gov.hk/english/reh/reh_overview/reh_mfrsc/reh_mfrsc.html

Correctional Services Department. (2023f, February 14). *Recidivism rate of local rehabilitated offenders*. https://www.csd.gov.hk/english/statistics/reh/recidivism_rate.html

Correctional Services Department. (2023h, February 9). *Overall passing rate and employment rate of persons in custody*. https://www.csd.gov.hk/english/statistics/reh/pass_rate.html

Fair, H., & Walmsley, R. (2022). *World female imprisonment list (fifth edition)*. https://www.prisonstudies.org/sites/default/files/resources/downloads/world_female_imprisonment_list_5th_edition.pdf

Garner, T. G. P. (1976). *Rehabilitation of drug addicts in a correctional setting (Presented at the 13th World Congress of Rehabilitation International, Tel Aviv, Israel, June 13–18, 1976)*. https://www.ojp.gov/ncjrs/virtual-library/abstracts/rehabilitation-drug-addicts-correctional-setting-hong-kong

Gray, P. (1999). Community corrections and the experiences of young male offenders in the Hong Kong youth justice system. *Journal of Social Policy*, 28(4), 577–594. 10.1017/S0047279499005772

The Hong Kong Government. (1999, November 10). *Gengsheng zhongxin tiaoli caoan er du zhifa zhongwen* [Second reading of the Rehabilitation Centres Bill (Chinese only)]. https://www.info.gov.hk/gia/general/199911/10/1110231.htm

The Hong Kong Government. (2015, February 25). *LCQ15: Rehabilitation services for persons in custody* [Press release]. https://www.info.gov.hk/gia/general/201502/25/P201502250529.htm

The Hong Kong Government. (2018, November 19). *CSD's Life Gym: First positive living centre for male persons in custody launched (with photos)* [Press release]. https://www.info.gov.hk/gia/general/201811/19/P2018111900243.htm

Hong Kong Police Force. (2023). *Crime statistics in detail*. Retrieved April 12, 2023, from https://www.police.gov.hk/ppp_en/09_statistics/csd.html

Hui, C. Y. T., & Lo, T. W. (2017). Hong Kong, corrections in. In K. R. Kerley (Ed.), *The encyclopedia of corrections* (pp. 1–9). John Wiley & Sons. 10.1002/9781118845387.wbeoc221

Lee, K. S. Y., Wong, W. K. W., & Kung, W. Y. (2017). Towards a safer society: Psychological assessment and treatment of serious violent offenders in Hong Kong. In H. C. (Oliver) Chan & S. M. Y. Ho (Eds.), *Psycho-criminological perspective of criminal justice in Asia* (pp. 142–159). Routledge.

Mak, V. W. M., Ho, S. M. Y., Kwong, R. W. Y., & Li, W. L. (2018). A gender-responsive treatment facility in correctional services: The development of psychological gymnasium for women offenders. *International Journal of Offender Therapy and Comparative Criminology, 62*, 1062–1079. 10.1177/ 0306624x16667572

Mak, V. W. M., Kwong, R. W. Y., Li, W. L., & Pau, B. K. Y. (2017). Gender-specific assessment and treatment for female offenders in Hong Kong. In H. C. (Oliver) Chan & S. M. Y. Ho (Eds.), *Psycho-criminological perspective of criminal justice in Asia* (pp. 126–141). Routledge.

Narcotics Division, Security Bureau. (2021a, September 10). *Compulsory placement programme.* https://www.nd.gov.hk/en/1.html

Narcotics Division, Security Bureau. (2021b). *Three-year plan on drug treatment and rehabilitation services in Hong Kong (2021–2023).* https://www.nd.gov. hk/pdf/three_year_plan_2021_2023_final_en.pdf

Security Bureau. (1998, November). *Legislative Council Panel on Security: Rehabilitation of offenders—A new short-term residential programme for young offenders (LC paper no. CB(2)748/98-99(04)).* https://www.legco.gov. hk/yr98-99/english/panels/se/papers/se0312_4.htm

Security Bureau. (1999). *Legislative Council Brief: Rehabilitation Centres Bill (Ref.: SBCR 11/2856/98).* https://www.legco.gov.hk/yr99-00/english/bc/bc53/ general/64_brf.pdf

Security Bureau. (2007). *Legislative Council Panel on Security: Latest developments in the provision of rehabilitative services by the Correctional Services Department (LC paper no. CB(2)2284/06-07(01)).* https://www.legco.gov.hk/ yr06-07/english/panels/se/papers/se0703cb2-2284-1-e.pdf

Security Bureau. (2017a, May). *Rehabilitative programmes for young offenders in correctional institutions (LC paper no. CB(4)1046/16-17(01)).* https://www. legco.gov.hk/yr16-17/english/hc/sub_com/hs101/papers/hs10120170523cb4-1046-1-e.pdf

Security Bureau. (2017b, June 22). *Subcommittee on Children's Rights: Follow-up to meeting on 23 May 2017 (LC paper no. CB(4)1293/16-17(01)).* https://www. legco.gov.hk/yr16-17/english/hc/sub_com/hs101/papers/hs10120170523cb4-1293-1-e.pdf

Security Bureau. (2021a, June 13). *Release under Supervision Board: The two early release schemes.* https://www.sb.gov.hk/eng/links/rusb/early_scheme.html

Security Bureau. (2021b, June 13). *Release under Supervision Board: Terms of reference.* https://www.sb.gov.hk/eng/links/rusb/term.html

Security Bureau. (2021c, January 24). *Long-term Prison Sentences Review Board: Establishment, functions and duties of the Board.* https://www.sb.gov.hk/eng/ links/ltpsrb/establishment.html

Security Bureau. (2021d, June 13). *Post-Release Supervision Board: After-care supervision services.* https://www.sb.gov.hk/eng/links/prsb/aftercare.html

Siu, B. W. M., Lai, E. S. K., Lam, J. P. Y., Chan, C., Chan, A. W. L., Chu, K. Y., Leong, S. L., Lui, S. H., Liu, A. C. Y., Tang, D. Y. Y., So, W. L., Leung, H. W., Mok, C. C. M., & Lam, M. (2022). Profiling mentally ill offenders in Hong Kong: A 10-year retrospective review study. *Asia-Pacific Psychiatry, 14*(3), e12505. 10.1111/appy.12505

Siu, B. W. M., & Lam, M. (2018). Forensic psychiatric services in Hong Kong. *East Asian Arch Psychiatry, 28*(4), 111–113. https://www.doi.org/10.12809/eaap1845

Social Welfare Department. (2022a, August 31). *Services for ex-offenders and discharged prisoners.* https://www.swd.gov.hk/en/index/site_pubsvc/page_offdr/sub_communityb/id_SRACP/

Social Welfare Department. (2022b, August 31). *Social Welfare Department – Services for offenders.* https://www.swd.gov.hk/en/index/site_pubsvc/page_offdr/

Social Welfare Department. (2022c, August 31). *Community service orders (CSO) scheme.* https://www.swd.gov.hk/en/index/site_pubsvc/page_offdr/sub_communityb/id_csoscheme/

Social Welfare Department. (2022d, August 31). *Probation service (PO).* https://www.swd.gov.hk/en/index/site_pubsvc/page_offdr/sub_communityb/id_PO/

Social Welfare Department. (2022e, December 28). *2021–22 annual service provision and statistics.* https://www.swd.gov.hk/en/index/site_pubsvc/page_offdr/sub_offdrsps/

Society for Community Organization. (2019). *Minjian jiancha chengjiao zhidu zhounian baogao (2019)* [Annual report on civil monitoring of penal system (2019)]. https://www.legco.gov.hk/yr19-20/chinese/panels/se/papers/secb2-461-1-c.pdf

United Nations Office on Drugs and Crime. (2022a, June 6). *UNODC research—Data portal—Intentional homicide.* https://dataunodc.un.org/dp-intentional-homicide-victims

United Nations Office on Drugs and Crime. (2022b, June 6). *UNODC research—Data portal—Violent and sexual crime.* https://dataunodc.un.org/dp-crime-violent-offences

Ward, T., & Fortune, C.-A. (2013). The Good Lives Model: Aligning risk reduction with promoting offenders' personal goals. *European Journal of Probation, 5*(2), 29–46. 10.1177/206622031300500203

Ward, T., Yates, P. M., & Willis, G. M. (2012). The Good Lives Model and the Risk Need Responsivity model: A critical response to Andrews, Bonta, and Wormith (2011). *Criminal Justice and Behavior, 39*(1), 94–110. 10.1177/0093854811426085

Case cited

Wong Chun Cheong v HKSAR (2001) 4 HKCFAR 12

Legislations cited

Community Service Orders Ordinance, Cap 378 (1984)
Drug Addiction Treatment Centres Ordinance, Cap 244 (1968)
Probation of Offenders Ordinance, Cap 298 (1956)
Probation of Offenders Rules, Cap 298A (1958)
Rehabilitation Centres Ordinance, Cap 567 (2001)

5

CURRENT ISSUES IN OFFENDER ASSESSMENT AND REHABILITATION IN JAPAN

Masaru Takahashi

Current Issues in Offender Assessment and Rehabilitation in Japan

Japan, located in East Asia, is over 3,500 km long and comprises several islands with a population of 125.5 million, as of 1 October 2021. Approximately 29% of the population is 65 years and above. This, combined with the low birth rate, high life expectancy, and low influx of immigrants, makes Japan one of the fastest super-ageing countries worldwide. Japan's official language is Japanese, and most of the population constitutes ethnic Japanese speakers, making it less diverse than other multi-ethnic countries. Although Japan's administrative divisions are divided into 47 prefectures, it has a uniform criminal justice system.

Japan is among the safest countries worldwide. Additionally, according to the 2022 White Paper on Crime (Ministry of Justice, 2022a), Japan is experiencing the lowest number of recorded crimes since World War II. This decrease in crime has drawn attention to repeat offenders and the need to prevent recidivism and enhance reintegration of people from prison into society. Evidence-based assessments and treatments have rapidly been promoted in correctional settings. In this chapter, Japan's status and crime trends and reviewed before the Japanese approach to the assessment and treatment of people who have committed offences is introduced. It discusses how Japanese criminal justice professionals incorporate and modify Western models as they work and considers the evidence for their effectiveness. Lastly, it discusses the challenges and prospects of the current Japanese correctional system. Unless otherwise

DOI: 10.4324/9781003360919-7

noted, the data in this chapter are drawn from the 2022 White Paper on Crime (Ministry of Justice, 2022a).

Crime Trends in Japan

Overall Trends and Organisational Overview

Figure 5.1 shows the trend in the number of reported cases for Penal Code offences since 1946. The number of reported criminal offences reached a post-World War II high of approximately 2.85 million in 2002. However, it has continually declined over the past 20 years, reaching approximately 570,000 in 2020, about one-fifth off its peak. Furthermore, since 2015, reported criminal acts have continually reduced. However, while the number of crimes has declined overall, the number of arrests for some crimes has increased or remained relatively high. For instance, in 2021, arrests for child abuse (2,174), intimate partner violence (8,703), cyber-crime (12,209) and special fraud such as bank transfer fraud (6,600) have at least doubled since 2011, with child abuse in particular increasing more than five-fold.

In Japan, the Ministry of Justice, manages and operates all correctional institutions nationwide, whether for adults or minors, institutional or community corrections. Correctional facilities (e.g., prisons, detention centres, juvenile training schools, and juvenile classification homes) are under the jurisdiction of the Correction Bureau of the Ministry of Justice.

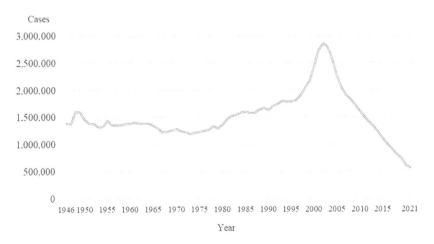

FIGURE 5.1   Number of Reported Cases for Penal Code Offences (1946–2021).

Source: Data from the 2022 White Paper on Crime (Ministry of Justice, 2022a).

Probation offices, responsible for community supervision and treatment of individuals on probation and parole, are under the jurisdiction of the Rehabilitation Bureau of the Ministry of Justice. The number of adults (including unsentenced persons) detained in correctional institutions (including prisons and detention centres nationwide) at the end of 2021 was 44,545.

Delinquency of Minors

The number of arrests for criminal offences committed by minors has declined since 2004, which can be attributed to the decline in the birth rate. However, even when viewed as a percentage of the population, the number of arrests of minors has sharply declined. For example, in 2021, the number of arrests of minors was approximately 186 per 100,000, which is nearly one-eighth of the 1,432 per 100,000 minors arrested in 1981, the highest rate of arrests for minors in recent years. The trend remains the same; the percentage of the population with criminal justice agency involvement is relatively higher for minors than for adults, but the gap between the two has narrowed in recent years. Several possibilities explain the rapid decline in juvenile delinquency. A marked decrease in 'biker gangs' and a consequent reduction in group delinquency have been recognised in official statistics, possibly due to the decline of this particular counterculture and the recent trend of disliking strict hierarchical relationships in antisocial groups among young people; however, these suggestions are speculative, and the real reason/s are unknown.

The age of adulthood under Japan's Civil Code had long been defined as 20 years but was lowered to 18 years in April 2022. Correspondingly, the Juvenile Law was also amended, and 18- or 19-year-olds began being referred to as 'specified juveniles' and treated differently. In principle, the family court handles juvenile delinquency cases. However, with this legislative change, those who have committed serious crimes are referred by family courts to adult criminal courts. Therefore, amendments to the Juvenile Law may result in harsher punishments for some juveniles owing to the more punitive focus of the adult criminal justice system.

Older Adult Offenders

Japan is a super-ageing society that maintains the highest ratio of the older adult population (65 years and over) worldwide. Consequently, the number of older adults involved in the criminal justice system has significantly increased, reaching the highest age distribution ratio (22.8%) among all age groups in 2013. While females account for one in five of all arrested persons, they account for one in three of all arrests of older adult offenders. One of the characteristics of older adult offenders is a markedly higher rate of thefts compared with offenders in other age groups. Theft constituted 48.2% of all arrests in 2021 and was 69.9% among older adults. Furthermore, approximately 90% of all arrests among female older adults were for theft, primarily shoplifting. The number of older adult offenders in prison has substantially increased over the past 20 years. The total number increased approximately 2.1 times from 2001 to 2020, while the number of female older people in prison increased 5.7 times. A dementia screening test is administered to inmates aged 60 and over on admission and efforts are made to ensure that people suspected of having dementia are examined by a doctor. Many older adult prisoners have been sentenced repeatedly, although 30% entered prison for the first time (aged 65 or older). It has been hypothesised that this is due to a loss of social placement and support, as well as financial burdens, may drive older people to commit theft.

International Comparisons

As countries differ in their definitions of crime and the activities of criminal justice agencies, comparisons in crime trends between countries is challenging. The United Nations Survey of Crime Trends and Operations of Criminal Justice Systems uses a standard questionnaire to tabulate each country's criminal justice responses. Using data from the United Nations Office on Drugs and Crime and the World Population Prospects (Ministry of Justice, 2022a), the White Paper on Crime showed that the number of homicide victims in Japan was 319 (0.3 per 100,000 people), which is low compared with that in Western countries (see Figure 5.2). This may be

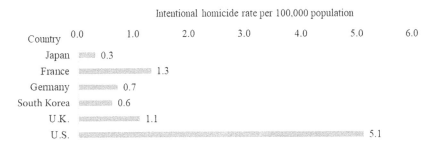

FIGURE 5.2 International Comparison of the Incidence of Intentional Homicide per 100,000 Population (2019).

Source: Data from the 2022 White Paper on Crime (Ministry of Justice, 2022a).

attributed to gun control in Japan, which is strict by global standards, and possession of firearms is prohibited, except when a person is legally required to be armed while performing their professional duties. According to the National Police Agency's statistics, only one fatal firearm incident and four injuries occurred in Japan in 2021.

Recidivism

The prevention of recidivism has long been a central issue in Japanese criminal justice policy. Previous research by the Ministry of Justice of Japan (2009) revealed that 30% of repeat offenders were responsible for 60% of crimes committed in Japan from 1948 to 2006. More recently, in 2016, the Re-offending Prevention Promotion Act was enacted to further promote recidivism prevention. Article 3 of the Act establishes the fundamental principles: In view of the fact that many persons who have committed offences face difficulties returning to society due to circumstances such as being unable to find stable employment and secure housing, initiatives to prevent recidivism need to be implemented; a successful reintegration relies upon the support of community members to prevent former offenders being isolated in the community. The Act stipulates that it is the responsibility of the national government to formulate and implement comprehensive initiatives to prevent recidivism based on the aforementioned principles. Characteristically, it not only states the responsibility of the state but also of local authorities in cooperation with the state in accordance with local conditions. It further stipulates that, when formulating reoffending prevention initiatives, the government should consider the results of empirical studies and examine the effectiveness of such initiatives.

Recidivism is indicated in Japan by considering the 'reincarceration rate within x years'. This indicator specifies how many people released from prison in a given year commit new crimes and return to prison. According to the latest figures, approximately 40% of people released from prison returned within five years, and about half returned to prison within two years. The recidivism rates are higher for those convicted of theft or who violated the Stimulants Control Act, for males than for females, and for the elderly (65 years old or older) than for the young (less than 30 years old). A gradual downward trend has been observed in recent years regarding changes in the reincarceration rate over time. As a key policy indicator, the national government has set a target of a two-year reincarceration rate of less than 16% by 2021; this target was achieved in 2019 (15.7%).

Securing Employment Opportunities for Persons Released from Correctional Institutions

In Japan, the Ministry of Justice, in cooperation with the Ministry of Health, Labour and Welfare, has been operating a policy of 'Dedicated Recruitment of Correctional Inmates' since 2014. This allows employers wishing to recruit people in correctional institutions to submit job openings to 'Hello Work' (a public employment security office) after designating the correctional facility. The aim is to facilitate a match for individuals in correctional facilities who desire to find employment with businesses following release. Additionally, to secure employment while incarcerated and to support early employment after release, the Correctional Employment Support and Information Centre offices, located in eight correctional jurisdictions across the country, centrally manage information on offenders' return destinations and qualifications. These centres provide consultations from companies wishing to employ people released from correctional institutions, and provide information on facilities that house and provide employment support for offenders that meet the needs of companies on a large scale.

Assessment and Treatment in Correctional Settings

In Japan, evidence-based assessments and treatments have been a feature of youth correctional institutions since World War II, when Juvenile Classification Homes and Juvenile Training Schools were established throughout Japan. Historically, most psychologists employed in correctional settings were assigned to Juvenile Classification Homes and here they developed psychological tests to assess young people who had engaged in antisocial behaviour. However, in adult prisons, the momentum to use behavioural science insights to rehabilitate people in prison lagged behind the work being undertaken in juvenile facilities. Over the past two decades, though, evidence-based treatment has been rapidly promoted in adult prisons, partly because of the enforcement of the Act on Penal Detention Facilities and Treatment of Inmates and Detainees in 2006, which focuses on educating and treating people in prisons. The Risk-Need-Responsivity (RNR) framework (Andrews & Bonta, 2010) and the introduction of cognitive behavioural intervention techniques have underpinned various developments in the adult correctional sphere.

The following section focuses primarily on initiatives created to rehabilitate people in correctional settings, including programmes for individuals in prisons with specific problems, research on outcome evaluations of these programmes, development and validation of risk assessment instruments, and other related practices and research.

Rehabilitation Programmes for Specific Problems in Prisons

Six different rehabilitation programmes are available to address specific problems in prison. They are numbered R1 to R6 as follows: R1: Relapse prevention programme for drug dependence; R2: Guidance on withdrawal from organised crime groups; R3: Guidance on prevention of repeat sexual offences; R4: Education from victims' point of view for persons who commit offences that result in the death of the victim or cause serious bodily harm; R5: Traffic safety guidance; and R6: Employment support guidance for acquiring the 'manners' and skills necessary for employment. As an example, R1 uses a combination of mandatory, specialised, and elective programmes, depending on the individual problems, risks, and length of the sentence, to help people understand their own drug use problems and consider ways to avoid drug use.

Recidivism Prevention Programmes for People with a History of Sexual Offending

Various treatment programmes have been introduced in Japanese prisons for people with a history of sexual offending. One of Japan's earliest evidence-based recidivism prevention programmes was *Seihanzai Saihan-Boushi Shidou* (Guidance on prevention of repeat sexual offences; R3 mentioned above), introduced in prisons nationwide in 2006. This programme was introduced after a tragic incident where a released offender, who had previously served a prison sentence for a sexual offence against a girl, kidnapped, sexually assaulted, and murdered a seven-year-old in 2004 (The Japan Times, 2004). This led to a public demand for measures to prevent recidivism among people who have sexually offended. With the assistance of the Correctional Service of Canada, intervention programmes based on the RNR principles were introduced on a large scale for the first time. Until then, efforts to prevent recidivism among people with a history of sexual offending had only been implemented in several facilities. However, this was the first time a unified programme was systematically implemented in Japanese prisons nationwide. This initiative is a good example of how Western practices and research are introduced directly into practice in Japanese correctional institutions.

Consistent with the risk and need principles, each individual's risk of recidivism for sexual offences is assessed and the treatment intensity was determined based on the results of the risk assessment. Accordingly, a treatment plan is formulated for each person after considering treatment suitability in such areas as intellectual ability, degree of motivation, and presence or absence of physical or mental problems. There are three levels of treatment intensity for this programme: high, medium, and low. Group work of 100 minutes per session is conducted twice a week for nine and seven months, for high- and medium-intensity programmes respectively, and once a week for four months for low-intensity groups. Besides group work, individual assignments and personal guidance are provided simultaneously, as needed. Other programmes have also been developed and implemented for participants with low treatment motivation or low intellectual capacity, or those who are unable to participate for a sufficient length of time due to short prison sentences. Currently, Japan does not have a registration and notification system for people who have sexually offended, and efforts are being made towards prevention and treatment. Regarding the application of Western programmes in Japan, the basic framework, treatment principles and methods are disseminated among staff through training. However, different cultures and crime situations may require some adaptations. For example, *Chikan,* or molestation on crowded commuter trains, is such a widespread problem that 'women-only' train carriages are provided in Japan. Recidivism rates for such individuals have been found to be particularly high, and effective treatment is needed for this type of high-risk offender.

Finally, in the field of offender rehabilitation, interest in strength-based approaches is growing, including the Good Lives Model (GLM), primarily to complement RNR principles. The GLM is an approach-goal-focused rehabilitation framework encouraging the identification and formulation of ways to prosocially achieve personally meaningful goals (Fortune, 2018). The RNR model can effectively determine the appropriate alloca-tion of human and material resources and treatment goals according to risk level. However, maintaining motivation for justice-involved people and treatment providers can be challenging when working to prevent recidivism. Considering these circumstances, sexual offender treatment programmes, revised in April 2022, focus on approach goals, strengths, and the risks of reoffending. Programmes utilise participants' positive motivation by making them think about their goal of not reoffending, future selves, desired goals, and their efforts to achieve them. This initiative has recently commenced, and evaluation is yet to be undertaken.

Outcome Evaluation in Correctional Settings

In recent years, the Japanese government has been urged to promote evidence-based policy making, actively utilising empirical data to ensure limited resources are used effectively so that justice administration/admin-istrators are trusted by the public. The Ministry of Justice of Japan has conducted outcome evaluation research on some programmes and published the results. For instance, an overview of a 2020 study on the above-mentioned sexual offender treatment programmes is hereby presented.

This study selected 1,444 participants who were required to attend sexual offender treatment programmes, and 324 comparison subjects who were released from prisons between 2012 and 2014 (Ministry of Justice, 2020). A comparison of recidivism (all types and sexual recidivism) within three years of release between the two groups showed statistically significant percentage differences: 27.3% and 38% for any kind of recidivism in the treatment and comparison groups, respectively; and 15% and 22.5% for sexual offence recidivism in the treatment and comparison groups, respectively. The Cox proportional hazards model controlled for recidivism risk scores for both groups and examined the association between programme attendance and recidivism. It reported a hazard ratio of 0.79 (95% CI = 0.64 – 0.96) and 0.75 (95% CI = 0.57 – 0.97) for any and sexual recidivism, respectively, showing significant treatment effects.

Another outcome evaluation study of a community relapse prevention programme for illicit drug users (Ministry of Justice, 2022b) employed propensity score matching to adjust for systematic differences between treatment and control groups, reporting significantly lower rates of recidivism in the treatment group after controlling for possible confounds. Future evaluation studies are expected to include methodological refinement, the use of diverse outcomes, and further analysis from a cost-effectiveness perspective.

Approaches in Juvenile Classification Homes

A Juvenile Classification Home is an institution with the primary role of detaining delinquent minors for a short period (approximately four weeks) until a hearing is held, a detailed psychological evaluation has been conducted, and recommendations are made to the family court for a final disposition. As of April 2022, 52 Juvenile Classification Homes were located throughout Japan. Most psychologists working in Japanese correctional facilities work in Juvenile Classification Homes where they prepare reports from psychological assessments and help judges make final decisions at family court hearings. Several recent initiatives in Juvenile Classification Homes are hereby presented.

Risk Assessment Instruments for Juvenile Delinquents

Although various personality tests have been developed and administered in Juvenile Classification Homes, no standard assessment tool has been specifically designed to identify a juvenile's likelihood of reoffending or determine their educational needs. Therefore, based on a literature review and field research on risk assessment in Western countries, the Ministry of Justice Case Assessment Tool was developed and introduced in 2013 to help practitioners to assess juveniles' risk of recidivism and to identify criminogenic needs. This instrument is based on RNR principles and was developed through statistical analysis based on a follow-up study of released youths (Ministry of Justice, 2013).

The Ministry of Justice Case Assessment Tool (52 items; 24 items in five static domains and 28 in four dynamic domains) was developed as follows (Ministry of Justice, 2013) using data from approximately 6,000 youths placed in Juvenile Classification Homes nationwide in 2010. The mean follow-up period was 473 days, and approximately 18% of the youth re-entered the Juvenile Classification Homes. The recidivism rate in this study may be slightly underestimated, as those who reached the age of 20 years during the follow-up period entered the adult criminal justice system rather than the juvenile system. Finally, the instrument development was completed by extracting only items related to recidivism. Besides confirming the rate of agreement among raters, the tool was found to have a moderate level of predictive validity, with an area under the curve of .66 (Ministry of Justice, 2013).

Psychologists use the tool at Juvenile Classification Homes to code items from interviews with youths, behavioural observations, psychological tests, and collateral information. The likelihood of reoffending and the need for education are indicated by four categories (Level I to IV), and the estimated recidivism rate increases from Level I to IV. The estimated reoffending rate for Level I is 10.1%, while the estimated rate for Level IV (corresponding to the highest level) is 78%. This tool determines the recommended disposition in Juvenile Classification Homes and examines the pre- and post-treatment effects for those who are subsequently sent to juvenile training schools.

Psychological Support and Consultation for Residents

In recent years, Juvenile Classification Homes have offered free psychological counselling and consultation services to residents and staff of related organisations, such as schools and foster homes. This initiative was implemented as per Article 131 of the Juvenile Classification Home Law, enacted in 2015. Juvenile Classification Homes respond to wide-ranging community needs by providing information, advice, and psychological support in response to requests from relevant organisations, and counselling to guardians and others who are troubled by their children's problematic behaviour. The support provided ranges from counselling on problematic behaviour to school adjustment for children with developmental issues, psychological testing for intelligence and personality, participation in case conferences of related organisations, and training and lectures for the public. In 2021, 5,610 persons received assistance. Furthermore, 9,239 consultations were provided by related institutions, mostly from educational institutions, such as elementary and junior high schools. In Japan, an official qualification system has been established for psychologists. However, not all psychologists are necessarily familiar with externalised problem behaviours such as theft, violence, drug addiction, and sexual addiction. This is because people with these behavioural problems appear less frequently in hospitals and clinics than in correctional institutions. In the future, it is necessary to determine whether continually implementing such initiatives will help prevent delinquency and crime in the community at an early stage.

The Role of Volunteers in Community Corrections

A unique feature of Japan's community correctional rehabilitation efforts is the extensive involvement of volunteers. Volunteer probation officers, known as '*Hogo-shi*' in Japanese, are citizens commissioned by the Minister of Justice to assist in rehabilitating offenders in cooperation with probation officers. Their main activities involve (a) assisting and supervising parolees and probationers, (b) coordinating and helping the inmates with their social circumstances, and (c) promoting crime prevention activities in the community. The involvement of community volunteers in supporting the rehabilitation of offenders is also practised in other countries. However, the Japanese system is unique as community volunteers are organised nationwide in cooperation with professional probation officers. As of 1 April 2022, 46,705 volunteers are registered to work in 886 districts nationwide. Volunteers engage with both juveniles and adults under the guidance of a probation officer. Training opportunities are provided, both nationally and regionally, to engage with individuals on probation, although training is not intensive. The involvement of community volunteers is helpful in guiding and supervising offenders in communities with scarce resources. These volunteer programmes help to foster positive attitudes amongst community members towards people returning from prison into society. In recent years, the number of volunteers has gradually declined due to an ageing volunteer population and a lack of new volunteers, making it a challenge to secure personnel for this role. In the future, researchers should examine the effectiveness of community volunteerism for reducing reoffending rates using various measurement indicators, and also whether volunteers help create more supportive community attitudes towards former prisoners.

Research on Recidivism Risk Factors

As discussed thus far, the development of Japan's sexual offender treatment programmes and risk assessment instruments has relied on research from North America. The introduction of programmes and assessment tools from foreign countries has been viewed with some scepticism. Questions have been raised about the extent to which risk-related psychological constructs are comparable (in North America and Japan) and whether these constructs can be measured similarly. Furthermore, questions have arisen about the extent to which Japanese culture and crime-specific factors are captured by Western instruments.

Takahashi et al. (2013) examined a cross-validation of the Youth Level of Service/Case Management Inventory (YLS/CMI), a recidivism risk assessment instrument developed in North America, and concluded that the overall findings supported the predictive validity of this instrument, but subscales, such as substance use, lacked content representativeness. Using a subsample from Takahashi's study, the predictive validity of actuarial risk assessment instruments (i.e., YLS/CMI) and clinical judgements in Japan were compared (Mori et al., 2017). Research in Western countries has consistently shown that actuarial measures are superior to unstructured clinical judgements in predicting recidivism (Grove et al., 2000; Hanson & Morton-Bourgon, 2009; Hilton et al., 2006). In Mori and colleagues' study of Japanese juvenile offenders there was no incremental predictive validity for clinicians' predictions over the actuarial risk assessment instrument. While this does not necessarily suggest the absence of risk factors specific to Japanese juvenile offenders, the results of this study at least suggest that such factors are not captured by clinicians' experience and judgement.

Furthermore, Takahashi and Nishihara (2017) conducted a post-release follow-up study of people incarcerated for sexual offences in prisons across Japan to examine recidivism risk factors. The recidivism rate of people who deny their sexual offences is perceived as high among members of the public. However, this study concluded that denial/minimisation does not contribute to predicting recidivism, despite controlling for potential confounding factors, such as known recidivism risk factors. These results are consistent with previous studies conducted in a Western context (Hanson & Morton-Bourgon, 2005). While the differences in definitions of crime and criminal justice systems preclude a strict comparison of research findings between Japan and the West, these studies show that some risk factors for reoffending are, at least to some extent, common across cultures.

Finally, while research findings from Western personality and clinical psychology have traditionally been utilised in offender rehabilitation practice in Japan, there has been less direct use of criminological theory. However, one of the reasons why the RNR model has gained traction in Japan in recent years is that it has provided a perspective for practical improvements in Japanese correctional services, such as the allocation of limited human and material resources. For better or worse, there has been an assumption, that Japan has a unique culture, which is reflected in its low crime rate; however, research using frameworks borrowed from the West suggests that, at least so far, there may be more commonality than heterogeneity. In the future, the accumulation of research findings from the East may reveal similarities and differences with the West and stimulate research on risk factors for recidivism that can assist in release decision making and rehabilitation planning.

Boosting Empirical Research in the Correctional Field

The momentum to apply empirical research results to criminal justice policy has grown in recent years. In 2019, the Center for Effectiveness Verification was established within the Training Institute for Correctional Personnel, Ministry of Justice. Here, experts in behavioural sciences are invited to systematically research the development and maintenance of treatment programmes, evaluate programme effectiveness, and develop and revise risk assessment instruments. Until recently, research in criminal forensic psychology has been conducted by psychologists within the Ministry of Justice through individual studies. However, future research is expected to be promoted in a systematic and organised manner, including data collection, analysis, and incorporation of findings into policy and practice.

An essential part of empirical research is developing databases. As such, the System for Crime and Recidivism Prevention was recently developed. This links the database information of prosecutors, correctional facilities, and probation offices that originally operated separately. This new system aims to (a) provide consistent and continuous recidivism prevention programmes based on considerable information, and (b) verify the effectiveness of programmes by identifying the status of recidivism, leading to treatment programme reviews. The system is expected to enable utilising 'big data' held by criminal justice agencies on a cross-departmental basis, enabling a detailed understanding of recidivism and potentially contributing to a reduction in the recidivism rate by reviewing measures and verifying their effectiveness. In the future, big data is highly anticipated to analyse crime patterns over the life course of individuals involved in criminal justice agencies.

Forensic Mental Health Services in Japan

Until the Act on Medical Care and Treatment for Persons Who Have Caused Serious Cases Under the Condition of Insanity was enacted in 2005, people who offended while mentally ill were treated in general psychiatric hospitals, rendering it difficult to provide specialised treatment. Furthermore, there was no institutional mechanism to guarantee ongoing medical care after the patient was discharged. The medical probation system under the aforementioned act intends to improve the condition of people who have committed serious criminal acts under the influence of mental illness. It does so by providing these people with continuous and intensive medical care, observation, and guidance to ensure prevention of similar acts and promote the rehabilitation of these people and their return to the community. Eligible people are those who have (a) committed the acts of arson, forcible indecency and sexual intercourse, murder, robbery (including attempts at these acts), or assault, (b) been found mentally incompetent and (c) not been prosecuted. Alternatively, people acquitted by reason of insanity or with a reduced sentence by diminished responsibility are also eligible.

Based on the results of the psychiatric evaluation, a decision is reached by agreement between two commissioners (a judge and a qualified psychiatrist) on whether to order inpatient or outpatient treatment (mental health supervision) or no treatment order. During hospitalisation, the designated inpatient healthcare provider or the patient may petition the court if they decide that the patient no longer needs to stay in the hospital. If this is granted, the court discharges the patient immediately. If the patient remains hospitalised, the court decides the necessity of hospitalisation at least once every six months. Contrarily, those receiving a discharge decision or an inpatient treatment order receive necessary medical care at a designated outpatient institution. In principle, the treatment period in the community under this system is three years from the date of the court's orders. Japan has 34 designated inpatient facilities and 850 beds available (Ministry of Health, Labour and Welfare, 2022). According to the White Paper on Crime, in 2021, 308 persons were processed at year-end, of which 237 (76.9%) were hospitalised, 24 (7.8%) were outpatients, 37 (12.0%) were deemed to not need medical treatment, and 10 (3.2%) were 'others'.

Empirical studies on the medical probation system are limited. Arai et al. (2017) examined Historical-Clinical-Risk Management-20's (HCR-20) predictive validity with 100 patients in Japan's forensic mental health inpatient units. They reported that the HCR-20 total score sufficiently predicted incidents of violence in forensic psychiatric units within three and six months after the initial assessment, supporting the predictive validity of the HCR-20 in Japan.

Challenges and Future Prospects for Japan's Offender Treatment System

First, one of the challenges to promoting evidence-based policies is to create a framework for using big data and developing human resources. From this perspective, the launch of the System for Crime and Recidivism Prevention database in 2017 is a promising initiative, and it is desirable to collaborate with academic researchers to evaluate the effectiveness of the programmes. Japanese bureaucratic organisations tend to emphasise generalists rather than specialists. However, developing specialists and improving scientific literacy within correctional organisations is imperative. Increasing the number of personnel with knowledge of psychology and criminology as high-level specialists is a useful option.

The second is the issue of continuity in offender treatment, which runs through treatment in institutions and communities. In order to unify management, it is advantageous to have a single organisation, the Ministry of Justice, managing correctional services. However, within the Ministry of Justice, the Correction Bureau has traditionally overseen institutional management and treatment, and the Rehabilitation Bureau that of community supervision and treatment; thus, a high degree of staff mobility is lacking between the two organisations. Accordingly, further interventions are required to increase staff mobility across both organisations.

Third, the ability to disseminate information internationally must be strengthened. While research is conducted within the Ministry of Justice's internal research institute, which can produce effective policies, results published in international peer-reviewed journals should be encouraged. The results of programme effectiveness evaluations may also benefit from review by experts outside criminal justice agencies. By establishing a more transparent system regarding the success or failure of policies and initiatives, it is hoped that public confidence in the criminal justice system will increase.

Conclusion

Japan is recognised as a relatively safe country with a low crime rate. However, the low rate of offenders in society may lead to their invisibility, exclusion, and isolation from society. In recent years, there has been growing momentum for cooperation between the national government, private sector, and local authorities regarding reintegrating those who have committed offences, including securing employment and continuing therapeutic treatment in the community. In 2022, Japan enacted a revision to the Penal Code to unify prison terms with and without labour. This can potentially bring about an important shift in the focus of criminal sanctions from 'punishment' to 'rehabilitation' by providing reintegration opportunities for those in prison. Further communication with the public on punishment and rehabilitation will be necessary, as myths and misrepresentations about the reality of people who have committed offences can lead to policies that are ineffective in reducing reoffending rates.

Finally, assessment and treatment in the Japanese criminal justice system has improved in recent years, influenced by research from Western cultures, and an increased familiarity with rehabilitation models including RNR and GLM. Assessment tools and treatment programmes developed in the West, including their philosophies and methods, seem to be generally accepted without major discrepancies, although elements unique to Japan may also need to be considered. It seems difficult for people of one country to recognise the uniqueness of their own criminal justice system without making comparisons with other countries. It is hoped that a comparison of the efforts of Japan with those of other countries will highlight the uniqueness of criminal justice in Japanese and other Asian cultures which, in turn, will lead to the improvement of rehabilitation services for people who have offended.

References

Andrews, D. A., & Bonta, J. (2010). Rehabilitating criminal justice policy and practice. *Psychology, Public Policy, and Law*, 16(1), 39–55.

Arai, K., Takano, A., Nagata, T., & Hirabayashi, N. (2017). Predictive accuracy of the Historical-Clinical-Risk management-20 for violence in forensic psychiatric wards in Japan. *Criminal Behaviour and Mental Health*, 27(5), 409–420.

Fortune, C. A. (2018). The good lives model: A strength-based approach for youth offenders. *Aggression and Violent Behavior*, 38, 21–30.

Grove, W. M., Zald, D. H., Lebow, B. S., Snitz, B. E., & Nelson, C. (2000). Clinical versus mechanical prediction: A meta-analysis. *Psychological Assessment*, 12(1), 19–30.

Hanson, R. K., & Morton-Bourgon, K. E. (2005). The characteristics of persistent sexual offenders: A meta-analysis of recidivism studies. *Journal of Consulting and Clinical Psychology*, *73*(6), 1154–1163.

Hanson, R. K., & Morton-Bourgon, K. E. (2009). The accuracy of recidivism risk assessments for sexual offenders: A meta-analysis of 118 prediction studies. *Psychological Assessment*, *21*(1), 1–21.

Hilton, N. Z., Harris, G. T., & Rice, M. E. (2006). Sixty-six years of research on the clinical versus actuarial prediction of violence. *The Counseling Psychologist*, *34*(3), 400–409.

Marshall, W. L., & Marshall, L. E. (2007). The utility of the random controlled trial for evaluating sexual offender treatment: The gold standard or an inappropriate strategy? *Sexual Abuse: A Journal of Research and Treatment*, *19*(2), 175–191.

Ministry of Health, Labour and Welfare, Japan. (2022). *Status of designated inpatient medical facilities*. (in Japanese) Retrieved March 30, 2023, from https://www.mhlw.go.jp/stf/seisakunitsuite/bunya/hukushi_kaigo/shougaisha-hukushi/sinsin/iryokikan_seibi.html

Ministry of Justice, Japan. (2013). *The Ministry of Justice case assessment tool (MJCA)*. (in Japanese) Retrieved March 30, 2023, from https://www.moj.go.jp/kyousei1/kyousei03_00018.html

Ministry of Justice, Japan. (2020). *Analysis of recidivism among participants in a sex offender treatment program in a penal institution*. (in Japanese) Retrieved March 30, 2023, from https://www.moj.go.jp/kyousei1/kyousei05_00005.html

Ministry of Justice, Japan. (2022a). *White paper on crime 2022*. (in Japanese)

Ministry of Justice, Japan. (2022b). *Research report on examining the effectiveness of relapse prevention program for drug offenders in probation offices*. (in Japanese)

Mori, T., Takahashi, M., & Kroner, D. G. (2017). Can unstructured clinical risk judgment have incremental validity in the prediction of recidivism in a non-Western juvenile context? *Psychological Services*, *14*(1), 77–86.

Research Division, Research and Training Institute, Ministry of Justice, Japan (2009). Comprehensive research on recidivism prevention. *Research Division Report*, *42*. (in Japanese)

Takahashi, M., Mori, T., & Kroner, D. G. (2013). A cross-validation of the youth level of service/case management inventory (YLS/CMI) among Japanese juvenile offenders. *Law and Human Behavior*, *37*(6), 389–400.

Takahashi, M., & Nishihara, M. (2017). Examination of the relationship between denial/minimization and recidivism among sex offenders. *The Japanese Journal of Psychology*, *88*(5), 460–469. (in Japanese)

The Japan Times. (2004). *Man held in girl's slaying. Suspect owns up to kidnapping, has record*. Retrieved March 30, 2023, from https://www.japantimes.co.jp/news/2004/12/31/national/man-held-in-girls-slaying/

6

REHABILITATION PRACTICES IN MACAO

An Overview of Approaches and Recent Developments

Donna Soi Wan Leong and Jianhong Liu

Introduction

Previously a Portuguese colony for over four centuries, Macau was handed over to Mainland China on 20th December 1999. Its land area is about 33.3 km², with a population of over 672,000 (Statistics and Census Service of Macao SAR [Portuguese: Direcção dos Serviços de Estatística e Censos, abbrev. DSEC], 2023). Since the Government of Macao Special Administrative Regions (SAR) ended the casino gaming monopoly system and liberalised casino gaming concessions in 2002 (DICJ, n.d.), Macao has become the world's largest gaming centre, sometimes referred to as the "Monte Carlo of the Orient" or the "Las Vegas of the East" (Gaming Inspection and Coordination Bureau of Macao SAR [Portuguese: Direcção de Inspecção e Coordenação de Jogos, abbrev. DICJ], n.d.). The economy is heavily dependent on gaming and tourism (DSEC, 2021b) and over the past two decades, tourists, mainly from mainland China, have significantly boosted the Macao economy (DSEC, n.d.). As a Special Administrative Region of China, Macao is administered under the "one country, two systems" policy. It has its own government, legal and financial affairs, as well as its own criminal rehabilitation system. Nevertheless, a dearth of academic literature exists concerning offender rehabilitation in Macao (Leong & Liu, 2022; Li & Ye, 2017; Liu & Zhao, 2014).

Recent Crime Trends and Patterns

The *Macao Penal Code* (Macao SAR Decree-Law No. 58/95/M, 1995) and the Criminal justice system primarily follow the Portuguese form

DOI: 10.4324/9781003360919-8

(Zhao, 2014). The *Macao Penal Code* classifies crimes into five major categories: crimes against persons, crimes against property, crimes against peacefulness and humanity, crimes against life in society, and crimes against the territory. In addition, some crimes, e.g., computer/cybercrimes (Macao SAR Law No. 11/2009, 2009) or drug-related crimes (Macao SAR Law No. 17/2009, 2009), are stipulated by particular laws in Macao. Zhao and Liu (2011) indicated that the classification of crimes in the *Macao Penal Code* differs from that in Western countries; for example, the Federal Bureau of Investigation in the United States categorises violent crime as murder, rape and sexual assault, robbery, and assault. However, the major violent crimes in Macao, such as homicide, assault, crimes against personal freedom, sexual offenses, libel, and crimes against privacy, are categorised into crimes against persons. These differences pose challenges when comparing crime rates between Macao and other jurisdictions.

The overall crime rate in Macao was between 2,086 and 2,253 per 100,000 inhabitants from 2013 to 2019, decreasing significantly to 1,472 per 100,000 inhabitants during the COVID-19 pandemic in 2020. After a slight rise (1,665 per 100,000) in 2021, the overall crime rate met the trough (1,456 per 100,000) in 2022, the lowest rate since the Macao handover. The rates of Crimes against property, Crimes against person, Crimes against life in society, and Crimes against the territory were broadly consistent with this trend after the COVID-19 pandemic. In contrast, the rates of the other crimes, including computer/cybercrimes and drug-related crimes, increased in 2021 (305 per 100,000). There are no official records of crimes against peacefulness and humanity during the past ten years (Table 6.1).

A total of 9,799 crime cases were reported in 2022, a decrease of 13.9% compared to the previous year (11,376 cases, 2021). Most crime types showed a significant decrease from 2020, believed to be primarily influenced by factors including the pandemic, border policies, and overall economic conditions; however, various computer-related crimes including cybercrimes that mainly focus on the theft of personal information increased. During the period of the pandemic, crimes, such as fraud and extortion have begun to be carried out more through the internet (Gabinete do Secretário para a Segurança [GSS], 2019-2023). Regarding specific types of crime in the past five years, property crimes, such as theft and fraud, and gambling-related crimes, frequently occurred in Macao; in contrast, violent crimes, such as homicide, arson, robbery, etc., were relatively rare. It is worth noting that theft (1,263 cases, –54.5%) and gambling-related crimes (413 cases, –80.1%) both decreased significantly in 2020 and stayed at lower levels for the

TABLE 6.1 Crime Rates in Macao (per 100,000 inhabitants), 2013–2022

	2013	2014	2015	2016	2017	2018	2019	2020	2021	2022
Overall Crime Rate	2,253	2,203	2,111	2,231	2,188	2,152	2,086	1,472	1,665	1,456
- Crimes against person	415	427	421	451	447	400	365	308	339	321
- Crimes against property	1,271	1,233	1,173	1,187	1,238	1,313	1,301	795	839	766
- Crimes against life in society	160	141	126	153	155	145	141	88	94	67
- Crimes against the territory	134	142	176	246	188	126	111	69	88	51
- Others	273	260	216	193	160	168	169	213	305	251

Source: Macao Yearbook of Statistics (DSEC, 2013-2021a); *Macao Full-Year Crime Case Statistics 2022* (Secretariat for Security of Macao SAR [GSS], 2019-2023).

following years than those before the outbreak of COVID-19. Conversely, computer crime/cybercrimes rose significantly (531 cases, +96.7%) in 2020 and met the peak (800 cases, +50.7%) in 2021, then dropped (–57.3%) to 342 cases in 2022, while fraud cases (1,007) decreased 34.0% in 2020 and then continuously increased during the post-pandemic period (GSS, 2019-2023).

Victimisation surveys also shed light on crime patterns in Macao. *The Victimization Survey of Macau Residents – Pilot Study* (Liu et al., 2022) was the first research project adopting the *Latin America and the Caribbean Crime Victimization Survey Initiative* [LACSI] Version 4.0 (United Nations Office on Drugs and Crime [UNODC], 2021) question-naire, revised by combining Macao's social, geographic, and demo-graphic characteristics variables into an integrated design on crime victimisation among Macao residents. One thousand one hundred and two telephone interviews with adult Macao residents were completed through the CATI technique (Computer Assisted Telephone Interview). Results showed that within the reference period of 12 months, 3.5% of respondents' households (n = 38) experienced household crime victimi-sation, while 11.9% of respondents (n = 131) reported that they suffered from personal crimes. Regarding household crime victimisation, van-dalism and theft of vehicle parts were most frequently experienced. Regarding personal crimes, respondents most frequently experienced cybercrimes in the past 12 months; the next most frequent were fraud and theft (larceny). Violent crimes (i.e., assault, robbery, and threats) were rarely experienced.

Current Mechanisms, Political and Statistical Contexts of Offender Rehabilitation

The establishment of Macao's prison legal system was derived from The *International Covenant on Civil and Political Rights* [ICCPR] (United Nations, 1966; Li & Ye, 2017). The *Macao Penal Code* stipulates many ways to facilitate rehabilitation processes, such as providing detailed clauses for probation (Macao SAR Decree-Law No. 58/95/M, 1995, Article 48 to 55) and parole (Macao SAR Decree-Law No. 58/95/M, 1995, Article 56 to 59), showing that sentencing in Macao is rehabilitation oriented (Zhao, 2014). Offender rehabilitation in Macao includes a range of institutional and community sanctions, treatment programmes, and rehabilitation services. The Correctional Services Bureau (Portuguese: Direcção dos Serviços Correccionais, abbrev. DSC), together with the Department of Social Reintegration under the Social Welfare Bureau (Portuguese: Instituto de Acção Social, abbrev. IAS) are responsible for implementing and overseeing services (Leong & Liu, 2022; Li & Ye, 2017; Zhao, 2014). The Coloane Prison under the DSC executes court-imposed custodial sentences; the Youth Correctional Institution under the same bureau is responsible for executing court-imposed measures of juveniles' detention. As for assisting the court to implement non-custodial sentences and sentence suspension orders, such as parole and probation, these are carried out by the Department of Social Reintegration. (DSC, 2023a; IAS, 2023a; Leong & Liu, 2022; Li & Ye, 2017; Zhao, 2014) Furthermore, the Social Reintegration Committee (Macao SAR Administrative Regulation No. 28/2015, 2015), formed by personnel of the stated accountable divisions, was committed to the formulation of all appropriate social reintegration plans for people with convictions, assisting them in the return to society and the launch of a normal and meaningful life so as to reduce the likelihood of reoffending (DSC, 2021).

Coloane Prison is the only prison in Macao. In 2021 it held 1,520 prisoners (1,359 convicted, and 161 remandees), representing about 75% of its maximum capacity of 2,041 prisoners (Government Information Bureau of the Macao SAR [Portuguese: Gabinete de Comunicação Social, abbrev. GCS], 2022). The prison population has increased significantly from 2012, when there were only 1,112 people in prison. In 2021, 197 prisoners were granted parole, which represented an increase (18.0%) compared with 2012, when only 167 prisoners were on parole (Table 6.2). According to the *Macao Penal Code*, prisoners can be granted parole by the court when the prisoner has served at least two-thirds or six months of his or her prison sentence. In other words, parole would not be applied to those with a custodial sentence of fewer than nine months. To be awarded parole prisoners must demonstrate that he or she is filled with remorse and shame from the convicted and have a low level of risk to society. The parole period equals the remainder of the prisoner's sentence length and is no more than five years (Kwan, 2010; Macao SAR Decree-Law No. 58/95/M, 1995, Article 56; Zhao, 2014).

Regarding the demographic characteristics of prisoners from 2015 to 2021 (DSC, 2016-2022), the prisoners were predominantly male (83.4% to 87.7%) and aged between 21 and 50 years (81.5% to 86.8%). Those with junior secondary education (40.8% to 47.0%) were the largest educational level group for seven consecutive years. It is worth noting that prisoners in Macao were mainly from Mainland China (41.0% to 50.2%), then Macao residents (25.7% to 35.1%). Since a considerable number of non-residents visit Macao, there is reason to believe there was a correspondingly large number of non-residents with convictions. In addition, in 2021, the DSC employed 922 people, including 593 correctional officers, 73 cadets, and 256 civilian staff;

TABLE 6.2 Macao Prison Population and Number of Prisoners on Parole, 2012–2021

	2012	2013	2014	2015	2016	2017	2018	2019	2020	2021
Prison Population (as at 31 December) *1	1,112	1,154	1,205	1,280	1,271	1,284	1,458	1,636	1,548	1,520
No. of prisoners on parole *2	167	197	162	179	157	149	117	169	207	197

Source: Yearbook of Statistics (DSEC, 2013-2021a).

*1 Including pre-trial detainees/remand prisoners, but not incorporate juvenile incarceration numbers.

*2 Not incorporate juvenile incarceration numbers.

the prisoner-to-correctional officer ratio was about 2.6 to 1. Moreover, the total number of crime incidents (e.g., 2,498 in 2021) was greater than the number of prisoners (e.g., 1,520 at year-end of 2021), as a person with a conviction might be convicted of more than one type of crime. For seven consecutive years (from 2015 to 2021), the most frequently cited crime for conviction was drug trafficking. Overall, the top five offences that led to convicted custodial sentences were drug-related, including drug trafficking and drug using, as well as fraud, theft, and illegal re-entry or assistance in crime (DSC, 2016-2022).

The Youth Correctional Institution is an educational facility established to provide guardianship for juvenile delinquents. Typically, the Institution caters to young individuals aged 12 to 16 years. However, under certain circumstances, its services may extend to individuals up to 21 years (GCS, 2022; Leong & Liu, 2022). The number of youths detained in the Institution were between 8 and 15 from 2016 to 2021. Most of them were male, between the ages of 12 and 19 years, with secondary education. They were mainly from Macao or Hong Kong. The most frequently cited crime for conviction of young individuals in the same period was drug trafficking, which was similar to the adult prisoners; the next most frequently cited was violent crime (e.g., bodily harm, sexual assault, and robbery) (DSC, 2016-2022).

The Department of Social Reintegration assisted and supervised in-dividuals with convictions under non-custodial measures; the Department also supported convicted persons and their families (IAS, 2023a; Leong & Liu, 2022). After a continuous downward trend (–1.7% to –7.4%) from 2017 to 2020, the number of adult cases intervened by the Department's social workers and counsellors showed a rising trend to 703 cases in 2022 (IAS, 2023b). Unlike the adults, youth cases fluctuated in previous years (–20.1% to +45.9%) and dropped by 5.1% to 187 cases in 2022 (IAS, 2023c). The categorisation of adult rehabilitative cases did not rely on the specific types of committed crimes but rather on the inherent nature of each case, taking into consideration the non-custodial measures or appropriate rehabilitation programmes assigned to the individuals. In 2022, the five most prevalent adult cases received by the Department were as follows: Probation (subject to drug treatment programme) (16.9%), Parole (15.1%), "Family Beyond the Wall" Project[1] (14.4%), Social Background Report[2] (13.5%), and Probation (others) (12.5%). Adult males accounted for 83.8% of the total adult cases. On the other hand, for youths in 2022, the most common case was the Probation Order (33.7%), followed by the Social Background Report (32.1%). The Rule-abiding Order and Halfway Home Order represented 13.9% and 12.3% of cases, respectively. Male youths constituted 84.0% of the total youth cases.

Individuals on community drug treatment programmes were the most common type of adult cases that were supervised by the Department of Social Reintegration, followed by individuals on parole. As for rehabilitation measures for juveniles, most cases were on probation orders. It is noteworthy that foreign nationals or non-residents who have committed a crime in Macao are subject to a monetary fine for misdemeanours or incarceration for more serious crimes. In case of conviction for serious crimes, such individuals would be required to serve a portion of their sentence in Coloane Prison. Their visas might be cancelled, and they may be deported after serving their sentence, with a prohibition on re-entry to Macao for a specified period. As a result, offender rehabilitation programmes in Macao primarily target residents who have been convicted (Leong & Liu, 2022; Li & Ye, 2017).

Rehabilitation Practices in Macao: An Overview of Prison-based, Community-based Programmes and Post-release Services

Numerous published outcome studies confirm the effectiveness of offender rehabilitation. The effectiveness relies on the theoretical underpinnings being adhered to and the design and delivery of services being based on a number of crucial principles of offender rehabilitation. For instance, the core principles of the Risk-Need-Responsivity (RNR) model are divided into risk, need, and responsivity. Previous research has demonstrated that implementing the RNR model has led to a more significant decrease in recidivism rates than programmes that did not follow the RNR model (Zhao et al., 2019). Besides, Desistance Theory outlines the process by which offenders cease their criminal behaviour, provides a conceptual framework for offender rehabilitation, and has practical implications for individuals under probation in the community (Farrall & Maruna, 2004). Desistance Theory accepts that desistance is a complex process, likening it to a journey without shortcuts to achieving the goal, which is linked to external and social factors, such as support from those around the individual, and internal psychological factors, such as beliefs and aspirations (LeBel et al., 2008). While the *Macao Penal Code* encompasses various provisions aimed at promoting rehabilitation processes, indicating a rehabilitation-oriented approach to sentencing (Zhao, 2014), the theoretical underpinnings of the rehabilitation model within Macao's criminal justice system have not been explicitly disseminated by the authorities.

Prison-based Rehabilitation Programmes

Prison-based rehabilitation programmes implemented by the Coloane Prison include social work and counselling support services, school education, vocational training, and various activities facilitating social reintegration. Prisoners are not compelled to engage in daily labour but can apply to work or study in prison according to individual interests and needs (DSC, 2016-2022; GCS, 2022; Leong & Liu, 2022; Zhao, 2014). Most programmes are jointly organised with the Social Welfare Bureau (abbrev. IAS) or social service organisations (DSC, 2023b, 2023c; Leong & Liu, 2022; Pun et al., 2019).

Regarding the social work and psychological counselling support services, the Social Assistance, Education and Training Division of Coloane Prison established the Social Assistance and Psychological Support Team (Portuguese: Grupo de Apoio Social e Assistência Psicológica, abbrev. GASAP) in 2014 to optimise the quality of professional counselling services in response to the increasing prison population; there are 12 social workers and six counsellors providing counselling services for prisoners (Choi et al., 2020). The prison arranges for social workers to meet with each newly admitted prisoner within 48 hours to understand their background and motives for the crime(s) and determine the support and assistance they need (Choi et al., 2020; DSC, 2023d; Leong & Liu, 2022). Prisoners with mental health disorders, inclination to sex crimes, or special psychological conditions are assigned to counsellors whereas all other prisoners are assigned a social worker. Normally, a prisoner is assigned to the same social worker or counsellor throughout his or her entire sentence. The social workers and counsellors continually follow each prisoner's case and provide counselling services for those in need to increase their mental wellness and adaptation. Meanwhile, they also promote contact between prisoners and their families and offer other practical assistance (Choi et al., 2020; Leong & Liu, 2022).

Offender rehabilitation in the Coloane Prison emphasises personal, familial, and community intervention and support (Choi et al., 2020). Such a frame is consistent with the concept of *Recovery Capital*. This concept is defined by three types of "capital" that are necessary to help prisoners re-join society smoothly upon release and support a person in their recovery journey: personal, family and social, and community (White & Cloud, 2008). The rehabilitation services conducted by GASAP directed at the personal aspect include identifying the specific reasons for offending and whether drug abuse or trafficking are involved; assistance is provided for prisoners in developing life plans that will guide them towards the "right track". Regarding the familial aspect, assistance is provided to prisoners to maintain and strengthen their familial relationships and promote family harmony, as support from family is a powerful boost to prisoners' confidence in their successful self-reform. Regarding the community aspect, GASAP helps prisoners to access social resources by communicating and collaborating with other authorities (e.g., IAS) and various social organisations (Choi et al., 2020). For instance, the Prison and the Department of Social Reintegration of the IAS collaborated in holding the "Employment Scheme for Pre-release Inmates", under which employers from various sectors were invited to interview soon-to-be-released prisoners for employment positions such as clerk, shop assistant, driver, cashier, waiter, and kitchen helper, to help prisoners secure employment and adapt to their new lives smoothly upon release (Choi et al., 2020; DSC, 2016-2022; Leong & Liu, 2022).

The prison has been launching activities and group counselling sessions incorporating artistic elements, story-telling theatre, sharing sessions, and the Narrative Therapy to promote prisoners' physical and mental development. Narrative Therapy is a mode of counselling that was applied to Macao's prison-based rehabilitation through collaboration with non-governmental organisations over the past decade (Choi et al., 2020). It is still a relatively novel approach to therapy that seeks to have an empowering effect and offer therapy that is non-blaming and non-pathological in nature (Vinney, 2019). During the counselling process, Narrative Therapy emphasises the idea that every person interprets the meaning of their own lives, which helps prisoners discover and appreciate their hidden strengths and potentials and enables them to understand that there are other possibilities in life besides committing crimes. Prisoners are encouraged to "rewrite the stories of their lives" through therapy. With more materials on positive psychology, prisoners are also guided to have increased confidence in life, rediscover their identity and regain control of their lives (Choi et al., 2020).

Rehabilitation Programmes for Detained Youths

The focus of the Youth Correctional Institution's work is on providing educational and reformatory services. Pursuant to the law *Education and Supervision Regime for Youth Offenders* (Macao SAR Law No. 2/2007, 2007), juvenile delinquents may be ruled by the court to undergo education and supervision during a custodial sentence. Upon admission, each detained youth is assigned a social worker and a counsellor who will assess the detainee's needs, closely monitor his or her adjustment to life in the institution and provide personalised counselling services for each detainee according to their actual problems (DSC, 2023e; Ieong et al., 2021; Leong & Liu, 2022). In addition, the performance of each detained youth will be subject to regular assessment and reports documenting their progress will be periodically compiled and submitted to the judge (Ieong et al., 2021).

Unlike adult prisoners, detained youths participate in systematic discipline training, including marching, physical fitness training, and a reward scheme, to strengthen their awareness of discipline and increase their willpower (DSC, 2023e; Ieong et al., 2021; Leong & Liu, 2022). Besides, vocational training programmes, cultural and recreational activities, interest classes, talks for small groups, and workshops are held for detainees to help develop a more positive attitude to life to help with their future social reintegration (DSC, 2023e; Leong & Liu, 2022). Moreover, the institution's supervisory and educational services concentrate on three aspects of counselling, which are personal, familial, and educational/vocational (Ieong et al., 2021). Regarding the personal aspects, most detained youths' problems lie within their self-awareness, emotional management, sense of right and wrong, and morality; as a result, counselling programmes dealing with various issues are tailored to each detained youth's background, educational level, and motives for the crime(s) (Ieong et al., 2021). Concerning the familial aspect, most cases stem from the relationship between the detained youths and their parents, including family discipline, parent-child communication, and parent-child education (Ieong et al., 2021). Therefore, the institution helps them re-establish and strengthen familial relationships through meetings, home visits, and family activities. It also helps some families develop a family support system and works to build parenting skills to enable the youths to receive more support and trust from their families (DSC, 2023e; Ieong et al., 2021; Leong & Liu, 2022). Regarding the educational and vocational aspect, the formal and recurrent education programmes and professional certificate courses are organised by the Institution and the Education and Youth Development Bureau (Portuguese: Direcção dos Serviços de Educação e de Desenvolvimento da Juventude [DSEDJ]) for the detained youths (DSC, 2016-2022; GCS, 2022; Leong & Liu, 2022). The institution also collaborates with the Department of Social Reintegration on the Employment Scheme for Juvenile Delinquents to set up recruitment interviews for soon-to-be discharged youths to increase employment opportunities after their release (DSC, 2016-2022; GCS, 2022; Leong & Liu, 2022).

The approach taken by the Youth Correctional Institution is to provide education and guidance to young people placed in their care. Chong (2022), an experienced psychological counsellor of the Institution, indicated that the custodial education of young people at the Institution coincides with the ideas proposed by positive psychology, and the five pillars of well-being; positive emotion, engagement, relationships, meaning, and accomplishment (Seligman & Csikszentmihalyi, 2000). The purpose of custodial education of the Institution focuses on helping detained youths develop their life goals, cultivate positive and happy emotions, and constantly break through and innovate with a spirit of dedication to fully display their potential, which shows that the blueprint for a happy life advocated by *Positive Psychology* and the connotation of custodial education are complementary (Chong, 2022).

Community-based Rehabilitation Programmes and Post-release Services

The Department of Social Reintegration provides non-custodial rehabilitation services for adults and youths; for instance, psychological counselling, preparing pre-trial social background reports to the courts, and supporting individuals previously incarcerated and those under non-custodial sentences. The Department is also responsible for providing family support for incarcerated persons and assisting families in resolving problems and restoring relationships (IAS, 2023a; Leong & Liu, 2022).

Regarding rehabilitation services for those convicted of non-custodial sentences and those on parole, the Department provides systematic correctional courses and activities for rehabilitated people according to the types of committed crimes and their needs, such as personal growth, legal education, civic education, treatment courses, skills training, and participation in social services, in order to raise their awareness of offence-free living and community caring to create a positive lifestyle (IAS, 2023a; Leong & Liu, 2022). For cases involving severe or particular crimes, the Department provides *Correctional Courses for Special Offenders* (IAS, 2023a) according to those clients' psychological and social needs, including systematic and tailored correctional courses and psychological counselling. Regarding counselling, recognition of criminal behaviour, personal emotional adjustment, self-esteem reconstruction and interpersonal skills focus to assist clients in improving social adaptability, avoiding reoffending, and establishing a healthy and law-abiding life (IAS, 2023a). In addition, the *Correctional Courses for Youth Offenders* enables youths who were involved in severe or particular crimes to receive diversified systematic correctional courses (IAS, 2023a; Leong & Liu, 2022).

Regarding sex crimes in Macao, the Department launched the *Heart Guidance Workshop* (IAS, 2023a) for cases involving sexual crimes. Sections include introducing the laws of sex-related crimes, cultivating healthy sexual attitudes, learning appropriate relief methods, and teaching clients to avoid deviant sexual preferences and behaviours. Furthermore, a *Sex Crime Case Follow-up Scheme* will be established in 2023 to provide various correctional counselling programmes for those who have committed sex crimes (IAS, 2023a).

Statistical Contexts of Recidivism and Social Reintegration in Macao

Three series of official surveys are crucial to offender rehabilitation in Macao. The *Report on Recidivism of Sentenced Macao Residents* (IAS & DSC, 2018) with its follow-up brief updated reports on Statistics of the *Recidivism of Sentenced Macao Residents – Recidivism Rate* (IAS & DSC, 2019-2023) have been reported to the public annually since 2018. These examine whether Macao residents re-offended within two years after completing their custodial or non-custodial sentences. Both the recidivism rate (5.3%) and the reimprisonment rate (3.0%) of individuals previously incarcerated in Coloane Prison who were released in 2020 met their troughs (Table 6.3). In contrast, both the recidivism rate (12.1%) and the percentage of imposed incarceration sentences due to reoffending (6.0%) of those who completed non-custodial sentences in 2020 reached their peaks (Table 6.4).

TABLE 6.3 Recidivism of Macao Residents Convicted of Custodial Sentences, 2015–2020

Year of Release	2015		2016		2017		2018		2019		2020	
	n	*%*	*n*	*%*	*n*	*%*	*n*	*%*	*n*	*%*	*n*	*%*
Re-offense within 2 years of release	25	14.6	24	13.6	17	9.9	14	12.4	13	9.2	7	5.3
- Sentenced to reimprisonment	10	5.8	12	6.8	13	7.6	7	6.2	9	6.4	4	3.0
Total*	171	100.0	176	100.0	171	100.0	113	100.0	141	100.0	133	100.0

Source: Report on Recidivism of Sentenced Macao Residents (DSC; IAS, 2018); *Statistics of the Recidivism of Sentenced Macao Residents – Recidivism Rate* (DSC; IAS, 2019-2023).
*The total of Macao residents released from Coloane Prison during 1 January to 31 December of the year.

TABLE 6.4 Recidivism of Macao Residents Convicted of Non-custodial Sentences, 2015–2020

Year of Measures Completion	2015		2016		2017		2018		2019		2020	
	n	*%*	*n*	*%*	*n*	*%*	*n*	*%*	*n*	*%*	*n*	*%*
Re-offense within 2 years of measures completion	33	10.4	21	7.6	14	6.7	10	5.1	8	4.9	22	12.1
- Sentenced to imprisonment	–	–	–	–	7	3.3	5	2.5	3	1.8	11	6.0
Total*	317	100.0	276	100.0	210	100.0	198	100.0	163	100.0	182	100.0

Source: Report on Recidivism of Sentenced Macao Residents (DSC; IAS, 2018); *Statistics of the Recidivism of Sentenced Macao Residents – Recidivism Rate* (DSC; IAS, 2019-2023).
*The total of Macao residents who have completed the measures implemented by the Department of Social Reintegration during 1 January to 31 December of the year.

Secondly, the *Report on the Survey of the Characteristics of Youth Offenders* (IAS, 2020), conducted by the Department of Social Reintegration reports juvenile delinquent statistics every four years. The most contemporary report revealed a significant decrease of about 33.8 percent to 149 cases. The report shows that cases were mainly males, aged 15 years old, born in Macao, and lived in the Zona Norte (i.e., the North District in Macao). The mean age for committing crimes or deviance was 13.9 years old, and the ratio of male to female was 3.9:1 (Leong & Liu, 2022). The youth cases mainly involved crimes against persons and crimes against property. The top three cited crimes for conviction were harm to bodily integrity, theft, and arson. Most of the youths who committed crimes were involved in gangs, and a majority of them were first-time offenders. The recidivism rate of those young persons has been reported in previous studies; however, the related contents were deleted in the up-to-date report due to the rearrangement of departments to undertake such analysis.

The *Report on the Survey of Characteristics of Rehabilitative Cases* (IAS, 2021) is conducted triennially; the last report indicated that a total of 735 rehabilitative cases undertaken by the Department of Social Reintegration were completed from 2018 to 2020, representing a decrease of 23.2% compared with those completed between 2015 and 2017. According to this Survey, voluntary cases refer to those people who proactively seek help from the Department when they encounter difficulties in life after completing the sentences or security measures. Except for voluntary cases, most individuals on parole and probation were involved in drug-related crimes, while those under community work orders were mainly involved in crimes against property and crimes against life in society. Additionally, the proportion of those who had drug-abuse records before the case intake was 57.6% (mainly using ketamine) and of those, 22.2% had abused drugs during the follow-up period (generally methamphetamine and cocaine). The results show that Macao's rehabilitation and reintegration processes strongly require drug treatment services. There are no statistics relevant to reporting on offenders with mental illnesses.

Current Challenges and Recent Developments in Macao's Rehabilitation Practices

The current rehabilitation in Macao focuses on helping convicted individuals reintegrate into society, which is consistent with that of Western developed countries. However, there is limited research regarding this topic in Macao (Leong & Liu, 2022; Li & Ye, 2017; Liu & Zhao, 2014). For instance, Malvas' (2014) quantitative research on parole decision-making found that when making decisions on conditional release, Macao prison managers were mainly concerned with protecting the community and maintaining internal order and security. Liu and Zhao (2014) have discussed the development trends of Macao's correctional system and relevant research from a comparative perspective. These were the rare studies investigating the topics related to offender rehabilitation in Macao. Even if a few papers involved related topics, most of them mentioned that incidentally or as part of the research, and those were mainly introductory (Leong & Liu, 2022; Liu & Zhao, 2014). In addition, there are a few book chapters (Kwan, 2010; Leong & Liu, 2022; Li & Ye, 2017) regarding rehabilitation in Macao. As Liu and Zhao (2014) suggested, evidence-based research regarding Macao's offender rehabilitation needs to be emphasised and developed. Comprehensive studies that help draw links between theories and practices are needed.

As previously stated, the prison population had increased by more than one-third over the past decade, which has created a heavy workload for Macau's prison's professional social workers and psychological counsellors. Meanwhile, prisoners in Macao are predominantly non-residents. These prisoners are from many countries and regions, each with a different language and cultural context; some prisoners have entirely different values and ideologies when compared with traditional Macao society (Choi et al., 2020). Historically, financial difficulties in the family and insufficient care from busy or less-educated parents were the primary issues faced by juvenile delinquents (Ieong et al., 2021). However, due to the rapid development of Macao, the issues faced by these individuals have shifted to issues such as being spoiled or neglected by parents who only provide material support, or being irrationally defended by parents despite committing offenses that result in their detention (Ieong et al., 2021). These issues complicate offender rehabilitation in Macao.

Regarding recent developments in Macao's offender rehabilitation, the Secretariat for Security, through the *Policy Address for Fiscal Year 2023 – Security Area* (GSS, 2022), has announced the Government's emphasis on "innovating community collaboration models to jointly assist in the reconstruction of a new life"; this initiative focuses on strengthening the connection and cooperation between the authorities concerned (i.e., DSC and IAS) and social service organisations, to provide more comprehensive community support to assist in the rehabilitation and reintegration of convicted individuals into society. The focal programmes include the first-ever "Assist in Offender Rehabilitation with Care and Inclusiveness" community promotion event, which aims to convey the importance of community support and facilitation of the social reintegration of rehabilitated persons to the public. Additionally, the new "Art Brut Therapy" is a prison-based services, which through painting, promotes and has been shown to develop interconnection between body and mind, and reduce emotional distress and negative psychiatric symptoms among prisoners in Guangdong, China (Qiu et al., 2017). Based on the current programmes' progress, the relevant authorities may consolidate the community-based rehabilitation services and make more efforts to deliver positive messages to the public to raise public awareness and support toward rehabilitation services.

Notes

1 The "Family Beyond the Wall" Project is designed to help Macao resident prisoners or youth detainees and their families solve familial issues and restore their relationships (IAS, 2023a; Leong & Liu, 2022).
2 One of the Macao non-custodial measures.

References

Choi, V., Lam, K., Kuok, S., & Lam, K. (2020). Social Workers as Companions in the Rehabilitation Journey – An interview of the Members of the Social Assistance and Psychological Support Team. *Correctional Services Newsletter*, (8), 24–37. Correctional Services Bureau of Macao SAR. Retrieved from https://www.dsc.gov.mo/CSN/issue_8/cn/mobile/index.html

Chong, W. (2022). 重塑幸福的再教育工作—從正向心理學角度看收容教育 (Re-education to Reshape Happiness – From the Perspective of Positive Psychology on Custodial Education). *Revista das Ciências Policiais de Macau (澳門警學)*, (1), 23–29. Retrieved from https://www.fsm.gov.mo/ESFSM/Media/Default/Journal/Science/S1.pdf

Correctional Services Bureau of Macao [DSC]. (2016-2022). *Annual Report of Correctional Services Bureau.* Author. Retrieved from https://www.dsc.gov.mo/siteen/journal.aspx?cid=42

Correctional Services Bureau of Macao [DSC]. (2021). Annual Meeting of the Socail Reintegration Committee – Continuously Optimizing Social Rehabilitation Services. In *Correctional Services Newsletter* (p. 12). Author. Retrieved from https://www.dsc.gov.mo/CSN/issue_11/cn/mobile/index.html

Correctional Services Bureau of Macao [DSC]. (2023a). *Responsibilities.* Retrieved from https://www.dsc.gov.mo/siteen/about.aspx?id=9

Correctional Services Bureau of Macao [DSC]. (2023b). *Activities Facilitation Social Reintegration.* Retrieved from https://www.dsc.gov.mo/siteen/SinglePage.aspx?id=53

Correctional Services Bureau of Macao [DSC]. (2023c). *School Education and Vocational Trainings.* Retrieved from https://www.dsc.gov.mo/siteen/service.aspx?id=18

Correctional Services Bureau of Macao [DSC]. (2023d). *Counseling Services.* Retrieved from https://www.dsc.gov.mo/siteen/service.aspx?id=17

Correctional Services Bureau of Macao [DSC]. (2023e). *Affairs on Facilitating Juveniles' Return to Society*. Retrieved from https://www.dsc.gov.mo/siteen/SinglePage.aspx?id=46

Correctional Services Bureau of Macao [DSC]; Social Welfare Bureau of Macao [IAS]. (2018). *Report on Recidivism of Sentenced Macao Residents (*被判刑澳門居民重犯狀況報告*)*. Retrieved from https://www.dsc.gov.mo/OtherPublications/2018/Report/mobile/index.html

Correctional Services Bureau of Macao [DSC]; Social Welfare Bureau of Macao [IAS]. (2019-2023). *Statistics of the Recidivism of Sentenced Macao Residents – Recidivism Rate in 2016–2020 (*被判刑澳門居民重犯狀況數據 *2016–2020*年重犯率*)*. Retrieved from https://www.dsc.gov.mo/siteen/others.aspx

Farrall, S., & Maruna, S. (2004). Desistance-Focused Criminal Justice Policy Research: Introduction to a Special Issue on Desistance from Crime and Public Policy. *The Howard Journal of Crime and Justice*, 43(4), 358–367.

Gaming Inspection and Coordination Bureau [DICJ]. (n.d.). *Macao Gaming History*. Retrieved from http://www.dicj.gov.mo/web/en/history/index.html

Government Information Bureau of Macao [GCS]. (2022). *Macao Yearbook 2022*. Author. Retrieved from https://yearbook.gcs.gov.mo/uploads/yearbook_pdf/2022/myb2022e.pdf

Ieong, T., Lei, H., & Chong, W. (2021). The Beacon Guiding Juvenile Delinquents Back to the Right Path – Interview of the Social Worker and Psychological Counseling Team, Youth Correctional Institution. *Correctional Services Newsletter*, (10), 12–26. Correctional Services Bureau of Macao SAR. Retrieved from https://www.dsc.gov.mo/CSN/issue_10/cn/mobile/index.html

Kwan, S. (2010). Macao. In G. Newman (Ed.), *Crime and Punishment Around the World* (Vol. 3, pp. 132–141). ABC-CLIO. Retrieved from https://ebookcentral.proquest.com/lib/umac/detail.action?docID=617100

LeBel, T. P., Burnett, R., Maruna, S., & Bushway, S. D. (2008). The 'Chicken and Egg' of Subjective and Social Factors in Desistance from Crime. *European Journal of Criminology*, 5(2), 131–159. 10.1177/1477370807087640

Leong, D.S.W., & Liu, J. (2022). Criminal Justice Rehabilitation in Macao, China. In M. Vanstone & P. Priestley (Eds.), *The Palgrave Handbook of Rehabilitation in Criminal Justice* (pp. 359–375). Palgrave Macmillan. 10.1007/978-3-031-14375-5_21

Li, S., & Ye, J. (2017). Macao, Corrections in. In K. R. Kerley (Ed.), *The Encyclopedia of Corrections*. John Wiley & Sons, Inc. 10.1002/97811188453 87.wbeoc214

Liu, J., Leong, D.S.W., Yu, P., Zhang, J., Tuo, Z., & Wang, Y. (2022). *The Victimization Survey of Macau Residents – Pilot Study (*澳門居民犯罪受害調查 - 先導研究*)*. Macau Society of Criminology. (Project No. G01790-2112) [Grant]. Macao Foundation.

Liu, J., & Zhao, R. (2014). Corrections in Macau: A Review from the Perspective of Comparative Criminal Justice (比較犯罪學視野下的澳門犯罪矯治及其發展趨勢). *Journal of Macau Studies (*澳門研究*)*, 73(2), 52–60.

Macao SAR Administrative Regulation No. 28/2015. (2015). *Organization and Functioning of the Social Welfare Bureau*. Retrieved from https://bo.io.gov.mo/bo/i/2015/52/regadm28_cn.asp?printer=1#28

Macao SAR Decree-Law No. 58/95/M. (1995). *Macau Penal Code.* Retrieved from https://bo.io.gov.mo/bo/i/95/46/codpencn/declei58.asp

Macao SAR Law No. 2/2007. (2007). *Education and Supervision Regime for Youth Offenders.* Retrieved from https://bo.io.gov.mo/bo/i/2007/16/lei02_cn.asp

Macao SAR Law No. 11/2009. (2009). *Law on Combating Computer Crimes.* Retrieved from https://bo.io.gov.mo/bo/i/2009/27/lei11_cn.asp

Macao SAR Law No. 17/2009. (2009). *Law on Prohibition of Production, Trafficking and Illicit Use of Narcotic Drugs and Psychotropic Substances.* Retrieved from https://bo.io.gov.mo/bo/i/2009/32/lei17_cn.asp

Malvas, C. M. (2014). The Paradigm of Parole Release in Macau: A Quantitative Analysis of Prison Recommendations (澳門的假釋模式：監獄建議的定量分析). *Journal of Macau Studies (澳門研究)*, 73(2), 72–80.

Pun, C., Lam, U., Kuan, S., & Wong, S. (2019). Community Support for Social Rehabilitation – Caritas Macau, the Women's General Association of Macau, YMCA of Macau & Macau Christian Prison Ministries. *Correctional Services Newsletter*, (7), 15–28. Correctional Services Bureau of Macao SAR. Retrieved from https://www.dsc.gov.mo/CSN/issue_7/cn/mobile/index.html

Qiu, H. Z., Ye, Z. J., Liang, M. Z., Huang, Y. Q., Liu, W., & Lu, Z. D. (2017). Effect of an Art Brut Therapy Program Called Go beyond the Schizophrenia (GBTS) on Prison Inmates with Schizophrenia in Mainland China – A Randomized, Longitudinal, and Controlled Trial. *Clinical Psychology & Psychotherapy*, 24(5), 1069–1078.

Secretariat for Security of Macao SAR [GSS]. (2019-2023). *Macao Full-Year Crime Case Statistics.* Author. Retrieved from https://www.gss.gov.mo/cht/statistic.aspx

Secretariat for Security of Macao SAR [GSS]. (2022). *Policy Address for Fiscal Year 2023 - Security Area (Linhas de Acção Governativa para 2023 - área da Segurança).* Author. Retrieved from https://www.policyaddress.gov.mo/data/policyAddress/2023/pt/3_2023SS_p.pdf

Seligman, M. E., & Csikszentmihalyi, M. (2000). Positive psychology: An introduction. *American Psychologist*, 55(1), 5–14. 10.1037/0003-066X.55.1.5

Social Welfare Bureau of Macao [IAS]. (2020). *Report on the Survey of the Characteristics of Youth Offenders (違法青少年特徵調查報告).* Retrieved from https://www.ias.gov.mo/wp-content/uploads/2013/10/2020-08-12_173149_26.pdf

Social Welfare Bureau of Macao [IAS]. (2021). *Report on the Survey of Characteristics of Rehabilitative Cases (更生個案統計調查報告).* Retrieved from https://www.ias.gov.mo/wp-content/uploads/2021/09/2021-09-29_112020_12.pdf

Social Welfare Bureau of Macao [IAS]. (2023a). *Social Reintegration Service.* Retrieved from https://www.ias.gov.mo/en/swb-services/rehabilitative_service

Social Welfare Bureau of Macao [IAS]. (2023b). *Reintegration Service for Adult Offenders.* Retrieved from https://www.ias.gov.mo/en/swb-services/rehabilitative_service/adult_offenders

Social Welfare Bureau of Macao [IAS]. (2023c). *Reintegration Service for Youth Offenders.* Retrieved from https://www.ias.gov.mo/en/swb-services/rehabilitative_service/young_offenders

Statistics and Census Service of Macao [DSEC]. (2013-2021a). *Yearbook of Statistics*. Author. Retrieved from https://www.dsec.gov.mo/en-US/Home/Publication/YearbookOfStatistics

Statistics and Census Service of Macao [DSEC]. (2021b). *Analysis Report of Statistical Indicator System for Moderate Economic Diversification of Macao*. Author. Retrieved from https://www.dsec.gov.mo/en-US/Home/Publication/SIED

Statistics and Census Service of Macao [DSEC]. (2023). *Macao in Figures 2023*. Retrieved from https://www.dsec.gov.mo/getAttachment/1a9589b1-d0e4-4268-9227-53421c0aff47/E_MN_PUB_2023_Y.aspx

Statistics and Census Service of Macao [DSEC]. (n.d.). *Tourism Statistics*. Retrieved from https://www.dsec.gov.mo/en-US/Statistic?id=401

United Nations. (1966). *International Covenant on Civil and Political Rights*. UN General Assembly. Retrieved from https://www.ohchr.org/en/instruments-mechanisms/instruments/international-covenant-civil-and-political-rights

United Nations Office on Drugs and Crime [UNODC]. (2021). *Latin America and the Caribbean Crime Victimization Survey Initiative [LACSI], Ver 4.0*. Author. Retrieved from https://www.cdeunodc.inegi.org.mx/index.php/lacsi-initiative/

Vinney, C. (2019). *What Is Narrative Therapy? Definition and Techniques*. Retrieved from https://www.thoughtco.com/narrative-therapy-4769048

White, W., & Cloud, W. (2008). Recovery Capital: A Primer for Addictions Professionals. *Counselor*, 9(5), 22–27.

Zhao, R. (2014). Official Responses to Crime in Macau. In L. Cao, I. Y. Sun, & B. Hebenton (Eds.), *The Routledge Handbook of Chinese Criminology*, pp. 325–341. Taylor & Francis Group.

Zhao, R., & Liu, J. (2011). A System's Approach to Crime Prevention: The Case of Macao. *Asian Journal of Criminology*, 6, 207–227.

Zhao, Y., Messner, S. F., Liu, J., & Jin, C. (2019). Prisons as Schools: Inmates' Participation in Vocational and Academic Programs in Chinese Prisons. *International Journal of Offender Therapy and Comparative Criminology*, 63(15-16), 2713–2740.

7

AN OVERVIEW OF CRIME TRENDS AND REHABILITATION PRACTICES IN SOUTH KOREA

Seung C. Lee, JeongSook Yoon, and Yongmyeng Keum

An Overview of Crime Trends and Rehabilitation Practices in South Korea

South Korea, officially known as the Republic of Korea, is an independent nation situated in the southern part of the Korean Peninsula in East Asia. It covers an area of 100,210 square kilometres (38,623 square miles) and, in 2021, had an estimated population of 51.7 million. As of 2021, children under 14 years old accounted for 11.8% (6.09 million) of the population, while 71.4% (36.9 million) were young and middle-aged adults aged 15–64, and 16.8% (8.71 million) were seniors aged 65 or older (Statistics Korea, 2022). The average age of the population has increased from 40 years old in 2015 to 43 years old in 2021. South Korea is widely recognised as one of the most homogenous societies globally, with ethnic Koreans comprising approximately 96% of the total population (Ministry of the Interior and Safety, 2022). The official language of South Korea is Korean, also known as Hangul.

South Korea has a centralised tripartite government structure comprising an executive, legislature, and judiciary. The central government oversees all aspects of the criminal justice system, including prosecution, courts, and prisons. There are no regional criminal justice systems. The Continental or Civil Legal System has been largely incorporated into South Korean law, with constitutional law and explicitly written legal codes serving as the main sources of reference. The Korean criminal procedure combines elements of both inquisitorial and adversarial systems, merging American and German criminal procedures.

DOI: 10.4324/9781003360919-9

South Korean culture shares similarities with Chinese and Japanese cultures due to geographic proximity, long history of contact, and the mutual influence of animism, shamanism, Buddhism, Confucianism, and Taoism. Despite some changes in contemporary society, traditional cultural characteristics such as collectivism and a hierarchical social structure influence South Korean society (de Mente, 2012; Niaz & Hassan, 2006; Yeh & Huang, 1996).

General Trends of Crimes in South Korea

From 2011 to 2016, the total number of crime incidents (i.e., cases involving criminal allegations from police or prosecutors) in South Korea slightly increased, but then decreased from 2017 to 2021. In 2015, the highest number of crimes in the previous decade was recorded, with 2,020,731 incidents and a crime rate of 3,921.5 per 100,000 people. However, in 2021, the number of crimes dropped to 1,530,511, with the lowest crime rate in the previous ten years (2,963.88 crimes per 100,000 people). Compared to other Western countries, the crime rate in South Korea is relatively low, for example, Canada's rate of 5,687 per 100,000 people [Statistics Canada, 2022]).

Major street crimes, such as murder, robbery, arson, and theft, have been steadily decreasing over the last few decades (Figure 7.1). However, fraud has been increasing. A total of 226,360 cases of fraud were reported in 2011, making the annual rate 453.3 per 100,000 people. In 2020, there were 354,154 recorded fraud offences, with an incidence rate of 683.2.

Sexual crimes in South Korea have increased by 49.0% from 22,168 in 2011 to 33,035 in 2021, with an incidence rate per 100,000 increasing 46.5% from 43.7 to 64.0. The sexual crime rate in South Korea is also relatively low when compared to Canada, which was 122 per 100,000 people in 2021. Violent sexual crimes like rape are declining, but there has been an increase in online sexual crimes such as non-consensual sharing of intimate images and videos, as well as distribution of illegally taken photos/videos of someone's body ("upskirting" Figure 7.2). In 2021, online sexual offences accounted for almost 35% of all sexual offences, making them a significant societal issue in South Korea. However, the increase in sexual crimes should be considered in light of the expanded scope of sexual crimes and possible changes in the reporting rate (Supreme Prosecutor's Office, 2022; Figure 7.2).

In 2021, 4% of sexual crimes were against children under 13 and 21% against those aged 13–20. About 90% of child victims were girls. There were 1,210 incidents of sexual offences against children under 13 in 2021, up 4.8% from 2020 and 14.5% from 2011, with an incidence rate per

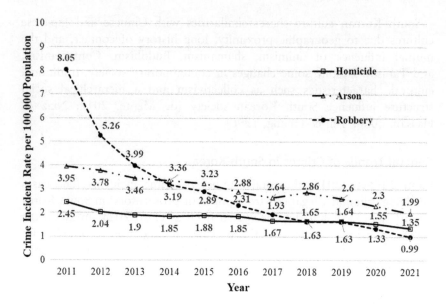

FIGURE 7.1 Major Violent Crime Incident Rates over Last 10 Years in South Korea.

Source: Analytics on statistics of crime (Supreme Prosecutor's Office: Republic of Korea, 2022).

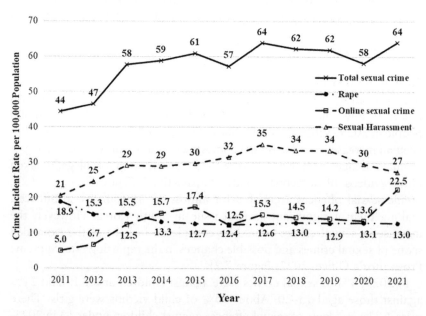

FIGURE 7.2 Sexual Crime Incident Rates over the Last 10 Years in South Korea.

Source: Analytics on statistics of crime (Supreme Prosecutor's Office: Republic of Korea, 2022).

100,000 people increasing by 44.0% from 16.3 to 23.5 (Supreme Prosecutor's Office, 2022).

Sexual offences against minors aged 13 to 20 years increased by 9.5% from 6,305 to 6,904 in the past year. The number of these crimes committed between 2011 and 2021 increased slightly by 0.3%, from 6,883 to 6,904, while the rate per 100,000 people in this age group increased significantly by 47.2%, from 142 to 209.

The number of alleged drug crimes in South Korea as reported by police or prosecutors has almost doubled over the past decade, with 9,174 cases in 2011 and 16,153 cases in 2021. Hallucinogens and stimulants (e.g., methamphetamine, LSD) were the most common (66%), followed by cannabis (e.g., marijuana; 23%) and narcotics (e.g., heroin, opium; 11%). Over half of the drug crime cases involved drug use (50.1%), followed by trafficking (21.9%) and smuggling (10.9%; Supreme Prosecutor's Office, 2022).

Under the Korean Act on the Safety Management of Firearms and Explosives, possession of firearms and related items without permission is prohibited, with only a few exceptions (Article 10). Additionally, anything that resembles a gun is prescribed by presidential decree and cannot be manufactured, sold, or possessed (Article 11). As a result, gun-related crimes are rare. There were only 46 criminal cases involving guns in 2021, with one homicide committed by a gun out of a total of 641 homicides (Korean Statistical Information Service, 2021).

In 2021, female offenders accounted for 21.4% of the total offender population (n = 287,839). Youth offenders under the age of 19 years made up about 4% of the offender population (n = 54,040),[1] with over 80% being male. Among the total number of arrestees in 2021 (N = 1,360,405), approximately 2.2% were non-Korean citizens, lower than their proportion (3.8%) in the general population.

Historical and Philosophical Perspectives on Rehabilitation of Offenders

The South Korean correctional system follows the United Nations Standard Minimum Rules for the Treatment of Prisoners, which prioritise rehabilitation and reintegration. Prisoners are classified and given a treatment plan based on their needs, abilities, and dispositions to facilitate their treatment and reintegration (rules 91, 92). These rules were established by the UN General Assembly in 1955 and continue to guide the modern correctional system in South Korea (United Nations Office on Drug and Crime, 1955/2015).

Risk Need Responsivity (RNR) principles for efficient corrective interventions are another important set of guiding concepts in the Korean correctional system (Andrews & Bonta, 2010; Andrews & Bonta, 2017). As per this model, the most successful interventions are those that target high-risk offenders (Risk), target criminogenic needs (factors that, when changed, reduce the likelihood of recidivism; Need), and administer the treatment in a way that is appropriate for the offender's culture and learning style (Responsivity; Andrews & Bonta, 2010).

Risk Assessment Tools Used in South Korea

Risk assessment tools used in the Korean criminal justice system include those imported from the West, including the Static-99, and those developed locally. The development of risk assessment tools for the Korean criminal justice system was based on reviews of existing literature and tools from the Western world. The following (actuarial) risk assessment tools are commonly used in South Korea.

Korean Offender Risk Assessment System-General (KORAS-G)

The Korean Offender Risk Assessment System-General (KORAS-G) is a risk assessment measure that was created in 2010 to evaluate the likelihood of reoffending among adult male offenders in South Korea. It was developed using data from 153 adult male prisoners and 52 adult male probationers who committed violent crimes. KORAS-G consists of 17 risk factors[2] with total scores ranging from 0 to 30. The evaluation of each factor is based on official records, including criminal background checks, investigative materials, and indictments, as well as interviews with the defendant and other related parties (Lee et al., 2010; Lee, 2011).

Lee (2011) evaluated the predictive validity of KORAS-G by following up on the development samples ($N = 189$) for up to 14 months. Recidivism was defined as any subsequent arrest, charge, or conviction for any crime. after being released into the community. KORAS-G significantly predicted recidivism (AUC = .684) with 61 recidivists; Lee, 2011; Lee & Ko, 2011).

Korean Sex Offender Risk Assessment Scale (KSORAS)

The Korean Sex Offender Risk Assessment Scale (KSORAS) was created in 2008 to assess the risk of sexual recidivism among adult male offenders and to help determine the use of electronic monitoring devices (Lee et al., 2008). The scale includes 15 static risk factors with total scores ranging from 1 to 29, and was developed using a sample of 81 adult male prisoners and 82 adult male probationers who had been convicted of sexual crimes in 2007).[3] The KSORAS total scores were highly correlated with Static-99 total scores (r = .548; Lee et al., 2010).

The predictive validity of KSORAS was evaluated by following up on the developmental samples (N = 163) from August 2007 to May 2010; sexual recidivism rates were 11.9% (n = 18), 31.1% (n = 47) for a new violent offence (including contact sexual offence), and 53.6% (n = 81) for any new offence. The predictive accuracy of KSORAS was significant, with moderate effect sizes for sexual recidivism (AUC = .676) and violent recidivism (AUC = .682).

Psychopathy Checklist-Revised (PCL-R)

The PCL-R manual was translated into Korean in 2009 and has been utilised in the Korean criminal justice system (Hare, 2003/2008) since. In South Korea, a PCL-R total score of 25 or higher is recommended for diagnosing psychopathy. In 2009, Lee et al. (2009) investigated the predictive validity of the PCL-R: Korean version with 153 adult male prisoners and 107 adult male probationers who were sentenced to various crimes. The average PCL-R total score was 22.08 (SD = 7.90). The PCL-R total scores showed good predictive accuracy for general recidivism with a range of follow-up periods between 7 and 11 months (AUC value of 0.70). In a study with 69 adult male prisoners and probationers, PCL-R was found to have moderate predictive accuracy (AUC = 0.675) for general recidivism (Lee & Kim, 2010). Recidivists had higher average PCL-R scores (M = 29.55, SD = 8.55) compared to non-recidivists (M = 21.44, SD = 8.21). In a study of 318 inmates who were released into the community from Korean prisons between 2005 and 2015, 10% reoffended and the predictive accuracy of PCL-R was moderate (AUC = .651; Ko et al., 2016).

Static-99/R

Static-99 (Hanson & Thornton, 2000) is an actuarial risk assessment tool developed to evaluate the risk of sexual recidivism among adult males who have been charged or convicted of sexually motivated offences. It is currently the most widely used risk assessment tool for adult male sexual offenders in Western countries and several East Asian countries (Helmus et al., 2022). In South Korea, Static-99 was adopted by the Ministry of Justice in 2014; scores are currently utilised to classify individuals for sex offender treatment (Yoon et al., 2020). The Korean criminal justice system still uses the older version of the Static-99 coding handbook (Harris et al., 2003).

In a prospective field study of 8,207 adult men (18 years old or older) convicted of a crime with a sexual motivation, the Static-99R demonstrated large effect sizes with respect to predictive validity (AUC = .721) and also exhibited good discriminating levels for violent and any recidivism, with moderate effect sizes (AUCs = .677 and .696; Lee et al., 2023). During an average follow-up period of 3 years, 9.9% (*n* = 816) of the overall sample were reconvicted for a sexual offence, 14.5% (*n* = 1,191) for a violent offence, and 26.9% for any offence.

Hallym Assessment Guide for Sex Offender Risk (HAGSOR)

Developed at Hallym University in South Korea, the Hallym Assessment Guide for Sex Offender Risk (HAGSOR) is a risk assessment tool consisting of ten static risk factors[4] and 13 dynamic risk factors.[5] It is used to assess the likelihood of sexual reoffending in individuals who have committed sexual offences (Jo, 2010). A study conducted on 765 inmates released between 2014 and 2020 evaluated the predictive accuracy of HAGSOR-Dynamic (13 items). Although HAGSOR-Dynamic did not predict sexual recidivism (AUC = .542), it predicted general recidivism (AUC = .594). Only two items, aggression towards people and social support, were significantly associated with sexual recidivism at the item level, whereas sexual compulsion was significant but in the opposite direction associated with sexual recidivism. Thus, further research is necessary to improve the ability of the HAGSOR-Dynamic factor items to predict sexual recidivism (Yoon, 2022).

Security Treatment Level Classification Index & Correctional Recidivism Prediction Index (CO-REPI)

The Korean penal system employs two different classification indices – the Security Treatment Level Classification Index (16 items) and the Correctional Recidivism Prediction Index (CO-REPI; 23 items) – to help with risk assessment, classification, and parole release (Yoon et al., 2021). These benchmarks have been in place since 2008 and 2012, respectively. A validation study including 9,929 individuals who were sentenced between 2012 and 2021 found that both indices were significantly associated with recidivism (AUC = .654 and .756, respectively; the recidivism rate was 16% [*n* = 1,592]). However, the indices do not account for any risk modifications resulting from prison-based treatments and interventions, as they primarily focus on static factors.

Crime Prevention and Rehabilitation Practice in South Korea

South Korea has been implementing harsh punishments for sexual offences since around 2000, resulting in an increase in the mandatory minimum sentence and the introduction of measures such as sex offender registration, electronic monitoring, and pharmacological treatment. However, to support successful reintegration, psychological treatment programmes have been developed in prisons and in forensic mental hospitals.

Sex Offender Registration and Notification

In 2006, South Korea established a sex offender registration system that initially only covered individuals who committed sexual crimes against children and adolescents. However, it was expanded in 2011 to include sexual offences against adults and then in 2013 to cover all sexual offences. The length of time an offender stays on the registry is based on their sentence. The Minister of Justice is required to keep registration information for 30 years for those given a death, life, or over 10 years sentence, 20 years for those sentenced to over 3 but not more than 10 years in prison, 15 years for those sentenced to 3 years or less, and 10 years for those given a fine. From 2008 to 2019, 87,764 new cases were recorded (Kim et al., 2020). The current process for selecting registration candidates disregards the risk of reoffending and relies on an automated procedure that determines registration eligibility after verifying a conviction for a registered sex offence. In 2015, South Korea's Constitutional Court ruled that the sex offender registration system was unconstitutional due to the excessive restriction of managing personal information for a uniform period of 20 years. Thus, a registration exemption system was introduced in 2016; by 2020, 739 individuals had applied for exemption, and 596 had been approved.

South Korean law specifies that individuals convicted for certain sex offences must be disclosed to the public. There are, however, exceptions for crimes against minors (sex purchase, prostitution, prostitution solicitation and sales, coercion, and the production of obscene materials) and offenders with disabilities based on their recidivism risk, which is left to the judge's discretion. The South Korean government discloses information about registered sex offenders to the public through mailed letters and online disclosures. This includes details needed to prevent crime and identifying information about the offender, such as name, age, address, physical characteristics, photograph, a summary of the sex offence, prior sex offences, and whether the offender is wearing an electronic device. From 2008 to 2019, only 17.1% of registered cases had the sex offender's identity disclosed through website, smartphone application, or notification via mail, mobile, or bulletin board. Most registered sex offenders (over 70%) were young adults aged 19 to 49, and the vast majority were native Koreans (97.5%) and men (99.0%).

Based on similar findings in Western countries (Zgoba and Mitchell, 2023), it is difficult to conclude that South Korea's sex offender registration/notification system effectively prevents sexual crimes, as the number of sexual crimes (especially those against children and adolescents) and crime rates have continued to rise since its implementation. Moreover, disclosing information may exacerbate the risk of recidivism for sex offenders, suggesting that the system has a negative impact rather than deterring reoffending (Kim et al., 2020).

Electronic Monitoring Device

The Act on the Attachment of Electronic Positioning Devices to Certain Sexual Violent Offenders was approved in 2007 and went into force in 2008, providing the legal foundation for electronic monitoring in South Korea. Originally, the Act only applied to crimes involving sexual assault but was later expanded to include kidnapping minors, murder, and robbery. The decision to require an offender to wear an electronic device is made during sentencing based on their risk of recidivism. In 2020, the system was expanded to include a system of conditional bail and electronic parole supervision for all crimes.

In the original Act, a 5-year attachment period was required but was extended to 10 years by the 2008 amendment. The 2010 amendment adjusted the upper limit of the attachment period to 10 years or more but not more than 30 years, 3 years or more but not more than 20 years, and 1 year or more but not more than 10 years, depending on the statutory sentence, and doubled the lower limit in the case of crimes against children under 13 years of age.

The prosecutor typically requests an attachment order from the court, and a pre-sentencing investigation is conducted to examine factors such as the suspect's motivation for the crime, their relationship with the victim, psychological state, and risk of reoffending. To assess the risk of reoffending, pre-sentencing investigations use the Korean Sex Offender Risk Assessment Scale (KSORAS) for crimes involving sexual assault, the Korean Offender Risk Assessment Scale-General (KORAS-G) for cases involving kidnapping, murder, and kidnapping minors, and the Psychopathy Checklist-Revised (PCL-R) under certain circumstances. The PCL-R is used for suspects who receive a KSORAS score of 13 or above or who committed a sexual crime against a child, denoting a "high" risk of recidivism.

According to Kim et al. (2021), the recidivism rate of sexual assault, murder, and robbery offenders under electronic supervision decreased significantly after the adoption of the electronic monitoring system in South Korea. In the 5 years following the system's implementation (2016–2020), only 2.1% of sexual assault offenders had committed sexual offences again, compared to an average of roughly 14.1% before the system's adoption (2003–2007; i.e., general deterrence). An empirical study to evaluate the effectiveness of psychological treatment (Yoon et al., 2020) found a decreased risk for general recidivism among the individuals wearing electronic monitoring devices compared to a control group who also received treatment but not electronic monitoring.

Pharmacological Treatment

In response to persistent public demands for implementing community safety measures, the Ministry of Justice of Korea passed a law in 2011 (the "Act on Sexual Impulse Drug Treatment of Sexually Violent Offenders") requiring chemical castration of adults (19 or older) who committed sexual crimes, were diagnosed as paraphilic and were at high risk of committing sexual violence crimes (Park, 2013).

By 2020, around 50 people have been treated in South Korea since the law's enactment in 2011, but no study has ascertained the measure's effectiveness. In a preliminary study, 38 male patients imprisoned for sexual offences at National Forensic Hospital were examined to evaluate the therapeutic effects and potential risks of chemical castration. The patients received androgen-deprivation treatment (ADT) monthly for three months, and their psycho-behavioural and clinical outcomes were studied. The study found that chemical castration led to a decrease in sexual desire, masturbation frequency, and sexual fantasies, making it a successful treatment for paraphilic sex offenders. The most common psychiatric diagnosis among the patients was paedophilia ($n = 17\%$; 45%; Koo et al., 2013), followed by Paraphilia NOS ($n = 8$; 24%).

Prison-Based Sex Offender Treatment Programme in South Korea

Psychological treatment programmes for sex offenders began in South Korean prisons in 2006, with a focus on child victims until 2013 (Yoon & Knight, 2013). Since 2014, basic, advanced, and intense psychological treatment programs have been compulsorily offered to sex offenders based on their risk of recidivism and the number of hours required by the court to attend the program (Yoon et al., 2020). The Classification and Examination Division evaluates the offenders' likelihood of reoffending

TABLE 7.1 Prison-Based Treatment Program in South Korea (example)

Modules		Goals
1	Motivation	Motivation to participate in the program
2	Self-esteem	Understanding and improving self-esteem
3	Self-understanding	Life graphs and autobiographies
4	Emotion	Understand emotion and management
5	Interpersonal relationship	Maintaining interpersonal relationships and problem solving
6	Sexual consciousness	Sex education and manage cognitive distortion on sex
7	Sexual trigger	Understanding and responding to sexual triggers
8	Empathy	Improve empathy on victimisation
9	Self-control	Control stress and addiction management
10	Good life	Planning for the future

Source: Yoon et al. (2020).

and determines their courses based on the combined results of Static-99, HAGSOR-S, and HAGSOR-total assessments.

The basic course is for low-risk offenders and lasts up to 100 hours, while the advanced course is for medium-risk offenders and lasts up to 200 hours (available in some facilities). The intense course is for high-risk offenders and lasts more than 200 hours, provided through the Psychological Treatment Centre in penal facilities as a 300-hour programme. The psychological services offered to sex offenders in prisons are context-specific, and the schedule structure is outlined in Table 7.1. The treatment plan consists of a minimum of two and a maximum of 12 distinct sessions, with pre- and post-tests used to monitor progress.

As of 2021, the number of sex offenders who completed either the basic, advanced, or intensive course since 2014 was 21,027 (16,933 for basic, 2,086 for advanced, and 1,911 for intensive; Ministry of Justice, 2022). In a study conducted by Yoon et al. (2020), the success of the basic, advanced, or intensive sex offender treatment programme was investigated using 6,028 inmates who had completed the programme since 2014, and a control group of 1,586 offenders who did not participate in the programme. With a follow-up of up to five years, and the impact of the programme on the CO-REPI (Correctional Recidivism Prediction Index) was examined; results showed that the psychologically-treated group had statistically lower CO-REPI scores than the control group.

The recent study also investigated the impact of a psychological treatment programme on the rate of recidivism among sex offenders following their release from prison (Yoon et al., 2020). The results revealed that individuals in the treatment group had a decreased risk of general recidivism compared to those in the control group. When controlling for other significant variables such as pre-treatment scores (self-esteem and child molestation), wearing an electronic device, and Static-99 total score, the treatment group had a 22% lower sexual recidivism risk than the control group. These findings suggest that the psychological treatment programme for sex offenders in prison has a beneficial effect on preventing repeat offences (Yoon et al., 2020). However, the treatment provided in this study did not ultimately lead to a significant decrease in sexual reoffending (Yoon et al., 2020).

Although the current treatment programme has been successful in reducing overall reoffending, it may not be as effective in preventing sexual offences. It may be necessary to assess the effectiveness of the sex offence-specific components of the programme to address this issue. The Korean correctional system has also implemented various other psychological treatment programs for crimes concerning substance abuse, mental illness, child abuse, and intimate partner violence, but their efficacy has yet to be examined.

Forensic Psychiatric Hospital

South Korea's criminal trial system does not have a separate court process for individuals with mental disabilities, unlike the mental health courts found in other countries like the United States. Instead, individuals with mental disabilities go through the general criminal trial process, which may result in a reduced sentence and therapeutic supervision through a psychiatric evaluation. However, recent amendments to the Treatment and Supervision Act have introduced court-ordered treatment, which functions similarly to a mental health court system. This system allows the court to require psychiatric treatment for individuals who have committed crimes and are deemed to have a risk of recidivism and a need for treatment (Kwon & Shin, 2015).

Therapeutic detention centres in South Korea provide therapy for individuals with mental and physical disabilities, drug and alcohol addiction, and those who have committed crimes and require treatment to prevent future offences. To apply for therapeutic commitment, a specialist such as a psychiatrist must diagnose or evaluate the individual. In the case of individuals with mental and sexual disabilities, a mental evaluation by an expert is required before medical treatment can be provided.

Therapeutic release/supervision as a form of security measure is granted based on the possibility of an individual reoffending and their need for treatment. The court may rely on medical examinations, evaluations, reassessments, and a professional assessor's expertise to determine the risk of reoffending before imposing therapeutic supervision.

Three categories of offenders have different requirements: 1) A person whose incapability to be punished results from incompetence or whose sentence is reduced as a result of limited responsibility; 2) A person who has committed a crime that is punishable by a sentence of at least three years, is addicted to drugs that can be abused or have a detoxifying effect, needs treatment in a therapeutic prison facility, and is at risk of recidivism; and 3) A person who has a mental and sexual disorder (e.g., paedophilia or sexual sadism), who has committed a crime of sexual assault that is punishable by a sentence of at least three years. Mental disorders officially used in Korea diagnosis and classification criteria used in Korea are the International Classification of Diseases (ICD-10) and the Diagnostic and Statistical Manual of Mental Disorders (DSM-5).

Rehabilitation Programmes in Prison

The programmes aimed at inmates' social rehabilitation include employment and vocational training, and education programmes, among others. The private sector is also actively involved in correctional services.

Education Programme in Prison

Inmates in South Korea have access to various educational opportunities, including General Education Development (GED) classes, high school and university courses in broadcasting and communication, self-study courses for obtaining a bachelor's degree, and commissioned education courses at vocational colleges. Additionally, they receive intensive personal development programming aimed at developing fundamental human traits, attitudes, and character. Trained volunteers from the community are involved in programmes covering topics, such as constitutional values, the humanities, communication, and group counselling. All prisoners have access to basic and advanced personal development courses.

Reformation Programme

Since 2005, the Ministries of Justice and Culture, Sports, and Tourism have been collaborating to offer cultural and artistic performances including theatre, music, art, and reading therapy programmes. Additionally, there are programmes to treat alcoholism, gambling addiction, and drug addiction. The Family Relationship Restoration Program includes the Family Meeting House programme and the Family Love Camp, which provide opportunities for offenders serving lengthy terms (since 1999) and their families to spend time together and repair family bonds. Family interviews are also conducted for people in prison experiencing a family crisis. Religious members of the public lead weekly gatherings for prisoners who practice many religions, including Buddhism, Catholicism, and other forms of Christianity. Experts from each religion offer religious counselling to people in prison about their religious beliefs, mental health, and life in prison.

Vocational Training

People in prison are provided with technical training tailored to their skills, interests, age, and education to help them develop job skills for post-release employment. Certification exams to earn various technical credentials, including those for industrial engineers and craftspeople are offered after vocational instruction. An annual exhibition showcases inmate work that is sold online or given to correctional institutions.[6]

Employment and Business Start-up Support Programmes

Various programmes are aimed at providing inmates with skills and knowledge about work and entrepreneurship to prevent recidivism. Examples of such programmes include the *Hug Job Support Program*, small business entrepreneurship training, and work-conditional parole. The Hug Job Support Program creates a job plan for potential inmates and offers a job success allowance if they find employment after release. The Start-up Instruction Program offers 20–40 hours of start-up education and information to inmates who are going to be released. Inmates who are not likely to reoffend and have demonstrated exceptional correctional performance are eligible for parole on the condition of employment. A Regular Job Interview is also conducted where employers describe the job and inmates attest to their talents, well-being, and willingness to work.

Visits

In Korea, family relationships are highly valued in the culture, and when a prisoner is detained in a correctional facility, family members and friends can come to visit and comfort them, helping them to maintain ties with the community. In particular, interview methods utilising IT technologies such as video interviews and smart interviews are used to help inmates' social rehabilitation by maintaining relationships with their families.

For a long time, video interviewing has enabled family members and friends to talk with people in other correctional facilities through a computer monitor deployed in a correctional facility close to their residence using a computer network installed in the correctional facility. Via smart interviewing, family members or friends use their smartphones (mobile devices such as tablets) or PCs to talk with inmates in correctional facilities. Combined, 331,625 video and smart interviews were conducted in 2021.

Furlough

Furloughs (i.e., an authorised temporary release granted to a prison inmate) serve the purpose of maintaining familial ties and enhancing social skills for successful reintegration into society after prison. They may be granted for various reasons such as attending to an ill or deceased parent, a child's wedding, outside hospitalisation due to sickness or injury, vocational training, or job search post-release. A regular furlough lasts up to 20 days per year, while a special furlough lasts up to five days per occurrence. Between 2012 and 2019, approximately 1,200 prisoners were granted annual furloughs to foster family connections and prepare for reintegration.

Civilian Correctional Advisors

The Volunteer Correctional Advisors Program appoints individuals from the public to support inmates in areas such as counselling, employment support, education, religious activities, as well as medical care. In general, there are four groups of correctional advisors, namely, correctional, religious, educational, and medical counsellors, with as many as 4,410 people participating as of 2021.

Conclusion

Since the beginning of 2000, the Korean Criminal Justice System has made significant efforts to successfully reintegrate and rehabilitate offenders into society by embracing models and programmes created in Western countries (e.g., RNR model, sex offender treatment programme). Additionally, South Korea has adopted and implemented the security measures that are frequently utilised in the West, such as sex offender registration, electronic surveillance, and drug treatment. However, additional research in the Korean context is necessary to demonstrate their effectiveness. In addition to these Western rehabilitation models, culturally specific Korean rehabilitation approaches have also been implemented (e.g., family-oriented programmes, and various spiritual and religious services). Nevertheless, more work should be put into determining whether there are any culturally-specific variables to help intervention programmes work better and whether risk assessment tools predict risks more accurately.

Notes

1 In South Korea, the age of legal adulthood is 19 years old. Minimum Age of Criminal Responsibility (MACR) is 14.
2 The 17 items contain age at release, level of education, marital status, age at first offense, incarceration occasion during juvenile, criminal history, number of prior violent crime, prior violent conviction, any violation during the sentencing period, school misconduct, drug and alcohol use history, index violent offence, spree crime during index offence, accept responsibility or denial in index offence, time free prior to index offence, antisocial attitudes (PCL-R, MMPI, PAI), and mental health history.
3 Fifteen items include age at release, marital status, age at first arrest, non-contact sexual offence, prior sexual offences, violent offences, total incarceration period, any violation during the sentencing period, victim types, relationship with victim, victim's gender, number of victims, age difference with victim, index violent offence, and accept responsibility or denial in index offence.
4 10 static items contain age at release from prison, age at first sexual offence, frequency of prior offences, frequency of parole and probation violations, frequency of convictions, any non-sexual offences, any extra-familial victims, any familial victims, any male victim, and any victim under the age of 13 years.
5 13 dynamic items contain sexually deviant lifestyle, Sexual compulsion, Criminal personality, Cognitive distortion, Aggression toward people, Emotional control, Insight, Substance abuse, Social support, Impulsivity, Treatment responsivity, Sexual deviance, and Intimate relationship problems.
6 https://www.corrections-mall.net/bbs/board.php?bo_table=gallery

References

Andrews, D. A., & Bonta, J. (2010). Rehabilitating criminal justice policy and practice. *Psychology, Public Policy, and Law*, 16(1), 39–55. 10.1037/a0018362

Andrews, D. A., & Bonta, J. (2017). *The psychology of criminal conduct* (6th ed.). London and New York: Routledge.

de Mente B. L. (2012). *The Korean mind: Understanding contemporary Korean culture*. Vermont: Tuttle Publishing.

Hanson, R. K., & Thornton, D. (2000). Improving risk assessments for sex offenders: A comparison of three actuarial scales. *Law and Human Behavior*, 24(1), 119–136. 10.1023/A:1005482921333

Hare, R. D. (2003). *Manual for the psychopathy checklist-revised* (2nd ed.). Toronto, Ontario: Multi-Health Systems.

Hare, R. D. (2008). *Manual for the Psychopathy Checklist-Revised (2nd ed.): Korean Version.* (E. Joe, & S. J. Lee, Trans.). Hakjisa. (Original work published 2003)

Harris, A. J. R., Phenix, A., Hanson, R. K., & Thornton, D. (2003). *Static-99 coding rules: Revised 2003.* Department of the Solicitor General of Canada.

Helmus, L. M., Kelley, S. M., Frazier, A., Fernandez, Y. M., Lee, S. C., Rettenberger, M., & Boccaccini, M. T. (2022). Static-99R: Strengths, limitations, predictive accuracy meta-analysis, and legal admissibility review. *Psychology, Public Policy, and Law, 28*(3), 307–331. 10.1037/law0000351

Jo, E. (2010). *Development of Hallym Assessment Guide for Sex Offender Risk (HAGSOR).* Ministry of Justice.

Kim, J., Kim, Y., Choi, J., Seong, Y., & Go, G. (2021). *An evaluation research on the effectiveness of punitiveness (II): Electronic Monitoring System.* Korean Institute of Criminology.

Kim, J., Kim, Y., Oh, H., Lee, J., & Kang, J. (2020). *An evaluation research on the effectiveness of punitiveness (I): Sex offender registration and notification.* Korean Institute of Criminology.

Ko, R., Sohn, S., Han, S., & Lee, S. J., (2016). Study on recidivism prediction capability of Korean version of PCL-R. *Korean Criminology Review, 27*(2), 263–289.

Koo, K. C., Shim, G. S., Park, H. H., Rha, K. H., Choi, Y. D., Chung, B. H., Hong, S. J., & Lee, J. W. (2013). Treatment outcomes of chemical castration on Korean sex offenders. *Journal of Forensic and Legal Medicine, 20*(6), 563–566. 10.1016/j.jflm.2013.06.003

Korean Statistical Information Service (2021). Number of accomplices and weapon in a homicide offense. https://kosis.kr/statHtml/statHtml.do?orgId=132&tblId=DT_13204_3209

Kwon, S., & Shin, K. (2015). *A study on the mental health court and forensic psychiatric ward.* Korean Institute of Criminology.

Lee, S. J. (2011). *A study on Establishing scientific prisoner treatment system for reducing recidivism (II): A study on the development of Korean Offender Risk Assessment System.* Korean Institute of Criminology and Justice.

Lee, S. C., Hanson, R. K., & Yoon, J. S. (2023). Predictive validity of Static-99R among 8,207 men convicted of sexual crimes in South Korea: A prospective field study. *Sexual Abuse, 35*(6), 687–715. 10.1177/10790632221139173

Lee, S. J., Hwang, E. K., & Park, S. Y. (2010). *A study on establishing scientific prisoner treatment system for reducing recidivism (I): A study on the development of Korean offender risk assessment system.* Korean Institute of Criminology and Justice.

Lee, S. J., & Kim, M. (2010). Study on recidivism prediction capability of PCL-R for criminals in South Korea. *The Korean Journal of Forensic Psychology, 1*(1), 43–55.

Lee, S. J., & Ko, R. (2011). A study on the validity evidences of Korean Offender Risk Assessment System. *Korean Criminology, 5*(2), 221–258.

Lee, S. J., Ko, R., & Choi, H. (2010). A recidivism follow-up study based on the Korean Sex Offender Risk Assessment Scale (KSORAS). *Korean Journal of Psychology, 29*(4), 999–1016.

Lee, S. J., Ko, R., & Kim, J. K. (2009). The study of construct validity on the Psychopathy Checklist-Revised (PCL-R): Korean version. *Korean Journal of Social and Personality Psychology, 23*(3), 57–71.

Lee, S. J., Ko, R., & Park, H. (2008). Development of the Korean Sex Offender Risk Assessment Scale (KSORAS) and its validity evidences. *Korean Criminological Review, 19*(4), 309–345.

Ministry of Justice, Republic of Korea. (2022). *2022 annals of correctional statistics.* https://www.moj.go.kr/bbs/moj/160/562125/artclView.do

Ministry of the Interior and Safety. (2022). *The number of foreign residents residing in Korea decreased by 2.13 million.* https://www.mois.go.kr/synap/skin/doc.html?fn=BBS_2022102902515673311&rs=/synapFile/202212/&synapUrl=%2Fsynap%2Fskin%2Fdoc.html%3Ffn%3DBBS_2022102902515673311%26rs%3D%2FsynapFile%2F202212%2F&synapMessage=%EC%A0%95%EC%83%81

Niaz, U., & Hassan, S. (2006). Culture and mental health of women in South-East Asia. *World Psychiatry: Official Journal of the World Psychiatric Association, 5*(2), 118–120.

Park, C. (2013). Implementation of medication for treatment of sexual impulse. *Korean Criminological Review, 24*(1), 265–297.

Statistics Canada. (2022). *Incident-based crime statistics.* https://www150.statcan.gc.ca/t1/tbl1/en/tv.action?pid=3510017701

Statistics Korea. (2022). *2021 population and housing census.* http://kostat.go.kr/portal/eng/pressReleases/8/7/index.board?bmode=read&bSeq=&aSeq=419981&pageNo=1&rowNum=10&navCount=10&currPg=&searchInfo=&sTarget=title&sTxt=

Supreme Prosecutor's Office. (2022). *Analytics on statistics of crime in Korea.* https://www.spo.go.kr/site/spo/crimeAnalysis.do

United Nations Office on Drug and Crime. (1955/2015). The United Nations standard minimum rules for the treatment of prisoners (the Nelson Mandela Rules). https://www.unodc.org/documents/justice-and-prison-reform/Nelson_Mandela_Rules-E-ebook.pdf

Yeh, C. J., & Huang, K. (1996). The collectivistic nature of ethnic identity development among Asian-American college students. *Adolescence, 31*(123), 645–661.

Yoon, J. (2022). Recidivism prediction of sex offender risk assessment tools: Static-99 and HAGSOR-Dynamic. *The Korean Journal of Forensic Psychology, 13*(2), 99–119.

Yoon, J., Kim, M., & Lee, T. (2020). *The effectiveness of prison-based sex offender treatment program in Korea (20-AB-02).* Korean Institute of Criminology.

Yoon, J., & Knight R. A. (2013). *Treating sexual offenders (II): Evaluation of the effectiveness of prison-based psychological treatment programs for sex offenders.* Korean Institute of Criminology.

Yoon, J., Seong, Y., & Lee, T. (2021). *Improving security treatment level classification index and correctional recidivism prediction index.* Korean Institute of Criminology.

Zgoba, K. M., & Mitchell, M. M. (2023). The effectiveness of sex offender registration and notification: A meta-analysis of 25 years of findings. *Journal of Experimental Criminology, 19*(1), 71–96.

8

OFFENDER REHABILITATION IN TAIWAN

Victor Tien-Cheng Cheng

Crime in Taiwan

In Taiwan, the Ministry of Justice (MOJ) oversees the rehabilitation of people who have offended, and there are two systems based on different processing environments, the Correctional system (correctional institutions) and the Judicial Protection system (community). The Correctional system is supervised by MOJ's Agency of Correction, which is responsible for the operations of 51 correctional facilities. These are categorised into different types based on custodial characteristics and include Prison Detention Centres, Drug Abuser Treatment Centres, Skill Training Institutes, Juvenile Correctional Schools, and Juvenile Detention Houses. The Judicial Protection system is supervised by MOJ's Department of Prevention, Rehabilitation and Protection, which is responsible for matters relating to probation, parole, deferred prosecution, and conditional suspension of prosecution, community service for offenders, as well as rehabilitation and reintegration services provided by the Taiwan Aftercare Association. There are 22 probation offices nationwide under the authority of the district prosecutor.

From the perspective of criminal policy, the Correctional system and the Judicial Protection system in Taiwan promote the rehabilitation of offenders, providing various resources and treatment measures to assist individuals reform and reintegrate. The goal is not only to help offenders adapt to social life and develop a law-abiding concept, but also to assess the needs of individuals during their sentence through risk assessment and case management, via a formulation of appropriate rehabilitation plans.

DOI: 10.4324/9781003360919-10

This aims to improve the specialised assessment and treatment for different types of offenders and special clients, provide individualised and appropriate medical treatment, as well as provide restorative justice, so as to reduce the risk of reoffending and establish a comprehensive social security net. These measures are consistent with relevant international norms including the International Covenant on Civil and Political Rights, the International Covenant on Economic, Social and Cultural Rights, and the Convention on the Rights of Children.

Taiwan's crime rate has decreased year by year in the past decade, from 1,308.77 crimes per 100,000 people in 2014 to 1,035.79 per 100,000 people in 2021. The total number of people in custody and the imprisonment rate have also decreased, from 283 per 100,000 people in 2012 to 248 per 100,000 people in 2020 (Academy for the Judiciary, 2022). According to the MOJ (Statistics of Justice, 2023), at the end of 2022, the total number of people in Taiwan's correctional facilities was 55,118, of which 49,720 were in prisons, accounting for 90.2% of all inmates.

The top four crime types among people in correctional facilities were: (1) violation of the Narcotics Hazard Prevention Act, 20,647 cases (41.5% of all prison inmates); (2) violent crimes (including homicide, serious injury, rape, robbery and piracy, theft, extortion, kidnapping for ransom, and the violation of the Anti-Robbery and Counterfeit Currency Act), 7,094 cases; (3) fraud, 5,177 cases; and (4) public endangerment crimes (including reckless driving), 5,123 cases. The Judicial Protection system that assists offender's reintegration had a yearly total of 59,125 probation and parole cases in 2022. Among ongoing cases, the largest proportion was for violation of the Narcotics Hazard Prevention Act, accounting for 8,925 (33.4%) cases, followed by fraud and sexual offences. As can be seen from these figures, the most common offence types in both custody and the community relate to drug violations. According to the Narcotics Hazard Prevention Act, relevant offenders can receive addiction treatment to help them avoid the deterioration of their condition or improve their capacity to prevent relapse.

Additionally, recent developments in legal responses to violence towards women and associated rehabilitation activities are noteworthy. A landmark criminal case in Taiwan in 1996 led to the drafting of laws concerning women's safety, receiving widespread attention from multiple sectors. With the active promotion of the Legislative Yuan and related civil society groups, the Sexual Assault Crime Prevention Act and the Domestic Violence Prevention Act were promulgated and implemented in 1997 and 1998, respectively, opening a new chapter for Taiwan in protecting the safety of women and children. In cases of sexual assault and domestic violence, offenders must receive treatment.

Furthermore, in recent years, Taiwan has seen a series of cases in which drunk driving has caused fatalities or serious injuries. The Road Traffic Management and Penalty Act also requires that relevant convicted individuals complete drunk driving prevention education or addiction treatment before applying for a driver's licence. At the same time, MOJ has promoted a judicial and medical cooperation treatment model to address the problem of drunk driving, allowing defendants who receive deferred prosecution to receive addiction treatment. Therefore, in Taiwan, the types of crimes that combine rehabilitation with treatment predominantly relate to the following types of criminal behaviours: drug abuse, sexual assault, domestic violence, and public danger (unsafe driving under influence). This chapter will focus on the implementation model of the current rehabilitation of inmates in the Taiwan correctional system. For an expanded discussion of forensic mental health legislation in Taiwan, see Kuo (1983) and Lin et al. (2022); rehabilitation of offenders with mental health problems is found in the section on Protective Rehabilitation.

Rehabilitation in Taiwan

History

Historically, Taiwanese society expected correctional institutions to achieve justice by restricting the freedom of criminals and punishing them. However, over time and with an expanded focus on human rights, the focus of prisons has shifted from retribution and punishment to education and rehabilitation. Initially, rehabilitation relied on individuals with knowledge and prestige entering prisons to provide educational services. For example, in the early 1980s, the MOJ included Religious Education and Edification for correctional education activities and allowed civilian groups to enter prisons to provide educational services for inmates. Christian, Buddhist, Catholic, and other religious groups entered various correctional institutions to carry out educational work, hoping to inspire the conscience and purify minds (mainly drug offenders at that time) through various religious activities and ceremonies such as teaching, counselling, prayer, Bible study, spiritual practice, witness, chanting, etc., to encourage abstinence from drugs and reform. To this day, Religious Education and Edification is ongoing in various correctional institutions.

Although Taiwan has implemented Religious Education and Edification for several decades, there is limited empirical research on the effectiveness of this intervention. Chang (2002) surveyed 208 prison managers, inmates, and members of the Buddha's religious group offered by the Fo Guang Shan Monastery at the Mingde Correctional Institution in

Tainan. Results showed overall satisfaction with the religious education activities and in terms of effectiveness, prison managers, religious group members, and inmates all gave high praise. However, this research was limited to a single prison, and the perceived positive effect of religious education on inmates' drug rehabilitation was subjective.

Lin and Yang (2008) report results from two questionnaires administered by MOJ to inmates in 1986 and 1989. Data from 1986 showed that 64.82% of prisoners believed that religious education was necessary and helpful to them; the 1989 survey results indicated that as many as 87.9% of prisoners believed that religious education was beneficial to their enlightenment and emotional stability. Wen and Wang (2013) also conducted an evaluation of the effectiveness of religious education in the Taipei Detention Center. They randomly selected 60 participants who received Buddhist religious education and administered a survey using an experimental method. When compared to a control group, those who received religious education showed significantly more positive attitudes towards religion, positive feelings, and willingness to share their experiences of enlightenment, improved physical health, positive self-concept, and calmness and emotional stability. Additionally, religious education helped rebuild social connections, including increasing attachment to volunteer teachers, enhancing interpersonal trust towards the prison managers, and a reduction in physical and mental stress associated with imprisonment.

Current Rehabilitation Activities and Approach

Taiwan implemented a revised Prison Act on July 15, 2020. Article 11 of the Act stipulates that prisons should develop individual treatment plans for inmates, based on investigative data, within three months of the person entering the correctional institution. Concurrently, prisons must follow the Inmate Information Investigation Regulations and provide personalised treatment based on the individual circumstances of each inmate. In 2021, to enhance the effectiveness of treatment and rehabilitation, the Agency of Corrections (2022) selected demonstration institutions to pilot the Using Professional Counselors in Individual Rehabilitation Work Program. This programme incorporates psychological and social work expertise in the planning and creation of a Risk-Needs-Responsivity (RNR) assessment model and differentiates rehabilitation programmes based on their therapeutic effect, protective effect and overall applicability; these are referred to as (1) Therapeutic Rehabilitation; (2) Protective Rehabilitation; and (3) General Rehabilitation.

Therapeutic Rehabilitation

Therapeutic Rehabilitation is designed for people convicted of sexual and domestic violence offences and crimes related to drug and alcohol use. These crimes are currently subject to legal regulations requiring corrective treatment.

Drug Offenders

Taiwan's drug policy has a long history and cultural context. Based on changing attitudes towards drugs from different time periods and ruling governments, Taiwan's approach to drug issues has differed over the years. The first recorded instance of opium use dates back to the Qing Dynasty in 1620. In 1729, the Qing Dynasty declared that opium smoking was harmful and issued a ban on its sale and use. At that time, Taiwan was under the rule of the Qing government. During the Japanese occupation period from 1895 to 1945, the government's regulations allowed the use of opium and the monopoly of opium sales. After the Kuomingtang (KMT) government moved to Taiwan in 1949, Taiwan's drug control policies were based on the laws and regulations established during the KMT government's rule on mainland China. The Act of Suppression of Smoking and Drug Abuse during the Period of Suppression of Communist Rebellion was enacted and became the legal basis for Taiwan's drug control policies. During this period, Taiwan's anti-drug policies were characterised by severe punishment for drug offenders and drug abusers, as Taiwan was in the midst of the anti-Communist fervour following the retreat of the KMT government to Taiwan after losing the Chinese Civil War. This was essentially a high-pressure drug control policy phase characterised by severe punishment (徐吉志，2022).

As Taiwan entered its democratisation phase various legal systems moved away from authoritarianism and as Taiwan's economic and cultural evolution accelerated, attitudes towards drugs also shifted. Currently, Taiwan's drug addiction treatment is mainly based on the Narcotics Hazard Prevention Act which classifies people who are addicted to drugs as "criminal patients" and "victims". Aside from those who are involved in drug trafficking, people who are dependent are considered criminals with a disease characteristic (i.e., a patient as well as a criminal identity) and must be offered treatment to assist their rehabilitation and reintegration. Taiwan has recently emphasised the development of diverse treatment and assistance programmes for relevant offenders to improve the effectiveness of drug addiction treatment through multiple approaches.

To further improve drug prevention and control efforts, the Executive Yuan launched the second phase of the New Generation Anti-Drug Strategy (2021–2024). In terms of rehabilitation of offenders charged with drug offences, efforts are made to enhance individualised treatment in correctional facilities with the goal of achieving a professional-to-inmate ratio of 1:300 for psychology, social work, and case management personnel. This is aimed at addressing the psychological and social needs of newly admitted users, providing counselling during incarceration, pre-release counselling, and follow-up after release to assist people with overcoming addiction and successfully reintegrating. Additionally, the Recidivism Prevention Program was established to intervene and provide comprehensive support and protection from the investigation stage onward, effectively reducing the high rate of recidivism for people convicted of relevant drug offences (Executive Yuan, 2020).

In order to implement the New Generation Anti-Drug Strategy and conduct evidence-based treatment, the Agency of Corrections issued the Scientific Evidence-based Drug Offender Treatment Model (SEDOM) project in December 2017. The treatment content of the SEDOM project is based on the 13 addiction treatment principles proposed by the National Institute on Drug Abuse (2006) for developing a comprehensive treatment programme. For the SEDOM project, (Huang et al., 2021), an initial assessment occurs within two months of admission into the correctional institution, and this includes individualised treatment (counselling strategies and suggestions) and information dissemination through verbal communication, mail, and poster campaigns to increase motivation for treatment. Additionally, in-prison counselling, which is aimed at increasing motivation and includes lectures, group therapy, and individual therapy, covers various dimensions affected by drug abuse, including: (1) addiction and quitting strategies, (2) family and interpersonal relationships, (3) career development and financial management, (4) drug hazards and legal responsibilities, (5) health education and AIDS prevention, (6) medication and medical detoxification consultations, and (7) education for successful drug rehabilitation.

Case management and family health education and counselling services, family relationship repair groups, family visits, family days, and other family counselling activities are also offered to the offender. During the pre-release phase, case management and counselling focuses on employment, health, and social welfare authorities to strengthen community support services and post-release community counselling. Collaborations with the Taiwan Aftercare Association, Drug Abuse Prevention Center, the Social Affairs Bureau, Employment Service Station, and with the correctional institution, create a four-way link to assist reintegration.

Yang and Tai (2022) were commissioned by the Agency of Corrections to conduct a three-year effectiveness evaluation study on the SEDOM project. Further to qualitative interviews and quantitative statistical analysis, they also conducted a programme review using RE-AIM-based 360-degree feedback analysis. Data from 844 individuals who participated in the SEDOM project were collected from 32 correctional institutions. Results showed that SEDOM had tangible benefits for correctional institutions and frontline workers and a positive impact on the lives of participants.

Further, the Crime Research Center at National Chung Cheng University (2023) published a summary evaluation of the SEDOM project. This evaluation found that the percentage of SEDOM completers increased annually from 3.7% in 2018 to 37.4% in 2021. This study compared outcomes for released drug offenders from 2018 to 2021, a total of 43,577 individuals, until the end of March 2022. Results showed that of the 6,577 people who received the treatment, 685 reoffended, with a reoffending rate of 10.4%, compared to 37,000 people who only "received lectures", with 9,121 reoffenders and a reoffending rate of 24.7%.

Driving under the Influence (DUI) Offenders

In Taiwan, accidents caused when driving under the influence of drugs and other substances are considered a form of offenses against Public Safety and fall under the category of Unsafe Driving Offenses. Those convicted of a custodial sentence must undergo treatment. In recent years, the number of people convicted of Unsafe Driving Offenses has increased due to the stricter punishment and enforcement regulations in the Criminal Code. According to the MOJ (Statistics of Justice, 2023), at the end of 2022, there were 4,495 inmates serving sentences for Unsafe Driving Offenses in prisons nationwide, accounting for approximately 9% of the total inmate population. Additionally, out of the total of 30,196 newly imprisoned inmates, 8,833 were convicted of Unsafe Driving Offenses accounting for approximately 29% of all new inmates.

To promote professional treatment for inmates with alcohol (or substance) addiction in correctional facilities, the Taiwan Agency of Corrections has been implementing the Treatment Implementation Plan for Inmates with drunk driving since 2018, based on the recommendations of the World Health Organization (WHO) European Region on alcohol-related issues in correctional facilities. The Plan is designed with a three-tiered prevention treatment framework, and utilises internationally recognised screening tools to assess inmates and arrange appropriate treatment.

For those with alcohol addiction, the rehabilitation implementation methods include: Primary (Developmental Prevention), Secondary (High-Risk Prevention), and Tertiary Prevention (Intervention Prevention) phases.

The Primary Prevention phase targets all newly admitted inmates through a drunk driving prevention course, with a main goal of strengthening the adaptive ability and self-health management skills of inmates through a comprehensive educational mechanism. In the Secondary Prevention phase people convicted of Unsafe Driving and high-risk groups with alcohol addiction are screened and counselling is provided. Counselling focuses on the participant's health, career and financial management plans, medical health education, life education, legal education, gender equality and violence prevention, family support to strengthen participants' health management, employment and financial planning, and disease awareness, to encourage and reinforce addiction cessation motivation. In the Tertiary Prevention phase, treatment focuses on inmates who have completed the secondary prevention course but who remain at risk of relapse; group therapy or individual treatment courses are also facilitated. Treatment focuses on disease awareness, motivation enhancement, and self-efficacy improvement, providing professional corrective counselling as well as physical and mental rehabilitation. Community resources are also provided before the person is released from prison. Moreover, the treatment process will involve coordinating employment and career development courses, arranging referrals to community medical resources, as well as connecting participants with the Aftercare Association to assist in follow-up and care services designed to ensure a smooth reintegration.

Recently, in order to avoid overcrowding in prisons and to address the goals of addiction treatment and recidivism prevention, the MOJ has promoted the expanded use of deferred prosecution with conditions or probation with conditions to provide community-based addiction treatment and rehabilitation for people who have committed less serious offenses related to drunk driving. An example is the use of the Brief Intervention model developed by the WHO at the Taipei City Hospital Songde Branch. This hospital provides clinical interventions for high-risk drinking cases and implements a range of addiction treatments for judicially referred offenders.

Liu and colleagues (2011) evaluated whether Brief Intervention could reduce unhealthy drinking behaviour in male hospitalised patients in Taiwan, using a randomised controlled trial. Of the 3,669 adult male hospitalised patients, 616 were identified as unhealthy alcohol users (>14 drinks/week) and were randomly assigned to either usual care ($N = 308$) or BI ($N = 308$). Results showed that brief in-hospital intervention can result in a reduction in alcohol intake by men who drink heavily or are diagnosed with an alcohol use disorder.

People Convicted of Sexual Offences

In Taiwan, treatment and rehabilitation for people convicted of sexual offences began with the amendment of the Criminal Code of the Republic of China in 1994 and has undergone several revisions, providing a legal basis for mandatory treatment. Subsequently, the Ministry of Health and Welfare successively promulgated the Sexual Assault Crime Prevention Act and The Regulation on Physical and Psychological Treatment, and Counselling Education for Sex Offenders. There are several models of treatment, including Pre-trial assessment, In-prison treatment, Community-based treatment, and Post-release treatment. This section focuses on treatment in correctional institutions.

The Taiwan Agency of Corrections has designated 10 institutions to specialise in the treatment of sex offenders. The designated institutions allocate funds, provide professional human resources, and can also hire external experts to supplement the treatment team. Currently, Taiwan's treatment adopts a cognitive-behavioural therapy framework focused on recidivism prevention. This approach helps offenders understand their criminal history, learn to identify and respond to high-risk situations, and use internal and external controls to reduce the likelihood of reoffending. After being referred to a designated correctional facility for assessment, sexual offenders treatment plans are determined through a Screening and Evaluation Meeting process. The main components of the treatment program include individualised assessment, which considers the offending, prison situation, family background, interpersonal relationships, educational history, physiological and psychological condition, treatment, and other related information for evaluation. The assessment report is then submitted to the Screening and Evaluation Meeting to make a decision on whether the person requires physical and psychological treatment or counselling education.

Treatment is either Basic or Advanced. The basic treatment courses are conducted in a group setting for a period of four months with two classes per month, a total of eight sessions. The content includes an introduction to the courses, legal education, life education, gender equality education, recidivism prevention, career planning, and other related courses. After completing the courses and based on the persons offence severity, and degree of risk, a decision will be made on whether advanced treatment courses are necessary. The Advanced treatment programme primarily focuses on group therapy. Inmates are assigned to different Advanced groups based on the length of their sentence, type of offense, cognitive function, and other individual differences. The groups are homogenous and can be categorised as: short-term, general, paedophilia, incest, homosexual, and special groups. The therapeutic groups mainly aim to prevent recidivism. The groups run once a week for three hours and are led by one therapist who is responsible for up to eight members. After one year of treatment, the therapist reports on the progress of all group members in the treatment assessment meeting. If approved by the committee, members can leave the group. If not approved, they will continue treatment.

In addition to group therapy, individual therapy is also provided for people who have difficulty adapting to group therapy or for those who have issues that are difficult to discuss in a group. Individual therapy sessions are held once every week to two weeks for 1.5 hours. After six months of individual therapy, the therapist can request a treatment assessment meeting, and if approved, the treatment will end. If not approved, the person will continue individual therapy or be assigned to a suitable group. At least one treatment assessment meeting must be held each year.

An alternative intervention is "Counselling education", a six-month group therapy programme led by a therapist with 12 to 15 participants in each group. The programme consists of 12 sessions, held twice a month. The content is expanded from the basic treatment programme and includes course introductions, legal education, life education, gender equality education, recidivism prevention, and career planning.

The Follow-up Treatment programme is designed for people who have passed the treatment evaluation meeting or counselling evaluation meeting but have not yet been released from prison. It involves a lecture course held once every three months, focusing on topics such as gender and marriage, parenting, legal knowledge, self-worth, career planning, interpersonal relationships and communication, emotional management and stress adaptation, life education, addiction to drugs and alcohol, and other related knowledge and skills. The goal of the programme is to enhance the capability to prevent re-offending, extend the effects of treatment or counselling, and connect people to community treatment.

Yeh (2018) examined 21 empirical studies evaluating sexual offender treatment in Taiwan, from 2002 to 2017, including 13 studies examining prison treatment and eight studies discussing the effectiveness of community treatment. Overall, whether treatment was provided in prison or in the community, there was evidence that some of the programmes are effective. Research on the effectiveness of sexual offending treatment in Taiwan is mainly focused on group therapy, there is scant evaluation of individual treatment.

Domestic Violence Offenders

Taiwan primarily relies on the Domestic Violence Prevention Act as the legal basis for the treatment and management of perpetrators of domestic violence. The Act allows the court to order the perpetrator to complete a treatment plan, while the MOJ is responsible for developing and implementing treatment plans for individuals convicted of domestic violence or violating protective orders. According to the Act, the treatment plan includes cognitive and parenting education, psychological counselling, mental health therapy, addiction treatment, or other counselling and therapy for perpetrators.

The Taiwan Agency of Corrections has selected ten correctional facilities to provide treatment for domestic violence offenders and has issued the Treatment Plan for Individuals Convicted of Domestic Violence or Violating Protective Orders as the basis for handling such cases. Currently, Taiwan's treatment model for domestic violence offenders is similar to that of some other countries, mainly using cognitive-behavioural therapy to change the offender's cognitive patterns and eliminate violent behaviour. In planning the treatment programme for domestic violence offenders, the Ministry of Health and Welfare's Regulations for the Treatment Plan for Domestic Violence Offenders is used as a reference, including addiction treatment, mental health therapy, cognitive counselling, and parenting education courses where necessary; the treatment programme is tailored based on whether the offender was convicted of domestic violence or violating protective orders. After completing the treatment and counselling programme, the therapist will complete a case closure report and conduct a risk assessment. Regarding the programme subjects, all inmates who have committed domestic violence or violated protection orders are considered for treatment participation. Treatment options focus on education, group or individual treatment and pre-release coordination. For those people who have completed their sentence for domestic violence offences and those who are released on parole, the county/city government social affairs bureau and the police station in the jurisdiction of the registered residence of the inmate and victim are notified in accordance with the law. The victim is also informed, and relevant treatment information is provided to the domestic violence prevention centre to facilitate follow-up counselling.

Protective Rehabilitation

Protective Rehabilitation includes specific treatments for four types of offenders: the Elderly, the Physically and Mentally Disabled, those with Serious crimes or a sentence of more than 10 years and not eligible for parole, as well as those at risk of suicide. In recent years, Taiwan's correctional facilities have experienced an increase in long-term detainees due to changes in criminal policies, resulting in an aging population in correctional institutions. Many elderly offenders have physical deterioration, are prone to chronic illnesses, are more likely to experience loneliness, depression, and despair in custody. Long-term detainees or those who are ineligible for parole may become institutionalised, leading to a lack of hope for the future. As their time in custody increases, they may also experience health problems. These people are vulnerable to bullying and mistreatment within correctional institutions. Therefore, appropriate planning is needed in terms of custody management, physical and mental health care, daily care, education, as well as work activities.

According to the MOJ (Statistics of Justice, 2023), the number of prisoners over 60 in 2022 was 4,696; representing 9.4% of all prisoners. To ensure elderly offenders can serve their sentences with peace of mind and stability, the Agency of Corrections collaborates with the Ministry of Health and Welfare and the National Health Insurance Administration to provide health insurance medical services, improving the quality of medical care for detainees, and enhancing accessibility of medical care. The measures taken for elderly prisoners (Agency of Corrections, 2018) include medical care (through outpatient visits coordinated with contracted hospitals under the National Health Insurance program); training courses for caregivers to assist elderly inmates in meeting their care needs; participation in work assignments (if appropriate); strengthened protection for elderly inmates to prevent bullying; enhanced hardware to create a safe confinement environment; activities and courses with entertainment and health functions to relieve the pressure of confinement and enhance interpersonal interactions; individual and group counselling, emotional support, and religious counselling according to individual religious beliefs and spiritual comfort need; and rehabilitation and resettlement counselling and referral services. For those with care and medical needs after release, referrals and placement are made by linking with social welfare agencies, aftercare association, private charitable organisations, and medical institutions.

For prisoners with a sentence of more than ten years, the Brief Symptom Rating Scale is used for assessment, with at least one screening assessment completed every six months. Based on the results of these assessments, emotional support, counselling, or medical referral services are provided. Health education is provided to improve the psychological health of prisoners and enhance their adaptability to long-term imprisonment. For other people convicted of serious crimes who are ineligible for parole, as well as for individuals with physical and mental disabilities in custody, each correctional institution is responsible for developing and constructing their own assessment and intervention approach based on the respective characteristics of the environment and its offenders.

In terms of the rehabilitation of prisoners at risk of suicide, correctional institutions implement assessment and intervention for people at risk of suicide in accordance with a common suicide prevention plan. The service targets include people who have attempted suicide or self-harm and those at risk of same (those who score 10 or above on the Brief Symptom Rating Scale or have a score of 1 or above on suicidal ideation, and score 15 or above on the Patient Health Questionnaire after rescreening). After observation by the prison education and counselling group, prisoners with self-harm or suicide risk are assessed for their mental status, personality traits, emotional symptoms, and life stress. Those who have self-harm or suicide risk are referred to the relevant professionals for suicide prevention and treatment.

General Rehabilitation

General Rehabilitation applies to all types of offenders in correctional facilities, and includes provision of psychological treatment, guidance and life counselling, work and skill training, education and reintegration into society, family support plans, as well as knowledge and competency courses. In practice, it is usually initiated at the inmate's request, or following referral by correctional staff to psychologists or social workers in the prison for psychological counselling. The correctional education and counselling manager will first seek to understand the person's situation before making a referral. If the person has special needs, s/he will be referred to the relevant departments or external resources. Assistance is also provided to stabilise the emotions of the individual and to adapt to life in prison.

In terms of General Rehabilitation programmes, correctional facilities have flexibility and autonomy in designing service plans and projects because there are no specific legal mandates or targets for treatment. Plans are aimed at understanding the individual or social resource needs of inmates or their families, linking them to relevant resources to provide family support services, or improving the social adaptability of individuals. Before the person is released from custody, a psychologist or social worker can provide a referral or notification to relevant social resources, such as job service stations (providing skills training or job matching), Aftercare Association (providing placement after release, travel expenses, assistance with medical treatment, or entrepreneurship loans), vulnerable families (reporting for care) or rehabilitation-related private sectors.

The General Rehabilitation courses provide individualised and appropriate treatment and resources to assist inmates with reintegrating.

Forensic Mental Health and Youth Justice Services

The criminal law in Taiwan adopts a dual-track system of "Punishment" and "Rehabilitative Disposition." The "Rehabilitative Disposition" includes preventive measures taken against the "future danger" of the person for the purposes of education and treatment, and are a supplementary system to punishment. These measures are set out in the Criminal Code and include Reformatory Education (§86), Custodial Protection (§87), Compulsory Cure (§88, §89), Compulsory Labor (§90), Compulsory Treatment (§91-1), Protective Measure (§92, §93), and Deportation (§95), each with its own purpose.

In the rehabilitation of offenders with mental illness, the person may be committed to a suitable custodial facility in the interests of public safety (Criminal Code §87). The custodial protection period is no more than five years, and the prosecutor may apply to the court for permission to extend. According to Article 46 of the Rehabilitative Disposition Execution Act, the prosecutor shall specify one or more of the following methods according to the situation of the person under custodial protection: (1) Order them to accept treatment in a judicial psychiatric hospital, hospital, or other psychiatric medical institution; (2) Order them to accept psychiatric care or rehabilitation in psychiatric rehabilitation institution or psychiatric care institution; (3) Order them to accept care or guidance in physically/mentally disabled welfare institution or another appropriate place; (4) Have them be cared by their statutory agents or most close relatives; (5) Accepting special outpatient treatment; and (6) Other appropriate treatment measures.

Pertaining to the rehabilitation of juvenile offenders (under the Juvenile Justice Act), for those juveniles who have committed a crime and those who are at risk of committing offenses, the court may order them to be placed in a reformatory education institution for reformation education (up to three years; Criminal Code §86). Reformatory education refers to all "educational measures" with the purpose and effect of correcting the harmful habits of juvenile inmates and persons subject to reformatory education through school education and encouraging them to reform and adjust themselves to their social lives. Currently, there are four "Juvenile Reformatory Schools" in Taiwan, with a total of 738 students at the end of 2022. The courses and curriculum materials of reformatory education are formulated by the MOJ together with the Ministry of Education and the Ministry of the Interior. Cross-agency resources and public-private cooperation are synergised to assist juvenile offenders/delinquents to reintegrate into society.

Experimental Practices

In addition to the aforementioned treatment measures, various experimental treatment programmes have been introduced in Taiwan's prisons over the years. These programmes include Introspection Therapy (Vipassana Meditation), Mindfulness-Based Practices (Mindfulness-Based Stress Reduction), Art therapy, Horticultural therapy, or Pet therapy (Prison Dog programme). Some of these experimental treatment programmes are brief and time-limited while others are ongoing courses lasting for several years. However, evaluations of the effectiveness of these experimental treatment programmes mostly rely on post-feedback analysis from the programme users in the prisons where the programs were implemented. There is still a lack of large-scale or systematic empirical research to determine whether these experimental treatment programmes have therapeutic effects or applicability for other offenders in Taiwan.

Taking Introspection/Naikan Therapy as an example, Taiwan introduced this therapy from Japan in 1987 and conducted trials in some correctional facilities prior to implementing it in all correctional institutions in 1990. Introspection/Naikan Therapy has been widely used to address psychological distress, alcohol and drug abuse, and stress relief, and its effectiveness has been recognised. Although Introspection therapy was applied to various offenders, its effectiveness was neither evaluated nor well-documented. Furthermore, the lack of systematic theory and methodology and the absence of professional guidance for inmates resulted in the therapy being limited to mere sitting meditation, with little substance to its introspective essence. Consequently, it began to be offered infrequently until 2003, when the MOJ re-introduced Introspection Therapy. Instead of the Japanese-style Introspection Therapy, a 10-Day Vipassana Therapy (meditation-sitting training method developed by the renowned Indian master Goenka) was introduced.

The Vipassana Therapy was trialled in several correctional institutions including the Yilan Prison and Taichung Women's Prison. It was run from 4 a.m. to 9 p.m., and the environment was kept dimly lit with only cushions, leg wraps, towels, and chair backs provided. Participation in Vipassana Therapy was voluntary and the willingness of participants to join was low. Additionally, the implementation of insight therapy requires participants to sit for long periods to train their minds, but coordination was difficult due to the correctional institution's scheduling for participants' daily lives. The choice of meditation location also created additional operational challenges (e.g., being alone, quiet, and in a well-ventilated space). Notably, this created a perception that it was unfair treatment for other inmates who did not receive this therapy, and most correctional institutions were overcrowded; there was no extra space available for the programme. Lastly, some human rights groups criticised the practice of long meditation as a form of punishment and called for its abolition. All of these factors made it difficult to widely implement the 10-Day Vipassana Therapy in other correctional institutions, and the programme was therefore discontinued (Chiu, 2007).

In addition, Chu (2019) pointed out that the use of positive psychology and related concepts (e.g., mindfulness, yoga) in substance abuse treatment is still in its infancy, most evaluations have been conducted in Western countries and empirical studies in Asian countries are uncommon. Chu et al. (2022) adopted a quasi-experimental intervention design to evaluate the effectiveness of implementing a positive psychology treatment programme for female inmates (i.e., 61 participants with 60 matched controls). The study that those women in the positive psychology programme group showed greater post-intervention scores in the dimensions of mindfulness and programme engagement when compared with the comparison group. Furthermore, the perceived stress levels of the experimental group were significantly lower than the control group. Although there was no significant difference between post-intervention and follow-up scores in the dimensions of optimism, depression, gratitude and well-being, the experimental group's scores were more positive than the control group.

Supporting System

The rehabilitation of offenders requires appropriate and individualised professional treatment for each case to be embedded in a well-designed and supportive system. Currently, Taiwan is strengthening the connection between correctional facilities and community-based correction by establishing an Individualized Transition and Referral Platform. Moreover, instead of the traditional Aftercare services, the Throughcare Judicial Protection approach provides for community resources not only after release from custody, but also early on during the period of incarceration or even during the investigation and prosecution stages, to provide resources that meet individual needs at different criminal justice stages. In addition, the treatment professionals are regarded as the most valuable assets in the rehabilitation plan, and are the key factors in the success of the programme. In recent years, Taiwan has been increasing the number of psychologists and social workers in its correctional and probation systems, and expanding the outsourcing subsidy programme to subsidise high-quality private organisations to invest in offender treatment and rehabilitation to increase the capacity of services. Through public-private sector collaboration and citizen participation, Taiwan aims to assist people successfully return to society and desist from crime, maintain social stability, and ensure Taiwan is one of the safest countries in the world.

References

Academy for the Judiciary. (2022). *2021 crime situations and analyses – crime trend reports. 27–38.* Academy for the Judiciary Press. https://www.cprc.moj.gov.tw/1563/1590/1592/37425/post

Agency of Corrections. (2018). *Correction white paper.* Agency of Corrections Press. https://www.mjac.moj.gov.tw/4786/4905/4907/92698/post

Agency of Corrections. (2022). *2021 annual report.* Agency of Corrections Press. https://www.mjac.moj.gov.tw/4786/4905/797768/1257601/post

Chang, J. L. (2002). Religious organizations and prison admonition: An evidential analysis of Fo Guang Shan's activity in Ming-Deh prison. *Pu Men Buddhist Studies Journal, 12,* Taiwan Kaohsiung: Fo Guang Shan Foundation for Buddhist Culture & Education. https://buddhism.lib.ntu.edu.tw/FULLTEXT/JR-MAG/mag202771.pdf

Chiu, M. W. (2007). The application of Vipassana meditation in correctional facilities for drug offenders rehabilitation. *Police Science Quarterly, 37*(4), 157–172.

Chu, D. C. (2019). The application of positive psychology to substance abuse treatment. *Journal of Criminal Policy and Crime Prevention Research, 20,* 24–33.

Chu, D. C., Chen, S. Y., Hsieh, P. Y., Chen, S. Y. & Zheng, Y. R. (2022). An evaluation of a positive intervention for female inmates. *Journal of Corrections, 11*(2), 31–64. https://www.mjac.moj.gov.tw/4786/4905/4909/1181588/post

Crime Research Center at National Chung Cheng University. (March 25, 2023). *Study: Evidence-based drug offender rehabilitation has a recidivism rate of 10.4%.* News section. https://deptcrc.ccu.edu.tw/index.php?option=module&lang=cht&task=pageinfo&id=776&index=8

Executive Yuan (2020). *New generation anti-drug strategy 2.0.* https://english.ey.gov.tw/News3/9E5540D592A5FECD/6d06eb32-bec0-4858-8ba4-eb5b0ae859a3

Huang, C. T., Chung, C. H. & Peng, W. N. (2021). Retrospect and prospect of institutional addiction treatment. *Journal of Corrections, 10*(1), 97–124. https://reurl.cc/MRXy2k

Kuo, S. H. (1983). Forensic psychiatry in Taiwan. *International Journal of Law and Psychiatry, 6,* 457–472.

Lin, C. H., Hsieh, W. C., Liu, H. W. & Chan, C. H. (2022). Psychiatric evaluations in offenders with mental illness: A case series. *Taiwan Journal of Psychiatry, 36,* 39–43

Lin, M. R. & Yang, S. L. (2008). *Prison studies – Principles and practices of crime correction and rehabilitation*. Wunan Publishers.

Liu, S. I., Wu, S. I., Chen, S. C., Huang, H. C. & Sun, F. J. (2011). Randomized controlled trial of a brief intervention for unhealthy alcohol use in hospitalized Taiwanese men. *Addiction*, *106*(5), 928–940.

National Institute on Drug Abuse. (2006). *Principles of drug abuse treatment for criminal justice populations: A research-based guide.* NIH Publication. https://nida.nih.gov/sites/default/files/txcriminaljustice_0.pdf

Statistics of Justice. (2023). *Monthly report on legal statistics.* (December, 2022). https://www.rjsd.moj.gov.tw/RJSDWeb/book/Book_Detail.aspx?book_id=571

Wen, M. N. & Wang, Z. H. (2013). *Rebuilding the social bond of inmates through religious education – A case study of the effectiveness of religious education in Taipei detention center.* 2013 Research Report of Taipei Detention Center, Agency of Corrections, Ministry of Justice. https://www.tpd.moj.gov.tw/media/97758/461617130633.pdf?mediaDL=true

Yang, S. L. & Tai, S. F. (2022) *The effective evaluation and policy promotion of the scientific evidence-based drug offender treatment model – 3rd phase.* 2022 Research Report Commissioned by the Agency of Corrections, Ministry of Justice. https://antidrug.moj.gov.tw/lp-1237-2.html

Yeh, Y. L. (2018) The effectiveness of treatment for sexual offenders: An etiological perspective of recidivism. *Essays on Criminal Policy and Crime Research*, *21*, 287–322. https://www.tpi.moj.gov.tw/public/Attachment/91101613381.pdf

SOUTH EAST ASIA

9

REHABILITATION OF PEOPLE WHO HAVE OFFENDED IN INDONESIA

Zora A. Sukabdi and Kim J. Wheeler

Introduction

As an archipelagic country, Indonesia consists of over 17,000 islands, including Bali, Java (the home to more than half of the country's population), Lombok, Sumatra, and parts of Borneo and New Guinea. By area, Indonesia is the 14th largest country in the world with a population of approximately 280 million people. It is the world's fourth most populous country and it is ethnically and religiously diverse, with 86.7% Muslims, 10.72% Christians, 1.74% Hindus, 0.8% Buddhists, 0.03% Confucianists, and 0.4% others. The country has a long history of colonialism, mainly by the Netherlands, and cultural as well as historical factors affect the country's criminal justice system.

According to the Central Statistics Agency/Badan Pusat Statistik (2015), the total number of criminal acts in Indonesia decreased during 2018–2020 (from 294,281 incidents in 2018 to 247,218 in 2020). The crime rate during 2018–2020 also declined, although some crimes, including substance-related offending, increased from 7.22% of all crimes in 2014 to 14.99% in 2018. In 2020, Police Registration Data suggests that Sumatera North had the highest total crimes (32,990 incidents), followed by Jakarta and beyond (26,585 incidents), and East Java (17,642 incidents); although West Papua had the highest crime rate, followed by Maluku and North Sulawesi. Meanwhile, West Sulawesi, North Kalimantan, and North Maluku had the lowest rates (1,704, 1,015, and 850, respectively). Indonesia uses Kitab Undang-Undang Hukum Pidana (KUHP) Republik Indonesia/the Criminal Code

DOI: 10.4324/9781003360919-12

and The International Classification of Crime for Statistical Purposes (ICCS) by the United Nations Office on Drugs and Crime (UNODC, 2015) for classifying crimes. Statistically, the most frequently recorded crime in Indonesia is robbery (Central Statistics Agency/Badan Pusat Statistik, 2021).

Of the 526 prisons in Indonesia, 399 are overcrowded (Resia, 2021). In 2021, prisons in Indonesia could only accommodate 135,561 prisoners, yet the total number of people in prison in August 2021 was 266,514 (97% overcapacity). The issue of prison overcrowding is significant and purportedly associated with prison riots (Sahara, 2021), creating concern among academics, correctional expert commentators, and government ministers. The Indonesian Minister of Law argues that prison overcrowding occurs because Indonesia detains both drug users and those convicted of offences who also have problems with drug use in prisons. This is because Indonesia views drug use as a crime (Marhaenjati, 2021). Drug users are only sent to drug rehabilitation centres if their lawyers propose it prior to prosecution and the judge approves. Moreover, 54.6% of people in prison are incarcerated for drug-related crimes. Conversely, the total number of people in drug rehabilitation programmes of the National Narcotics Agency (BNN/ Badan Narkotika Nasional) is unsatisfactory (only 32,706 people since 2012). Hence, the Minister of Law has asserted that Indonesia should focus on rehabilitation instead of incarceration for people who use drugs (Marhaenjati, 2021).

Next, we seek to describe Indonesia's stance on people who offend, and current practices and preferences regarding rehabilitation within both correctional and forensic mental health services. The chapter is divided into six sections: Indonesia's perspectives on criminal behaviour, the criminal justice system, correctional population, rehabilitation of people in prison, other instruments of law (e.g., indigenous laws based on local wisdom) used in the country for rehabilitation, and the implementation of the Risk Need, Responsivity (RNR) and Good Lives Model (GLM) in Indonesia.

Indonesia's View on Criminal Behaviour

Indonesian scholars view *crime* as behaviour that disobeys social norms and regulations. Accordingly, crime is regarded as "any behaviour that is opposed against humanity, disadvantageous, anti-social, and violating laws and regulations" (Kartono, 2003, p. 122). According to Kartono (2007), crimes are explained via three categories (jurisdictive, social, and economic) as follows:

1 In the legal sense, crime is when a person violates laws and regulations and is charged as "guilty" by legal authorities and sentenced.
2 In the social sense, crime is when a person fails to adjust to society or shows delinquent behaviours which oppose social norms.
3 In the economic sense, crime is when a person is financially harmful or imposes a financial burden on others and disrupts others' contentment.

In line with the above description, Kartono (2007) defines criminal behaviours in the following ways:

1 *Formal jurisdiction:* Criminal behaviours are behaviours that are inconsistent with morality, are harmful to society, and violate laws and regulations.
2 *Sociology:* Criminal behaviours are all statements and behaviours which are socially, psychologically, economically, and politically harmful to society and violate social norms.

Furthermore, criminal behaviours are seen as deviant behaviours, which are explained as: (1) uncommon behaviours that are not in line with social norms that attract attention, and intervention from the authorities (Lawang in Rahmat, 2013), (2) deviate from social norms and principles (Soekanto, 1999, 2000), and (3) deviate from central tendencies or the average behaviours of society (Kartono, 2000, 2003, 2007).

According to Indonesian scholars, factors motivating crimes are considered either internal (i.e., personality traits and temperament) (Kartono, 2007; Santoso & Zulfa, 2013) or external (i.e., modelling, physical and the psycho-social environment, such as limited opportunities to generate law-abiding behaviours, social interaction, peers, and family dysfunction) (Soedjono, 1977; Soekanto, 2000). Wiriaatmadja (in Kartono, 2007) argues that criminal behaviours result from the ineffectual nature of social units and a lack of opportunities in acquiring economic resources (i.e., poverty, low income), socio-economic discrepancies amongst people, and foreign cultures/influences that disrupt harmony in society (e.g., media).

Indonesia's Criminal Justice System

In terms of the formal guidance to prosecute criminal offenders, Indonesia remains under the influence of the Dutch colonial justice system by referring its prosecution to *Wetboek van Strafrecht voor Nederlandsch Indie (WvS NI)*. In Indonesia *WvS NI* is known as "Kitab Undang-Undang Hukum Pidana" (KUHP) or the Criminal Code (Aminullah & Arief, 2020). The Code does not make a clear statement about the objectives of prosecution (Arief, 2016, 2017), which arguably requires revision (Aminullah & Arief, 2020; Mudzakkir, 2010; Sholehuddin, 2003; Tongat in Susetyo et al., 2012). Aminullah and Arief (2020) argue that prosecution based on the colonial system, as seen in KUHP/the Criminal Code, focuses on repression against criminal offenders rather than rehabilitation. For instance, the sentences mentioned in Article 10 KUHP/the Criminal Code are centred on execution, imprisonment, detention, fines, and taking the rights of offenders, not rehabilitation (Aminullah & Arief, 2020).

Some Indonesian scholars suggest the importance of implementing customary/organic/indigenous laws (*hukum adat*) based on local wisdom before the arrival of the colonial forces, referring to the fact that Indonesia consists of many islands, cultures, and ethnicities (Zulfa, 2010). Scholars argue that customary laws through traditional/indigenous institutions can play an important role in the Indonesian criminal justice system, give recognition to Indonesian local wisdom, and oppose the lingering domination of European colonial influences on Indonesia (Zulfa, 2010).

Indigenous courts existed before the colonial era although there is very limited information on the way these indigenous courts functioned (Dinnen, 2003; Engelbrecht & Engelbrecht, 1950; Zulfa, 2010). Their key principles were based on local wisdom applied in the villages where the courts were located. These key principles across villages in Indonesia were later abstracted into *"Pancasila"* by Indonesian independence proclaimer, Mr. Soekarno, on June 1st 1945. *Pancasila*, Indonesian national philosophy and the Indonesian constitution provided a foundation for rehabilitation in Indonesia (see below). During colonial times the indigenous courts were "replaced" with village courts, which were controlled by colonial forces; for example, *Regeling van de Inheemsche Rechtsspraak in rechtsstreeks bestuurd gebied* (indigenous court) in Staadsblad No. 80/1932, *Zelfbestuursregelen* 1938, and *Reglement Ordonantie* in Staatsblad No. 102/1935 (Dinnen, 2003; Engelbrecht & Engelbrecht, 1950; Zulfa, 2010).

Zulfa (2010) argues that consideration of indigenous laws could help resolve the problem of mass incarceration and prison overcrowding since most criminal cases can be effectively and rapidly "solved" in the communities before the intervention of formal law enforcement institutions (yet still meeting people's sense of justice; for example, the agreement between victims and offenders of crime is reached even before police come to record and investigate the incident). Moreover, instead of involving legal officials or police, unwritten indigenous laws practiced in villages only require the initiatives of offenders and their families, victims and their families, and advice of reputable leaders (i.e., religious, tribal, or senior leaders) in the villages where the behaviour has occurred (Dinnen, 2003; Zulfa, 2010).

Rehabilitation of General Inmates

Indonesia's rehabilitation approach is determined by both law and the country's universal philosophy, termed *Pancasila*. *Pancasila* is based on an abstraction of Indonesian ancestral universal wisdom, consisting of Five Fundamental Commandments or Principles (Amir, 2013). The Five Principles have become the blueprint of the Indonesian nation in every aspect of life including rehabilitation of offenders. In the constitution of the Republic of Indonesia the Five Principles of *Pancasila* are listed as:

1 *The belief in God the Almighty:* This principle includes religiosity and spirituality, beliefs in higher goals and the afterlife, tolerance and harmony amongst different believers, and beliefs in the purposes and meanings of life. This explains the vital role of religion and spirituality in nearly all aspects of life (Aditya et al., 2021). Indonesia is one of the most religious countries in the world (Iswara, 2020).
2 *Just and civilised humanity:* This principle includes respect for humanity (e.g., equality of humans, recognition of human values and dignity), love, empathy, pro-social behaviours, altruism, integrity, relationships, and gratitude towards others. This principle emphasises the importance of human rights.
3 *The unity of Indonesia:* This principle includes prioritising societal well-being over one's personal agenda/interests, nationalism, national altruism, generosity, patriotism, cooperation, and collaboration for the greater good. This principle emphasises the importance of unity in diversity amongst the heterogeneous people of Indonesia. Indonesia consists of 1,340 ethnic groups (Aditya et al., 2021; Central Statistics Agency, 2015; Naim & Syaputra, 2011) and more than 700 spoken languages (Lewis, 2009). The founding fathers of Indonesia have highlighted the importance of having a unity of spirit in the country. The principle also stresses cooperation and coordination among local governments, sectors (i.e., private and public sectors), and non-governmental organisations within Indonesia.
4 *The democracy under the wise guidance of representative consultations:* The principle includes the pursuit of virtues and wisdom, righteousness, genuineness, patience, mindfulness, consciousness, ethical behaviours, self-efficacy, positive involvement in society, social responsibilities, collective decision making, and togetherness in problem-solving. This principle underscores the democracy based on ethics and wisdom rather

than the number of votes. This also stresses communal coping ("musyawarah" and "gotong royong").

5 *Social justice for all the peoples of Indonesia:* The principle includes the desire for independence and self-autonomy, well-being, inner and outer peace, noble behaviours, prosocial attitudes, justice, law-abiding behaviours, respect for civil rights, thoughtful minds, humble attitudes, proper planning, excellence of professionalism, quality of results, appraisal for others' works, and continuous learning. This principle is also related to socio-cultural and economic equality in Indonesia.

Detaining inmates without any rehabilitation programme is seen as opposing the spirit of *Pancasila* (Sujatno, 2008a, 2008b). The Preamble to The 1945 Constitution rules that the state of Indonesia shall protect all the people of Indonesia, improve public welfare, educate the life of the people, and participate in the establishment of a world order based on freedom, perpetual peace and social justice.

Indonesian scholars support the concept of "reversion to initial situations" when explaining the word "rehabilitation" (Astutik, 2014; Dau, 2015; Siallagan et al., 2021). Suparlan (1993), for example, suggests that rehabilitation is an activity to "restore" a person's situation and develop their mental and physical skills to be able to overcome problems. Partodiharjo (2006) also suggests that rehabilitation is physical and psychological recovery to return to the original state where an individual was still free from negative characteristics and physical and mental harms. Similarly, Soewito (in Sri Widati, 1984, p. 5) explains that "Rehabilitation is all efforts in the field of medical, psychosocial, education, economy, or others, managed as a continuous process and aimed to physically and psychologically recover targeted people so that they 'revert to their initial positions' in society as productive, independent, and helpful members of society and the country". Furthermore, Banja (1990, p. 615) defines rehabilitation as "a holistic and integrative approach to manage medical, physical, psychosocial, and vocational interventions for an individual so that he/she can obtain achievements, social mindfulness, effective interaction, and positive contribution to the world".

The Indonesian correctional system is juridically regulated under Law No. 12/1995 on Correctional (Khotimah, 2016), the Code of Criminal Procedure/KUHAP (Dau, 2015), and Government Regulation (PP) No. 31/1999 (Khotimah, 2016). Rehabilitation, according to Article 1 Section 23 of the Code of Criminal Procedure/KUHAP is a person's right to make a recovery in skills, position, values and dignity in the process of investigation, litigation, or trial (Dau, 2015). Law No. 12/1995 describes the Indonesian correctional system as an integrative arrangement in terms of directions, limitations, and approaches for the correctional population's rehabilitation. This is based on *Pancasila* with the involvement of practitioners, inmates, and society, for the inmates to admit mistakes, modify behaviours, and maintain consistency of positive changes. This creates the capability to reintegrate into the broader community, contributing to Indonesian development, and being responsible citizens. Moreover, the primary purpose of rehabilitation according to this law is "to shape behaviours of inmates, so they perform as holistic human beings, admit mistakes, modify behaviours, maintain positive changes, to be able to reintegrate to broader society, actively contribute to Indonesian development, and function as free and responsible citizens" (Khotimah, 2016). Hence, according to the former Minister of Law, Mr Sahardjo (in Susetyo et al., 2012), the function of correctional centres is to rehabilitate inmates for them to "re-gain" self-confidence and be "re-accepted" by society. In terms of mental health, an eminent psychiatrist in Indonesia, Professor Hawari (Hawari, 2006a, 2006b) explains that rehabilitation consists of four functions: prevention (of recidivism), restoration, maintenance, and development.

The Correctional Director's Decision Letter No. K.P.10/3/7 on February 8/1965 mentions the concept of correctional as a healing process in a correction centre which shows progress from a condition where inmates are unwanted by the community and incapable of building peaceful relationships with society to a state where they are healed from negative behaviours and able to contribute to the harmony of society (Khotimah, 2016).

Article 14 of Law No. 12/1995 describes that all inmates have fundamental rights, as follows: (1) to pray according to their beliefs and religions, (2) to achieve both physical and psychological well-being, (3) to receive education and teachings, (4) to receive decent foods and health facilities, (5) to file complaints, (6) to receive reading materials, (7) to receive working incentives, (8) to receive visits from families and others, (9) to receive opportunities for assimilation, (10) to be granted parole, (11) to be granted holidays before release, and (12) to be granted other rights according to laws and regulations (Sari & Nuqul, 2014). According to Article 5 of Law No. 12/1995 on Inmate Rehabilitation there are ten fundamental principles of the Indonesian correctional system; these are as follows (Khotimah, 2016; Paramarta et al., 2004, pp. 35–36; Priyatno, 2006):

1 Nurturing and providing inmates with life skills so that they can reintegrate and perform as good citizens in society.

2 Sentencing is not an act of revenge by the country; hence no verbal and physical torture against inmates is acceptable, even in treatment and placement.
3 Giving inmates guidance, not pain, so they repent, understand social norms and activities, and develop competencies in societal life.
4 Not entrapping inmates or setting up conditions where inmates become worse after being detained (not showing positive changes).
5 Not alienating inmates from society during their incarceration; hence, they deserve visits, meetings, or other social entertainment from families or society.
6 Providing inmates with integrative education and helping them realise their potential. This means not merely paying lip service to the idea of education or providing materials only for short-term occupation.
7 Referring rehabilitation of inmates to *Pancasila*.
8 Leading inmates to the right things.
9 Limiting inmates' freedom only for a certain period of time based on the sentence.
10 Providing inmates with infrastructure needed during rehabilitation.

In terms of categories of rehabilitation, Government Regulation (PP) No. 31/1999 mentions that rehabilitation of inmates consists of three areas of development: (1) mental and spiritual (called "self-independence" and "personality" rehabilitation), (2) vocational (by providing skills), and (3) physical (e.g., sports, exercise). The detailed objectives of rehabilitation and guidance for people in prison in Indonesia are to improve the quality of life (Khotimah, 2016): (1) faith in God the Almighty, (2) intellectual capacity, (3) attitude and behaviours, (4) skills and professionalism, and (5) physical and mental health (Khotimah, 2016). Furthermore, the indicators of an effective correctional system (for evaluation purposes) are (Khotimah, 2016):

1 The number of inmates is less than the maximum capacity of each correction centre.
2 The decreasing crime rates each year.
3 The increasing number of inmates receiving early release (i.e., through parole, assimilation, or reintegration programs).
4 The decreasing number of recidivisms each year.
5 The increasing number of institutions helping the rehabilitation of any inmates.
6 Former inmates working in industrial and maintenance fields reach 70% of the total correctional population.

7 The death and sickness percentages of inmates in prisons are similar to those of people in society.

8 The treatment costs for inmates are similar to the minimum costs for basic needs of most Indonesians in the country.

9 The sustained cleanliness and hygiene of correctional centres.

10 The internalisation of social norms, values, and wisdom into correctional centres.

Nonetheless, rehabilitation activities in Indonesian prisons (i.e., sewing, drawing, sports, automation, cooking) are optional activities. Official programmes in the community (outside prisons) are unheard of, except those initiated by non-government organisations which may lack sustainability. Other challenges are centred on the limited numbers of competent practitioners to deliver interventions and availability of suitable methods to conduct risk assessments and guide intervention.

Rehabilitation of People Convicted of Extraordinary Offences

Indonesia regulates inmates who commit extraordinary crimes (such as drug crimes, corruption, and terrorism) with separate laws (e.g., rehabilitation for terrorist offenders, referred to as "deradicalisation", is regulated in Law No. 5/2018 and Government Regulation (PP) No. 77/2019, whereas rehabilitation for people convicted of drug offenders is regulated in Law No. 22/1997, Law No. 35/2009 on Narcotics (Article 45, Article 46, Article 47, Article 48, Article 49, and Article 50), and Presidential Decision No. 17/2002).

Since the total number of people in prison involved in substance abuse cases is 54.6% of the overall prisoner population, this section will focus on this group. Rehabilitation of these people is defined as integrative and includes medical, mental, psychosocial, and educational approaches to improve capability in adjustment, independence, growth, and other life skills based on the person's physical, social, and economic potentials (Dau, 2015). Therapies aim to heal inmates so they do not depend on narcotics, psychotropics, and other addictive substances. This needs the involvement of multidisciplined practitioners and professionals (e.g., doctors, therapists, psychologists, religious counsellors, psychiatrists, social workers, trainers) and the contribution of broader society to guarantee the sustainability of outcomes (Dau, 2015).

Drug offenders are rehabilitated in specific rehabilitation centres for narcotics (e.g., Cipinang Prison) (Dau, 2015). The National Anti-Drugs Agency (BNN) collaborates with other government and non-government organisations to rehabilitate drug offenders (Dau, 2015). Regulation of the

National Anti-Drugs Agency (Peraturan BNN) No. 11/2014 states that drug offenders can appeal for rehabilitation to prosecutors (during a lawsuit) or judges (during trial). The prosecutors or judges will then request the assessment team to conduct an examination (Dau, 2015). Accordingly, the assessment team provide the examination results to prosecutors or judges, who will determine the placement of the person. There are four stages of rehabilitation in relation to drug offenders: medical check-up, detoxification, psychological therapies by counsellors (individual and group), and recovery (i.e., empowerment, socialisation, and reintegration programs with the community) (Dau, 2015). Moreover, some rules for rehabilitation of people convicted of drug offences in correction centres are: (1) the rehabilitation process runs for six months, (2) families cannot visit the residents of rehabilitation centres following admission during detoxification, and (3) families are required to inform BNN if the residents escape from rehabilitation centres, and they should then return them to the centres (Dau, 2015).

Indigenous Laws as an Alternative Approach to Rehabilitation

Indonesian scholars and practitioners in the field of law believe that the correctional system in Indonesia has been ineffective, and this is evidenced by prison riots, overcrowding/overcapacity, the lack of infrastructure and facilities, unsatisfying outcomes of rehabilitation, and recidivism (Aminullah & Arief, 2020; Susetyo et al., 2012; Widodo, 2015; Zulfa, 2010). In 2022 Indonesia launched the New KUHP/Criminal Code which emphasises "restorative justice" (for instance, the death penalty is removed from this New Criminal Code). It is believed by Indonesian scholars and practitioners of law that the Old Criminal Code, which was developed by Dutch colonials, used a retributive, rather than restoration/prevention paradigm (Aminullah & Arief, 2020). Unlike traditional/Indigenous laws which support restorative justice, the Old Criminal Code was seen as supporting colonial principles of punishment. By contrast, the New Criminal Code seeks to adopt indigenous laws in a hybrid justice system.

Restorative justice focuses on restoration and prevention (Mudzakir, 2013; Prayitno, 2012; Waluyo, 2017). It is "a process in which everyone involved in a criminal case (i.e., victim and family, offender and family, community seniors/leaders) collectively work to find solutions for problems, reconcile, and overcome possible effects that may raise in future" (Susetyo et al., 2012, p. 16). Restorative justice in Indonesia is rooted in traditional values and collective wisdom (Zulfa, 2010). *KNorth Manawa* (the ancient criminal code) by the Majapahit Empire in 1293

(Mulyana, 1979) and *Qonun Mangkuta Alam* by Sultan Iskandar Muda in Aceh in 1607 (Wiranata, 2005) are examples of the operation of the restorative justice system in Indonesia. Indigenous sanctions in these guidebooks include: (1) immaterial agreement such as marrying the victims, (2) providing physical and psychosocial services for victims, (3) reconciliation and religious rituals, (4) admitting mistakes and apologising, (5) physical redemption, and (6) alienation from people (Wiranata, 2005). Nowadays, restorative justice is performed through penal mediations, reconciliations/conflict resolutions, legal process terminations, and diversions, especially for child offenders, based on the needs of all related parties: victims, offenders, and society, not only of offenders (Aminullah & Arief, 2020; Amrullah, 2008; Dewi, 2021; Muladi, 1995, 1997; Susetyo et al., 2012; Widodo, 2015; Zulfa, 2010). These historical practices are manifested in the New Criminal Code, which will be implemented in 2025.

Risk-Need-Responsivity

The Risk-Need-Responsivity (RNR) model is a well-known model of correctional assessment and rehabilitative programming used in many Western countries. The RNR Model involves general personality and cognitive social learning perspectives on human behaviour and includes all efforts to prevent crime in clinical, social, and human services provided to individuals and groups (Andrews & Bonta, 2010). While there is little recognition of the RNR Model in Indonesia (although some scholars have tried to introduce the model, see Arham & Runturambi, 2020), there are common features in Indonesia's criminal justice system. For example, assessments for criminal offenders performed by the Indonesian Forensic Psychological Association during investigations and detention encourage examination of seven aspects of offenders: (1) intellectual capacity, (2) personality (including assessments to determine insanity), (3) motives, (4) risks (i.e., abilities in self-harming, aggressiveness, risks of recidivism), (5) malingering behaviours, (6) deceiving behaviours, and (7) substance abuse. Overall, it appears that Indonesian forensic psychologists take into account the importance of identifying risk and a number of criminogenic needs of offenders before embarking on rehabilitation. Nonetheless, the lack of valid risk-assessment tools in Indonesia is noted. There is no systematic use of Western-developed and validated tools or locally developed risk and needs assessment instruments; hence, Indonesian clinicians use traditional techniques such as interviews, observation, tests of intelligence, and general personality inventories to conduct risk assessment. For people charged with terrorism offences, forensic psychologists in the Indonesian Forensic Psychological Association use MIKRA (Motivasi-Ideology-Capability Risk Assessment), an instrument designed especially for examining terrorist offenders' risks and needs (Amelia et al., 2020; Indonesian Forensic Psychological Association, 2020a; Salsabila, 2020; Slamet, 2020; Sukabdi, 2018, 2020a, 2020b, 2021a, 2021b, 2021c).

Implementation of the Good Lives Model (GLM) in Indonesia

As mentioned earlier, the preamble to the 1945 Constitution mandates that the Indonesian government protect humanity, improve welfare, provide education, and participate in the establishment of a world order based on freedom, perpetual peace and social justice. Therefore, any other models of rehabilitation (i.e., the GLM and RNR Models) implemented in Indonesia should be consistent with the principles stated in *Pancasila* and the 1945 Constitution.

Ward and colleagues' GLM emphasises human rights, well-being, and freedom (Willis et al., 2013) and encourages initiatives that seek to improve offenders' well-being whilst also seeking reduction of risks for re-offending (Willis et al., 2013). Ward and Brown (2004) propose nine comprehensive primary human goods that motivate human behaviour and which, when left unsatisfied, may contribute to criminal behaviour. Although there is no formal adoption of GLM in Indonesia's criminal justice system, there are overlaps between the primary human goods delineated by Ward and colleagues and the principles of *Pancasila*:

1 *Life:* This area is consistent with the fifth principle of *Pancasila*. Several medical and (physical) health interventions are delivered to people in Indonesian correctional centres.

2 *Knowledge:* This area parallels the fifth principle of *Pancasila*. Education is provided on topics such as basic parenting, traditional medicine (i.e., herbal, tibu nabawi), marketing, business, and accounting.

3 *Excellence in play and work:* This area is consistent with the fifth principle of *Pancasila*. Several vocational training programmes such as barista/coffee making, cooking, yoghurt making, sewing, tempe (soya cake) making, home industry, soap making, interior decorating, handicrafts making, even boat making, are offered to improve inmates' skills. Moreover, although *Pancasila* does not mention play, however, correctional programmes at prisons in Indonesia contain various

recreational activities (e.g., musical drama, wayang show, ketoprak, karaoke, costume events, drawing, paintings and sports).

4 *Excellence in agency:* This area is in line with the fifth principle of *Pancasila*. To address this area, correctional centres in Indonesia invite several non-governmental organisations, professionals, and rehabilitation practitioners to conduct counselling and mentoring for people in prison. These interventions seek to develop confidence, independence, self-efficacy, and become responsible human beings.

5 *Inner peace:* This area is in line with the first, fourth, and fifth principles of *Pancasila*. As mentioned earlier, Indonesia is a religious country and religions and associated belief systems are seen as the remedy for any stress and turbulence in life; hence, various programmes in correctional centres of Indonesia always involve religious leaders as mentors for people in prison.

6 *Relatedness and community:* This area is consistent with the second, third, fourth, and fifth principles of *Pancasila*. As a communal society that conducts all aspects of life based on collective values, Indonesian people place more importance on family relations and togetherness as indicators of happiness than other indicators of success such as income (The Jakarta Post, 2014). Therefore, correctional centres always welcome visits from families and significant others of inmates. Nonetheless, for offenders in maximum security prisons (i.e., terrorists, drug dealers), prison authorities typically suspend this privilege to avoid the spread of ideology or further criminal behaviour.

7 *Spirituality:* This area is consistent with the first, second, and fifth principles of *Pancasila*. As explained earlier, correctional programs in Indonesia involve spiritual leaders/figures to be mentors for inmates at all times.

8 *Happiness:* This area is consistent with the first, fourth, and fifth principles of *Pancasila*. Indonesians base their activities on collectivism and spirituality; hence, people perceive contentment and relatedness under the same theme as happiness. Happiness is addressed in correctional centres through spiritual counselling and empowerment, reintegration, resocialisation, and recreational programs that involve families and people outside correctional centres.

9 *Creativity:* This area is implicitly in line with the fifth principle of *Pancasila*. Activities that support creativity and innovation include displaying and selling products made by people in prison including handicrafts, drawings, and paintings. Furthermore, correctional institutions also welcome any creative contributions of NGOs in rehabilitation.

Conclusion

Despite the decline of total crimes and the crime rate in 2020, Indonesia is still facing a severe challenge in regard to prison overcrowding. Indonesia is caught between adopting the principles of *Pancasila*, which encourages rehabilitation, and applying a justice system that was established by former colonial powers which encourages punitive responses to crime. Indonesian legal scholars argue that indigenous laws could be the answer for prison overcrowding in Indonesia, as agreement between victims and offenders' families can repair the harms done by crime and achieve satisfaction prior to the interventions of law enforcement officials. Against this background, in 2025 Indonesia will embrace a New Criminal Code, which combines modern and indigenous laws. Diverting people who have a history of drug use away from prisons towards rehabilitation may also reduce overcrowding.

The Indonesian Code of Criminal Procedure describes the Indonesian correctional system as an integrative arrangement in terms of directions, limitations and approaches for the correctional population's rehabilitation, which is based on the universal philosophy of *Pancasila*. This requires the involvement of practitioners, offenders, and society to encourage and facilitate prisoners to admit mistakes, modify their behaviours, and establish and maintain positive changes, so that they are capable of reintegration into the broader community. Even though Western models such as RNR and GLM have not received much attention in Indonesia, their basic ideas are apparent in Indonesia's criminal justice system. These basic ideas are not however models overt nor are they systematically applied throughout the archipelago. Reliable and valid assessment tools and effective intervention strategies need to be developed to improve rehabilitation practices in the criminal justice and forensic mental health systems in Indonesia.

References

Aditya, Y., Martoyo, I., Nurcahyo, F.A., Ariela, J., & Pramono, R. (2021). Factorial Structure of the Four Basic Dimensions of Religiousness (4-BDRS) among Muslim and Christian College Students in Indonesia. *Cogent Psychology*, 8(1), 19746.

Amelia, F., Widodo, P., & Budiarto, A. (2020). Women's Motivation as Perpetrators of Terrorism in Indonesia. *Journal of Asymmetric War*, 6(1), 23–42.

Aminullah & Arief. (2020). Penerapan Mediasi Penal Dengan Pendekatan Restorative Justice Dalam Upaya Penanggulangan Kejahatan di Indonesia. *Jurnal Meta Yuridis*, 3(1). http://journal.upgris.ac.id

Amir, S. (2013). Pancasila as Integration Philosophy of Education and National Character. *International Journal of Scientific & Technology Research*, 2, 54–57.

Amrullah, M. A. (2008). *Ketentuan dan Mekanisme Pertanggungjawaban Pidana Korporasi.* Paper Presented at the National Seminar on Corporate Social Responsibility (CSR), Organized by PUSH-AM-UII Yogyakarta in collaboration.

Andrews, D. A., & Bonta, J. (2010). *The Psychology of Criminal Conduct* (5th ed.). Matthew Bender & Company, Inc.

Arham, L., & Runturambi, A. J. S. (2020). Kebijakan Perlakuan Narapidana Teroris Menggunakan Risk Need Responsivity (RNR) di Lembaga Pemasyarakatan Kelas I Cipinang [RNR in Cipinang Prison]. *Deviance: Jurnal Kriminologi*, 4(1), 45–66.

Arief, B. N. (2016). *Kebijakan Formulasi Ketetntuan Pidana dalam Peraturan perundang- Undangan.* Pustaka Magister.

Arief, B. N. (2017). *Tujuan dan Pedoman Pemidanaan (Perspektif Pembaharuan & Perbandingan Hukum Pidana).* Pustaka Magister.

Astutik, S. (2014). Rehabilitasi Sosial 3. *UIN Sunan Ampel Press*, 5–11. http://digilib.uinsby.ac.id

Banja, J. D. (1990). Rehabilitation and Empowerment. *Archives of Physical Medicine and Rehabilitation*, 718, 614–615.

Central Statistics Agency. (2015). *Mengulik Data Suku di Indonesia.* Central Statistics Agency. https://www.bps.go.id/news/2015/11/18/127/mengulik-data-suku-di-indonesia.html

Central Statistic Agency. (2021). *Statistik Kriminal 2021.* https://www.bps.go.id/publication/2021/12/15/8d1bc84d2055e99feed39986/statistik-kriminal-2021.html

Dau, Y. (2015). *Putusan Rehabilitasi dalam Konsep Pemidanaan di Indonesia [Airlangga University].* https://repository.unair.ac.id/30724/

Dewi, D. K. (2021). *Upaya Menghentikan Penuntutan Demi Rasa Keadilan Dalam Masyarakat Berdasarkan Peraturan Jaksa Agung Nomor 15 Tahun 2020 [Pancasakti Tegal University].* http://repository.upstegal.ac.id/3567/

Dinnen, S. (2003). *Interfaces between Formal and Informal Justice Sistem to Strengthen Access to Justice by Disadvantaged Syystem*, , Makalah disampaikan dalam Practice In Action Workshop UNDP Asia-Pasific Rights and Justice Initiative, Ahungala Sri Lanka, 19-21 November 2003, hlm.2-4.

Engelbrecht, W. A., & Engelbrecht, E. M. L. (1950). *Netherlands & Indonesia: De wetboeken, wetten en verordeningen van Indonesie: benevens de Grondwet voor het Koninkrijk der Nederlanden en de ontwerp constitutie voor de Republik der Verenigde Staten van Indonesie.* Sijthoff.

Hawari, D. (2006a). *Manajemen stress cemas dan depresi* (2nd ed.). Balai Penerbit Fakultas Kedokteran Universitas Indonesia.

Hawari, D. (2006b). *Penyalahgunaan dan ketergantungan NAZA: narkotika, alkohol dan zat adiktif* (2nd ed.). Balai Penerbit Fakultas Kedokteran Universitas Indonesia. http://lontar.ui.ac.id/detail?id=120699

How Happy are Indonesians, Really? (2014). The Jakarta Post. https://www.thejakartapost.com/news/2014/04/17/how-happy-are-indonesians-really.html

International Classification of Crimes for Statistical Purposes. (2015). *United Nation Office on Drugs and Crime (UNODC)*.

Iswara, M. A. (2020). *Indonesia Ranks among Most Religious Countries in Pew Study*. The Jakarta Post. https://www.thejakartapost.com/news/2020/07/30/indonesia-ranks-among-most-religious-countries-in-pew-study.html

Kartono, K. (2000). *Hygiene Mental*. CV. Mandar Maju.

Kartono, K. (2003). *Patologi Sosial*. Raja Grafindo Persada.

Kartono, K. (2007). *Patologi Sosial*. Raja Grafindo Persada.

Khotimah, K. (2016). *Proses pembinaan warga binaan pemasyarakatan di lembaga pemasyarakatan kelas iia wirogunan Yogyakarta [Universitas Negeri Yogyakarta]*. http://eprints.uny.ac.id/id/eprint/41648

Lewis, M. P. (2009). *Ethnologue: Languages of the World* (16th ed.). SIL International.

Marhaenjati, B. (2021). *Indonesian Prison System at More Than Double Its Capacity*. The Jakarta Globe. https://jakartaglobe.id/news/indonesian-prison-system-at-more-than-double-its-capacity/

Mudzakir. (2013). *Analisis Restorative justice: Sejarah, Ruang Lingkup, dan Penerapannya*. PT. Macanan Jaya Cemerlang.

Mudzakkir. (2010). Kebijakan Kodifikasi (Total) Hukum Pidana Melalui RUU KUHP dan Antisipasi terhadap Problem Perumusan Hukum Pidana dan Penegakan Hukum Pidana di Masa Datang. *Lokakarya Perencanaan Pembangunan Hukum Nasional Perkembangan Hukum Pidana Dalam Undang-Undang Di Luar KUHP Dan Kebijakan Kodifikasi Hukum Pidana*.

Muladi. (1995). *Kapita Selekta Sistem Peradilan Pidana*. Badan Penerbit Universitas Diponegoro.

Muladi. (1997). *Hak Asasi Manusia, Politik dan Sistem Peradilan Pidana*. Badan Penerbit Universitas Diponegoro.

Mulyana, S. (1979). *Nagarakretagama Dan tafsir Sejarahnya*. Bhatara Karya Aksara.

Naim, A., & Syaputra, H. (2011). *Nationality, Ethnicity, Religion, and Languages of Indonesians*. Bendan Duwur Semarang: Universitas Katolik Soegijapranata.

Paramarta et al. (2004). *40 Tahun Pemasyarakatan Mengukir Citra Profesionalisme*. Direktorat Jenderal Pemasyarakatan Departemen Kehakiman dan Hak Asasi Manusia RI.

Partodiharjo. (2006). *Kenali Narkoba dan Musuhi Penyalahgunaannya*. Esensi.

Prayitno, K. P. (2012). Restorative Justice Untuk Peradilan di Indonesia (Perspektif Yuridis Filosofis dalam penegakan Hukum In Concreto). *Jurnal Dinamika Hukum*, 12(3), 404. 10.20884/1.jdh.2012.12.3.116

Priyatno, D. (2006). *Sistem pelaksanaan pidana penjara di Indonesia*. Refika Aditama.

Rahmat, D. (2013). Problematika Geng Motor di Kabupaten Kuningan dalam Prespektif Sosiologi. *Jurnal Unifikasi*, 1(1)(ISSN 2354-5976).

Resia, E. (2021). Menakar Kebutuhan Penambahan Kapasitas Penjara [Evaluating the Need to Build More Prisons]. Kemenkeu.go.id. https://www.djkn.kemenkeu. go.id/kpknl-pekanbaru/baca-artikel/14256/Menakar-Kebutuhan-Penambahan-Kapasitas-Penjara.html#:~:text=Dari%20526%20penjara%20dan%20rumah, 399%20diantaranya%20mengalami%20over%20kapasitas
Sahara, W. (2021). *9 Lapas dengan Kelebihan penghuni Terbesar di Indonesia.* Kompas.Com.
Salsabila, P. (2020). The Hidden Face in Every Terror Action. *International Relation Journal.* 10.19165/2018.2.06
Santoso, T., & Zulfa, E. A. (2013). *Kriminologi Jakarta.* Raja Grafindo Persada.
Sari, I. N., & Nuqul, F. L. (2014). *Criminal Thinking pada Narapidana Wanita.*
Sholehuddin, M. (2003). *Sistem Sanksi Pidana.* Rajawali Press.
Siallagan, M. J. R., Aulia, M., & Anita, S. (2021). *Rehabilitasi: Pengertian, Jenis, Bentuk, Fungsi Dan Metode.* Universitas Negeri Medan.
Slamet, A. W. (2020). *Lone Wolfs in Indonesia.* Universitas Indonesia.
Soedjono. (1977). *Ilmu Jiwa Kejahatan.* Karya Nusantara.
Soekanto, S. (1999). *Sosiologi.* Grafindo Persada.
Soekanto, S. (2000). *Pengantar Penelitian Hukum.* UI Press.
Sujatno, A. (2008a). *Pencerahan Di Balik Penjara dari Sangkar Menuju Sanggar Untuk Menjadi Mandiri.* Teraju.
Sujatno, A. (2008b). *Pencerahan Dibalik Penjara dari Sangkar Menuju Sanggar Untuk Menjadi Manusia Mandiri.* Jakarta: PT. Mizan Publika.
Sukabdi, Z. A. (2018). Terrorism Criminogenic Risk Factors. *The 2nd International Conference on Social and Political Issues*, Bali, Indonesia.
Sukabdi, Z. A. (2020a). Indonesian Forensic Psychological Association. *Psifor-Talks.*
Sukabdi, Z. A. (2020b). Measuring the Effectiveness of Deradicalisation: The Development of MIKRA Risk Assessment. *The International Conference on Pandemics Crisis Risks, Impacts, and Mitigation: Global Perspectives of Social, Humanities, and Resilience*, Indonesia, conference presentation.
Sukabdi, Z. A. (2021a). Measuring the Effectiveness of Deradicalisation: The Development of MIKRA Risk Assessment. *Elementary Education Online*, 19(4), 3417–3434.
Sukabdi, Z. A. (2021b). Psychological Risk Factors of Terrorist Offenders in Indonesia. *Journal of Psychological Research*, 3(3), 3299. 10.30564/jpr. v3i3.3299
Sukabdi, Z. A. (2021c). Risk Assessment of Women Involved in Terrorism: Indonesian Cases. *International Journal of Social Science and Human Research*, 4(9), 2495–2511. 10.47191/ijsshr/v4-i9-32
Suparlan, P. (1993). *Agama: Dalam Analisa dan Interpretasi Sosiologi, Penerjemah Achmat Fedyani Saifuddin.* Raja Grafindo Persada.
Susetyo et al. (2012). *Laporan Tim Pengkajian Hukum tentang Sistem Pembinaan Narapidana Berdasarkan Prinsip Restorative Justice.* Kementerian Hukum dan Hak Asasi Manusia Republik Indonesia or Ministry of Law and Human Rights, Republic of Indonesia (in English).
Waluyo, B. (2017). *Penegakan Hukum di Indonesia.* Sinar Grafika.

Ward, T., & Brown, M. (2004). The Good Lives Model and Conceptual Issues in Offender Rehabilitation. *Psychology, Crime, & Law*, *10*(3), 243–257.

Widati, S. (1984). *Rehabilitasi Sosial Psikologis*. PLB FIP IKIP.

Widodo. (2015). Diversi dan Keadilan Restoratif dalam Sistem Peradilan Pidana Anak di Indonesia: Urgensi dan Implikasinya. *Rechtldee Jurnal Hukum*, *10*(2).

Willis, G. M., Prescott, D. S., & Yates, P. M. (2013). *The Good Lives Model (GLM) in Theory and Practice*. https://unafei.or.jp/publications/pdf/RS_No91/No91_10VE_Prescott.pdf

Wiranata, I. G. A. B. (2005). *Hukum Adat Indonesia: Perkembangannya dari Masa ke Masa*. Citra Aditya Bakti.

Zulfa, E. A. (2010). Keadilan restoratif dan revitalisasi lembaga adat di Indonesia. *Jurnal Kriminologi Indonesia*, *6*(II), 182–203.

10

SINGAPORE'S MULTI-PRONGED APPROACH IN THE REHABILITATION OF PERSONS WHO HAVE OFFENDED

Carmelia Nathen, Melvinder Singh, and Kala Ruby

Introduction

Overview of Singapore

Singapore is a relatively small city-state located in the Southeast Asia region with a population of 5.64 million. The state's ethnic distribution stands at about 74% Chinese, 14% Malays, 9% Indians and 3% 'Others'. Singapore is a multi-cultural and multi-lingual society with four official languages – English, Chinese, Malay and Tamil. It is a secular state with one criminal justice system.

Prior to independence from Malaysia in 1965, Singapore was a British colony under the British Military Administration. While elements of the Western system, including legal, education and government structures, continue to be a part of Singapore, post-independence nation-building efforts have been grounded in Asian values. The five Shared Values, adopted in 1991, helped forge Singapore's identity, which included: (i) family as the basic unit of society, and (ii) community support and respect for the individual.

In this chapter, we will discuss Singapore's approach to the rehabilitation of people who have offended, showcasing how the adoption of models such as the Risk-Needs-Responsivity (RNR) principles, are complemented by local research, and how values such as family and community involvement are central to Singapore's rehabilitation approach.

Crime Trends

Singapore's crime rates have remained consistently low over several years, ranging between 23,980 physical crime cases in 2019 to 20,193 cases in

DOI: 10.4324/9781003360919-13

2022 (Singapore Prison Service, 2023) and its recidivism rates have also remained relatively low, −13.7% for people on probation orders,[1] 25% for young people[2] in the residential homes, and 20.4% for those who have been incarcerated.[3]

While the crime situation in Singapore has remained relatively stable and seemingly under control, effortful vigilance and holistic intervention approaches to tackling crime have remained the hallmark of Singapore's approach to a safe and peaceful nation. This has resulted in Singapore being rated as one of the safest countries in the world (Economist Intelligence Unit, 2021). Singapore's criminal justice system is anchored on a coherent set of principles, rule of law, robust policies, and effective implementation. It includes a whole of government effort on its offender management strategies, of which rehabilitating the person who has offended is an important component. Rehabilitation and the prevention of reoffending are effected through various sentencing options and practices and community-based, institutional, and correctional services.

Overview of the Criminal Justice System

Singapore's criminal justice system comprises several key stakeholders including the Courts, Attorney-General's Chambers, government agencies such as the Ministry of Home Affairs which includes law enforcement (e.g., Singapore Police Force, Central Narcotics Bureau) and correctional services such as the Singapore Prison Service, and the Ministry of Social and Family Development's Probation and Community Rehabilitation Service and Youth Residential Service. The National Committee on Prevention, Rehabilitation and Recidivism oversees efforts to prevent offending and enhance rehabilitation. The law defines the types and range of punishment that the Courts may impose for specific offences. In deciding the appropriate sentence, the Court will usually consider the following four key principles: *Proportionate Punishment, Deterrence, Rehabilitation and Prevention* and how much weight should be placed on each principle, based on case-specific facts.

Management of Youth and Adult Offenders

In the sentencing and management of youths who offend (those aged below 21 years), Singapore's guiding principle is rehabilitation. The criminal justice system recognises that these youths need guidance, and this philosophy undergirds the various stages of the criminal justice system. In both youth and adult offender management, this principle is translated to differentiated management strategies such as: (i) community rehabilitation without exposure to the Court system; (ii) community-based sentencing options; and (iii) comprehensive rehabilitative regimes in the community and within institutions. People who complete probation and community-based sentences do not have a conviction record. This facilitates their reintegration into the community as they can legally declare they do not have a criminal record, thus increasing their chances of securing employment or returning to education.

The next few sections will outline the various options available for youths and adults who commit offences.

Pre-Court Diversion

Youths below the age of 19 who offend are, as far as possible, diverted away from the Court system. However, police warnings without any form of intervention or support have been found to be insufficient, with one in three youths returning to offending (Ministry of Social and Family Development, 2019). Hence, efforts have been made to fund and upskill social service agencies within the community (since 1997) to support the rehabilitation of youths who have been diverted from the Court system.

The Guidance Programme, a six-month rehabilitation programme, was introduced for youths who commit minor offences. Efforts have yielded positive outcomes with close to 86%[4] of youths completing the Guidance Programme. The re-offending rates for youths, three years after completing the programme, have remained relatively low at about 7%,[5] indicating success in delaying youths from further contact with the Courts. Other community-based programmes targeting specific offending behaviours are delivered by these agencies, including the Streetwise/Enhanced Streetwise programme for youths engaged in gang-related activities, and the Youth Enhanced Supervision Scheme, for youths arrested for first-time drug consumption or inhalant abuse. In 2018, a triage system was also formalised to support the police and prosecutors in their decision-making, through social reports prepared by social workers following interviews with youths and their families at police divisions. More information on these programmes can be found in the Report on Youth Delinquency (Ministry of Social and Family Development, 2019).

On 1 April 2018, the Integrated Service Providers, comprising appointed social service agencies running a suite of services for youth offenders, were established. This effort strengthened government-community partnerships and ensured a coordinated and consistent approach to delivering community rehabilitative services. The framework is underpinned by evidence-based practices, rigorous capability-building, and supervision.

Similar diversion approaches exist for certain categories of higher-risk or older drug offenders. Those between the ages of 16 to below 21 who are caught for minor offences involving consumption of drugs may be sent to a Community Rehabilitation Centre run by an appointed social service agency. Likewise, adults caught for drug consumption offences may be placed on an Enhanced Direct Supervision Order (community-based rehabilitation provided by the Singapore Anti-Narcotics Association) or sent to a Drug Rehabilitation Centre, depending on their risks and other circumstances, without being prosecuted. Upon completion of their residential phase, they will undergo supervision within the community to aid reintegration. In the above instances, offenders will not have a criminal record for their drug abuse. This approach does not apply to offenders caught for other drug-related or criminal offences given Singapore's tough stance on drugs. These people will be charged in court under the Misuse of Drugs Act 1973.

Prosecution and Rehabilitation – Youth Court

The Youth Court presides over those aged 10 to, pending the operationalisation of the age raise to below 18 under the Children and Young Persons Act (see next paragraph). Assessments for suitability for Probation Orders within the community commence when an offender pleads or is found guilty. Those found unsuitable by the Youth Court for probation are committed to institutions, known as Juvenile Rehabilitation Centres, run by the Ministry of Social and Family Development, Youth Residential Service, or other social service agencies.[6] The Court takes on a collaborative approach to decision-making, considering the assessment of the Probation Officer and views of the Panel of Advisors[7] to the Youth Court before it decides on the most appropriate dispositional order that is in the youth's best interest.

The Children and Young Persons Act was amended in 2019 to include youths below age 18 (from below 16) under the youth justice framework, instead of treating them as adult offenders. This was to enable youths aged 16 to below 18 who may lack the cognitive maturity of adults to benefit from more targeted and age-appropriate rehabilitation in the community and residential settings. However, exceptions are made for those who commit serious offences or are repeat offenders for whom firmer treatment is warranted. These rehabilitation-related amendments have yet to manifest.

Prosecution and Rehabilitation – State Courts

The State Court has jurisdictions over offenders aged 16 and above who are charged in court (unless the law prescribes otherwise; for example,

TABLE 10.1 Sentencing Options for Offenders Charged in Court

	Youth Court[8] *(for offenders below the age of 16)*	*State Courts (for offenders 16 and above)*
Sentencing Options	Probation Order[9]	Probation Order **Community Based**[10] **Sentences:** • Day Reporting Order • Community Service Order[11] • Community Work Order • Mandatory Treatment Order • Short Detention Order
	Community Service Order Detention Order/Juvenile Rehabilitation Centre[12]	Fine Reformative Training Centre
		Incarceration

serious offences might be dealt with before the Supreme Court). Probation Orders, and Reformative Training instead of imprisonment, are considered more readily for younger offenders aged 16 to below 21 as part of their rehabilitation.

In 2010, Community-Based Sentences were introduced to provide the Courts with greater flexibility in sentencing offenders who commit minor crimes, instead of traditional sentences (imprisonment or a fine). Table 10.1 provides a summary of these options.

Court Orders/Sentences

Probation Orders – Youth and State Courts

Probation is a community sentencing option typically considered for people under 21 years old. While the most common offence among those on probation is theft, probation has also been considered for violence, drug, and sexual offences. Seen primarily as a rehabilitation option, the probation regime harnesses the rehabilitative potential of offenders with community support. It seeks to tap into their motivation and capacity to change and effect positive changes in their attitudes, lifestyle, and behaviour. The probation officer is an important change agent in the rehabilitation process and works with the probationer, his/her family, community partners and stakeholders to facilitate rehabilitation. Each year, about 450 to 500 people are placed on Probation Orders. Outcomes are consistently positive with completion rates averaging over 80% with an all-time high of 87% in 2021.

Probation Orders typically include a condition of community service to enable probationers to make amends for their actions and to learn new skills. Other conditions include time restrictions, electronic monitoring, or hostel residency. Probationers are also required to undergo general or offence-specific rehabilitative programmes. All people on probation can continue to go about their daily routines in education or employment so long as they abide by probation conditions.

Juvenile Rehabilitation Centres – Youth Court

The Youth Court has generally applied the principle of rehabilitation (Lim, 2023). As such, placement in institutions is considered a last resort after family care arrangements and community-based options are exhausted or assessed as ineffective. Youths with significantly higher risk/ needs issues are ordered to reside in institutions that provide a structured and safe place for rehabilitation. The Singapore Boys' and Girls' Home are closed institutions and serve as Juvenile Rehabilitation Centres. Rehabilitation plans are designed to be relevant to each youth's risk and needs, with reintegration of the youth offender in mind. Youths are enrolled in either mainstream or vocational education within the Homes while undergoing other programmes targeted at general skills building and/or offending behaviour. Mainstream education for the larger population was made possible because of the set-up of an Education Centre in 2013, an initiative that saw teaching staff from the Ministry of Education seconded to the Homes. Post-care supervision was introduced in 2020 for up to 12 months post-release, to sustain the youths progress and strengthen their reintegration into the community.

Community-Based Sentences

Community-Based Sentences are alternative sentencing options for those aged 16 years old and above. A person may be sentenced to one or a combination of the Community-Based Sentences (see Table 10.1).

Reformative Training Centre

Reformative Training is a sentencing option for those aged 16 to below 21.[13] The sentence comprises a residential phase of up to 36 months (with a minimum detention period of 6 or 12 months), and a statutory supervision phase. Reformative training, including any period of statutory supervision, can last up to 54 months. The regime addresses the rehabilitation needs of the youths, and their reintegration needs as they progress to the community supervision phase.

Imprisonment

When sentenced to prison, people usually serve a part of their sentence (usually two-thirds) in custody before completing the remainder in the community. This forms part of the throughcare approach to rehabilitation. In 2022, there were 7,660 people in prison, with another 2,920 under community corrections. During the In-Care (custodial) phase, various programmes and services are available to facilitate rehabilitation (e.g., Psychology-based Correctional Programmes, Family, Religious, Vocational, Academic, Arts and Befriending programmes). Before being released, offenders go through the Pre-Release phase where they are provided additional programmes and services (e.g., skills training for employment, job coaching and placement, and referral and case management). In the Aftercare phase, which facilitates gradual reintegration into the community, they are placed in various community-based programmes and come under the supervision of the Singapore Prison Service. Finally, in the Reintegration phase, where people are discharged from their sentence, support is continued through a range of services (e.g., employment support, educational assistance, addiction treatment, financial support, and residential support).

The various options available underscore the different pathways to rehabilitation, sensitive to the different profiles of offenders and offences. While each option has its unique nuances, the offender rehabilitation space in its entirety is guided by data and research, evidence-informed frameworks and guiding principles that harness the strength of families and the community.

Offender Rehabilitation

The Ministry of Social and Family Development's Probation and Community Rehabilitation Service and Youth Residential Service and the Ministry of Home Affairs' Singapore Prison Service work in collaboration with key agencies such as the Singapore Police Force, Attorney-General's Chambers, Central Narcotics Bureau, the Courts and the Institute of Mental Health and social service agencies, to deliver its offender rehabilitation services.

Since the early 2000s, the Risk-Needs-Responsivity (RNR) framework has guided assessments, interventions, and practices with offenders under the various programmes and Court Orders mentioned above (see e.g., Thevathasan & Singh, 2023). The introduction of the RNR framework has allowed for a more structured and systematic way to identify and assess risks and needs and develop a common language among correctional professionals.

Assessment

Risk-Needs-Responsivity (RNR) Framework

Both the probation and correctional services adopt the RNR framework in their offender management strategies. Structured risk assessment tools such as the Youth Level of Service/Case Management Inventory (YLS/CMI) and the Level of Service/Case Management Inventory (LS/CMI) were introduced, along with training and supervision, as part of the adoption of the RNR framework (Chua et al., 2014). In addition to these tools, other risk assessment tools to determine sexual and violent offending risk are also used (e.g., the Historical-Clinical-Risk-20 [HCR-20] and the Sexual Violence Risk-20 [SVR-20]). Risk assessments are conducted just prior to the start of orders, or upon commencement. Re-assessments are conducted at various other milestones as part of the tracking of the person's progress and to ensure case plans are reviewed.

To determine and maintain the relevance of these assessment tools to Singapore, studies have been conducted to examine their reliability and validity. Norms have been established and a review of the scoring of items that are sensitive to the local population has been considered in collaboration with the tool's authors. Local studies have found the YLS/CMI to have good predictive accuracy in Singapore (Chu et al., 2015). Similarly, local norming studies on the LS/CMI have confirmed the relevance of the criminogenic needs identified by the LS/CMI for general adult offenders in Singapore (Kaur et al., 2016).

Structured assessment tools on risk and needs provide an objective and consistent way of determining the nature, intensity, and duration of intervention. To illustrate, the different grades of probation (i.e., administrative probation, supervised probation, and intensive probation) allow for differing intensity of interventions according to risk and needs. Cases with higher risk and needs are monitored more closely within the community and provided with higher levels of support and services to lower their likelihood of re-offending. This includes more regular reporting and monitoring, more restrictive conditions (e.g., electronic monitoring or hostel residency) and targeted rehabilitative programmes. The YLS/CMI and LS/CMI assessments also provide information on areas for intervention that reduce the risk of reoffending. These translate to targeted case plans and customised programmes to address risks. For instance, it could be to equip them with decision-making and conflict-resolution skills or to address cognitive distortions and anti-social thinking.

In prisons, similarly, people with higher risk of reoffending are provided with higher-intensity programmes. Psychology-based correctional programmes are designed to target criminogenic needs. Before programmes are designed or reviewed, needs analyses are conducted to ensure that programmes address the appropriate needs across various populations of inmates (e.g., penal, drug and women offenders). To address responsivity issues, inmates are assessed on their language proficiency and mental health to identify potential barriers. As programmes are group-based and mostly conducted in English, inmates who are deemed unsuitable will receive treatment individually. In addition, a motivational primer called *Looking Forward* is provided to increase intrinsic motivation (Loh & Cheng, 2021).

Good Lives Model

The risk-needs-centric approach has benefited Singapore in building the foundation for an evidence-based offender assessment and management approach. Beyond the emphasis on criminogenic needs and risk factors, it spearheaded efforts to develop a comprehensive intervention framework to guide officers in their work. While the RNR framework remains the cornerstone for assessments and rehabilitation, the Good Lives Model (GLM) was also adopted, given its strength-based focus. According to the proponents of GLM, risk factors indicate problems in the way offenders seek to achieve valued goods (Ward & Brown, 2004). Offenders seeking primary goods such as relatedness and sense of achievement may adopt anti-social approaches to acquire such goods. The GLM adds to the understanding of offending behaviour by going beyond risk factors to a larger appreciation of intrinsic motivations and aspirations of the offender that perpetuate offending behaviour.

The application of GLM in the RNR approach provides probation and correctional officers with a framework to understand the offender's motivation and design alternative pathways for offenders to achieve their primary goods. In Singapore, the integration of the GLM into the RNR paradigm is reflected in the offender's case management plans (Chu et al., 2013). Officers use these plans to organise the rehabilitation goals and to match interventions according to the varying needs of the person to achieve the desired rehabilitation outcomes. For example, recognising the importance of achievement as a source of motivation, and providing opportunities to discover interest areas and excel in them are emphasised during the rehabilitation process. This includes learning a new skill or sport instead of only encouraging offenders to stay away from unhealthy activities and peers.

Approach to Intervention

Offender rehabilitation services recognise the need to scaffold the offender with a strong network of support to sustain their progress and serve as a safety net for an offender when he/she is faced with challenges. As such, partnerships with families remain integral to rehabilitation. While front-line officers play a significant role in facilitating change, volunteers, employers, schools, and other stakeholders are also rallied to support the offender. Offenders participate in various general and offence-specific programmes that are based on cognitive behavioural therapy and motivational interviewing. Development of narratives to facilitate a positive self-identify is also incorporated into programmes (Loh & Cheng, 2021).

Restorative practices were introduced to provide a platform for offenders to resolve conflicts and understand the impact of their actions on others. As an illustration, in 2016, restorative practices were introduced within the Reformative Training Centres, to help youths learn ways to communicate feelings and reflect on how their offending behaviour has impacted others. Restorative circles are facilitated by staff to promote engagement and ensure a fair process for all people involved. Similarly, restorative practices were instituted in the Singapore Boys' Hostel in 2016 to help probationers recognise the impact of their behaviours on others in a communal setting and learn socially acceptable ways to deal with conflict and restore relationships.

Forensic Mental Health

Youths and adults have access to clinical and forensic psychologists and psychiatrists to address mental health issues. Based on general inmate population statistics in 2018, the most common psychiatric conditions diagnosed amongst people in prisons were adjustment disorder, major depressive disorder, and schizophrenia. Inmates with mental health disorders are regularly reviewed by psychiatrists and if they are stable, are housed within the general inmate population and undergo the same rehabilitation pathways as other inmates (Kwek et al., 2023). Inmates requiring intensive psychiatric treatment are housed in the Psychiatric Correctional Unit where psychiatric and psychological care are provided by the Institute of Mental Health. Beyond this, a dedicated unit of clinical psychologists provides psychological consultations to inform policies and operations for inmates with mental health issues and provide intervention to those with significant mental health issues who are at risk of violent and/or sexual reoffending (Kwek et al., 2023).

Youths in Juvenile Rehabilitation Centres and on probation who have mental health issues are referred to the Institute of Mental Health or community mental health services depending on need. These youths are frequently also supported by psychologists from the Ministry of Social and Family Development's Clinical and Forensic Psychology Service. Common treatment modalities employed are Dialectical Behavioural Therapy, Schema Therapy, Acceptance and Commitment Therapy, and Cognitive and Behavioural Therapy.

Role of Families in Offender Rehabilitation

In Singapore, the family is regarded as the building block of society. Family is considered in all rehabilitative measures as part of a holistic approach to breaking cycles of offending. Family factors have been shown to have significant impact on offending and rehabilitation in Singapore. A local study found that dysfunctional family patterns were predictive of recidivism (Chu et al., 2015) and that youths from poor family circumstances had poorer outcomes than their counterparts. Another Singaporean study of protective factors also found that family supervision and involvement in an offender's behaviours and experiences also impacted rehabilitation outcomes. This study noted that youth offenders with high family supervision were 3.47 times more likely to complete their probation orders as compared to youths with low supervision (Li et al., 2018). Other protective factors were also observed to impact outcomes. For instance, connectedness to school or work enhanced outcomes (i.e., booster factor) among those with high family supervision, while self-control among youths served as both a booster factor among those with high levels of supervision and buffered the impact of having low levels of family supervision. These findings further supported Singapore's ongoing focus on strengthening protective factors such as family involvement and supervision throughout rehabilitation processes.

Families are engaged throughout the rehabilitation process, during visitations, family sessions or as part of structured programmes. One example of a structured programme for families is the Functional Family Therapy (FFT). FFT is an intensive family-centric programme that aims to ameliorate behavioural and emotional problems in youths through restoring healthy patterns of interaction within their families. FFT was introduced for probation cases in 2014 and evaluation showed that youths who received FFT were more likely to complete probation than those who did not (Gan et al., 2021). FFT was subsequently made available for high-risk youth offenders served by both the Probation and Community Rehabilitation Service and Youth Residential Service.

While the current initiative shows some success, working with multi-stressed families is a challenging task that impacts a person's rehabilitation and reintegration. A local study noted that youth offenders from criminally involved families and parents who were in constant conflict, or those with parental neglect or poor supervision, were more likely to offend at a younger age and re-offend at a higher and quicker rate (Ministry of Social and Family Development, 2019). Agencies working with offenders from multi-stressed families will have to continue to work with different systems to coordinate and strengthen their approaches and seek creative ways to resolve problems and work within challenging circumstances.

Volunteers and Community Partnerships

Involving the community to support the rehabilitation process remains fundamental in Singapore's rehabilitation approach. Key partners and service providers in the community are partnered to ensure the continuity of support for offenders during and post-order. This includes volunteers and various community agencies coming together to facilitate change. Some of the areas volunteers support offenders include mentoring and be-friending programmes, coaching on life skills such as resume writing and job seeking, supervising younger offenders on community service, and supporting their families. Individuals can also volunteer their time to support agencies to conduct checks at night to ensure offenders abide by their curfews. Volunteers supporting former and current inmates have grown from 200 in 1999 to at least 3,800 (Shanmugam, 2023). Apart from volunteers, Community Service agencies also guide and support probationers when they are required to perform community service. The role of Volunteer Probation Officers is also provided for under the Probation of Offenders Act 1951, complementing Probation Officers in their supervision of offenders.

Education and Vocational Training

Offenders within the community are encouraged to continue with school, seek employment, or attend vocational training to build their skills and improve employability. Case conferences are conducted with schools, offenders, and their significant family members to facilitate reintegration, or to discuss ways to support offenders to adopt positive behaviours and improve their school experience. Offenders in residential facilities are also able to continue their education either within the institution or in public schools during their community supervision phase.

Nation-wide Efforts to Support Reintegration and Rehabilitation

Wider government and non-government initiatives are also undertaken to support rehabilitation and re-integration. One such initiative is the Community Action for the Rehabilitation of Ex-Offenders (CARE) Network. This brings together both government and non-government agencies to support inmates, ex-offenders, and their families. The CARE Network was established in 2000 to coordinate aftercare rehabilitation and reintegration services, and increase community engagement and support for ex-offenders. The CARE network had various initiatives since its establishment; one such community engagement effort was the Yellow Ribbon Project, a national public engagement campaign aimed at changing society's mindset in giving ex-offenders a second chance.

Yellow Ribbon Project

The Yellow Ribbon Project was launched by the former President of Singapore, Mr. S. R. Nathan, in 2004 with the following three 'A's as its aims:

a Raise **Awareness** of the need to give ex-offenders and their families a second chance.
b Generate **Acceptance** of ex-offenders and their families in the community.
c Inspire community **Action** to support the rehabilitation and reintegration of ex-offenders.

Since then, the project has developed into a year-long movement that peaks in September with the Yellow Ribbon Run, which usually sees about 10,000 runners annually, with participation from organisations, ex-offenders and well-wishers. The run has been extremely successful in furthering the cause of ex-offenders and their families with 5,634 employers signed up in Yellow Ribbon Singapore's job portal in 2019 (Yellow Ribbon Singapore, 2019), up from 1,344 in 2004 (Wee, 2020). This job portal matches ex-offenders seeking employment with prospective employers. The Yellow Ribbon Run has since expanded beyond Singapore to other countries like the Czech Republic, Hong Kong and the Philippines.

Besides the run, other activities include a community arts festival, a songwriting competition and a culinary competition, which are diverse platforms that allow inmates and ex-offenders to showcase their talents. The Yellow Ribbon Awards are given out to recognise individuals, organisations and ex-offenders for championing second chances for ex-offenders. Together, the Yellow Ribbon Project highlights that close partnership between the government, community partners and civil society is vital to effect a mindset change and move Singaporeans to give ex-offenders and their families a second chance (Wee, 2020).

Conclusion

Singapore's rehabilitation frameworks and approaches are grounded in theories and data that have been developed and adopted from a wealth of best practices locally and internationally. Over time, Singaporean government departments and local services have ensured that these approaches remained responsive to evolving challenges. The success of its offender management strategies continues to be backed by a strong commitment to quantitative research, evaluation and feedback from practitioners, offenders, and stakeholders, and a coordinated whole of society's response. Singapore values family and community and these underpin rehabilitation efforts and are firmly embedded in success stories and translated into rehabilitation and reintegration approaches. While the outcomes for offender rehabilitation have been promising, there is no room for complacency. Continuous improvements to practice and policies remain vital, also informed by the evolving context in the local and international offender management landscape.

Notes

1 Based on a five-year average of re-offending rates 3 years after completion of probation.
2 Based on the three-year recidivism rate of youths discharged from the Youth Residential Homes in 2017. As the number of youths in the Homes are small (<100), the recidivism rates do appear higher.
3 Based on the two-year recidivism rate of Singaporean and permanent resident offenders released from the Singapore Prison Services' custody in 2020 (Singapore Prison Service, 2023).
4 Based on a five-year average of completion rates of youths discharged from the Guidance Programme between 2017 and 2021.
5 Based on a five-year average of the recidivism rates of offenders discharged from Guidance Programme between 2013 and 2017.
6 In very rare circumstances, the Youth Court may within the prescribed legislative provisions, also order for a youth to be transferred to the Adult Court, to be considered for Reformative Training.
7 The Youth Court typically sits with two advisors from a panel of advisers appointed by the President. They serve to inform and advise the Youth Court on any matter or consideration which may affect the treatment of any child or young person or any order that may be made in respect of any child or young person brought before the Youth Court.

8 Dispositional options under the Youth Court fall under the Children and Young Persons Act 1993. The Act was amended in 2019 to raise the age for youth offenders from below 16 to below 18.
9 All Probation Orders are managed by the Probation and Community Rehabilitation Service (PCRS), Ministry of Social and Family Development (MSF). Apart from supervising offenders on probation, probation officers also assess the suitability of offenders for probation and prepare probation suitability reports for the Court. The Probation of Offenders Act 1951 provides for the probation of offenders in the community.
10 These sentences are provided for under the Criminal Procedure Code 2010.
11 Community Service Orders, are managed by PCRS, MSF and undertaken by Probation Officers who are also appointed as Community Service Officers, under the Criminal Procedure Code.
12 These are managed by the Youth Residential Service, MSF.
13 In very rare circumstances, Youths aged 14 to 16, can be ordered to the Reformative Training Centre, within the prescribed legislative provisions.

References

Chu, C.M., Lee, Y., Zeng, G., Yim, G., Tan, C.Y., Ang, Y., Chin, S., & Ruby, K. (2015). Assessing youth offenders in a non-western context: The predictive validity of the YLS/CMI ratings. *Psychological Assessment*, 27, 1013–1021
Chu, C.M., Ward, T., & Wills, G.M. (2013). *Practising the Good Lives Model (GLM): Understanding penal practice*. Routledge
Gan, D.Z.Q., Zhou, Y., Abdul Wahab, N.R., Ruby, K., & Hoo, E. (2021). Effectiveness of functional family therapy in a non-western context: Findings from a randomized-controlled evaluation of youth offenders in Singapore. *Family Process*, 60(4), 1170–1184. 10.1111/famp.12630
Kaur, J., Addison, J., & To, W. (2016). Assessing the validity of the LS/CMI in Singapore. Manuscript submitted for publication
Kwek, B.S., Zain, R.M., Tay, G., & Yeung, J. (2023). Working with offenders with mental health issues. In *Correctional Rehabilitation and Psychological Interventions in Singapore: Practitioner's experiences in Singapore Prison Service* (pp. 199–215). Singapore: World Scientific. 10.1142/9789811267369_0010
Li, D., Chu, C.M., Xu, X., Zeng, G., & Ruby, K. (2018). Risk and protective factors for probation success among youth offenders in Singapore. *Youth Violence and Juvenile Justice*, 17(2), 194–213. 10.1177/1541204018778887
Loh, E., & Cheng, X.L. (2021). Introduction to correctional rehabilitation in Singapore Prison Service. In *Correctional Rehabilitation and Psychological Interventions in Singapore: Practitioner's experiences in Singapore Prison Service* (pp. 3–19). Singapore: World Scientific. 10.1142/9789811267369_0001
Ministry of Social and Family Development. (2019). Probation Service's Annual Report 2019: Retrieved from: https://www.msf.gov.sg/research-and-data/Research-and-Data-Series/Pages/default.aspx
Shanmugam, K. (2023). In *Correctional Rehabilitation and Psychological Interventions in Singapore: Practitioners' Experiences in Singapore Prison Service* (pp. v–vi). Foreward, Singapore: World Scientific

Singapore Prison Service. (2023, February 9). *SPS Annual Statistics Release for 2022*. https://www.sps.gov.sg/resource/media-releases/sps-annual-statistics-release-for-2022/

The Economist Intelligence Unit. (2021). Safe Cities Index. Safe Cities Index 2021 – Home (economist.com). Retrieved from: https://safecities.economist.com/#:~:text=What%20are%20the%20top%20ranking,%2C%20Tokyo%2C%20 in%20that%20order

Thevathasan, T., & Singh, K.P. (2023). Working with offenders: An overview. In *Correctional Rehabilitation and Pscychological Interventions in Singapore: Practitioner's experiences in Singapore Prison Service* (pp. 37–52), Singapore: World Scientific. 10.1142/9789811267369_0003

Ward, T., & Brown, M. (2004). The good lives model and conceptual issues in offender rehabilitation. *Psychology, Crime & Law*, *10*(3), 243–257. 10.1080/10683160410001662744

Wee, M. (2020). *The Yellow Ribbon Project Singapore: Reaching out and touching a nation*. UNAFEI Public Lecture Series. https://www.unafei.or.jp/english/activities/lecture2020.html

Yellow Ribbon Singapore (2019), *Beyond Second Chances*, Annual Report 2019. http://www.yellowribbon.gov.sg/docs/default-source/module/annual-reportfiles/ea3a4672-f364-476a-83af-891918d2eb2a.pdf

11

FORENSIC REHABILITATION AND PROCESSES IN THAILAND

Weerapong Sanmontree and Apichat Saengsin

Introduction

Thailand is situated in Southeast Asia at the centre of the Indochinese Peninsula. It spans 513,120 square kilometres, with a population of almost 70 million. Thailand borders Myanmar and Laos to the north and Laos and Cambodia to the east. The south is bordered by the Gulf of Thailand and Malaysia, and to the west is the Andaman Sea and Myanmar. The historical name of Thailand is Siam and its official name is The Kingdom of Thailand. The capital and largest city is Bangkok.

Buddhism is Thailand's dominant religion and approximately 95% of Thais identify as Buddhist. There is complete freedom of worship in Thailand with Christianity, Hinduism, Islam, and Sikhism all freely practiced. From the past to present, Buddhism has unified all Thai Buddhists mentally and spiritually, and hence Thai temples have served as a centre for Thai people from a wide range of backgrounds. Temples have also functioned as schools, orphanages, meeting halls, theatres, and crematoriums. Buddhism encourages respect for every person, and non-maleficence (do no harm to others). Buddhism has strongly influenced Thai lifestyle, traditions, mannerisms, and characters.

The institution of the monarchy in Thailand is unique. It has more than 700 years of history and maintains its relevance in contemporary Thai society. The institution is deeply respected by Thais, and functions as a guiding light and unifying force for the country. It also serves as a focal point that brings together people from a wide variety of backgrounds and shades of political thought and provides them with a strong awareness of

DOI: 10.4324/9781003360919-14

TABLE 11.1 Prisoners Classified by Crimes

Crimes	Male	Female	Total	Percentage
Property related crimes	10,505	2,155	12,660	6.01
Drug/Volatile Substances Act	156,144	21,021	177,165	84.11
Death-related crimes	9,464	286	9,750	4.63
Body-related crimes	930	26	956	0.45
Sexual crimes	5,405	162	5,567	2.64
Threats to the public	40	2	42	0.02
Other crimes (e.g., deforestation, gambling, guns, immigrants and light punishments)	3,961	526	4,487	2.13
Total	186,449	24,178	210,627	100.00

being Thai. Thailand is a constitutional monarchy with a democratic government. The Thai monarch reigns but does not rule the country. Thai kings are above politics whilst continuing to contribute to the development of the Thai kingdom as well as the well-being of Thai people.

Crime in Thailand

In Thailand, criminal behaviour is regarded as a social threat. Personal crimes, which threaten the lives and well-being of other people (e.g., acts of physical violence including murder, sexual assault) and public policy-related crimes, widely affect society. Imprisonment is regarded as necessary to punish criminals, to incapacitate by preventing known offenders from committing further criminal acts – thereby temporarily enhancing community safety and deterring other people from committing similar crimes. The number of people imprisoned in Thailand and their criminal offences, as classified by the Department of Corrections (2022) is shown in Table 11.1.

As can be seen from Table 11.1, most crimes committed by people in custody in Thailand concern illegal drug use (84.11%). Therapeutic responses for these people have been the focus of recent developments in Thailand's criminal justice system. Accordingly, the concept of "decriminalisation" for people in prison who are drug dependent and who have been convicted for drug-related crimes where the quantity of drugs involved is small, may receive a therapeutic response (e.g., in-custody or in the community) rather than a simple punishment-oriented sentence. If the quantity of drugs found on the person is higher than that specified by law, then the person would be considered the owner of the substance, somebody involved in distribution or sale of drugs, and therefore, they would be imprisoned. It is broadly accepted that a therapeutic response in addition to more formal legal sanctions, including incapacitation and punishment, has benefits not only for individual prisoners but also for society more generally.

Moreover, Thailand has recently changed the methods for controlling some previously illicit substances. For example, the revised Narcotics Act (No. 8) B.E. 2564 (2021), removed Kratom, a psychoactive plant with opiod-like characteristics, from the list of prohibited substances, partly on the basis that its consumption is part of traditional Thai cultural norms. Following the enactment of the Act and public registration, Kratom was classified as a medical and household herb and more than 12,000 people who had been convicted for Kratom-related offences were granted amnesty. Furthermore, in 2022, Thailand became the first country in Asia to decriminalise cannabis. Thailand's Health Minister and Deputy Prime Minister Anutin Charnvirakul argued that decriminalisation would help reduce poverty among rural farmers.

For crimes other than those involving drugs, punishment and incapacitation, as well as rehabilitation determine sentencing. Various behavioural therapies and rehabilitation programmes seek to reform prisoners, reducing their propensity for criminal behaviour and preparing people to "walk on the right paths and be good people in society". According to the reports of the Department of Corrections (2022) and the Bureau of Rehabilitation, Department of Corrections (2022), rehabilitation programmes seek to help change the physical, mental, and social capabilities and functioning of people in custody.

Carceral settings in Thailand include prisons, penitentiaries, houses of relegation and confinement, and detention centres. Houses of confinement are used to detain people serving sentences for three months or less whereas habitual offenders are detained in a house of relegation, according to the Habitual Criminal Relegation Act. Thailand has 143 prisons and people are sent to particular prisons with consideration to gender, a prisoner's status, security level, and prison characteristics. Thai prisons can be divided into the following four categories:

- A central prison is a prison that normally accepts convicted people. Currently, there are 34 central prisons, with two having the power to detain inmates serving sentences of 15 years or more and those on death penalty sentences: Bang Kwang Central Prison and Klong Prem Central Prison.
- Provincial prisons are those with detention powers for inmates sentenced to imprisonment not exceeding 15 years, except for Trang Provincial Prison which has the power to detain inmates sentenced to imprisonment not exceeding 25 years. There are currently 49 provincial prisons.

- Special prisons accept similar people to a provincial prison but exist in areas where there is no provincial prison. Special prisons may detain people serving a term of imprisonment of not more than seven years (two prisons) or 15 years (28 prisons). Currently, there are 30 special prisons.
- District prisons are provincial prisons with detention powers for people serving prison sentences of ten years to not more than 15 years. Currently, there are 26 district prisons.

Many prisons in Thailand hold men and women, who are segregated in different parts of the prison. There are a small number of prisons (eight) exclusively for women. Women comprise 11.6% of the Thai prison population.

Rehabilitation Programmes for People in Prisons

There has been little adoption of novel Western practices and models for offender rehabilitation (e.g., Risk-Need-Responsivity and Good Lives Models) in Thailand. Rehabilitation approaches tend to focus on education and employment. Some rehabilitation programmes are designed for people who have committed certain offences, for example, people who sell drugs, people convicted of sexual or violent offences, or those who have caused death. Prisoners' risks and needs are evaluated by a multidisciplinary committee that selects which rehabilitation programme is suitable for the prisoner. There is no systematic use of structured risk assessment instruments to determine the intensity of treatment or to assist placement or release-decision making. Some people on parole will be monitored with electronic monitoring bangles in order to monitor their behaviour and to prevent parole violations. Rehabilitation programmes for prisoners with mental illness receive specific rehabilitation programmes based on the Bio-Psycho-Social Model, designed by multidisciplinary teams working in the forensic psychiatric field.

Projects under the Royal Guidelines

Several projects are described as examples of Thailand's prisoner rehabilitation practice.

1 *The Corrections Project of Sharing Happiness and Doing Good Things for the Country, Religions and King:* This project, according to the intention of King Rama X, focuses on helping people in prison access medical and health services, including mental health services. In 2020

His Majesty King Rama X donated 128 million baht (approximately USD4,000,000) for the purchase of medical equipment and supplies to help improve medical care for people in prison. The latest donation is earmarked for the second phase of the Ratchathan Pansuk (Corrections Department Sharing Happiness) project for 19 prisons and the hospitals which provide health care for these prisons.

Currently, mental health services for people in prison are limited. Mental health services in prison include periodic screening for five mental health conditions: depression, suicide, psychosis, substance abuse, alcohol withdrawal syndromes. There is only one forensic psychiatric hospital – Galya Rajanagarindra Institute of Forensic Psychiatry, which provides forensic mental health services for another 17 psychiatric hospitals across Thailand.

2 *The King Rama X's Khok Nong Na Royal Project of Kindness and Hopes, the Department of Corrections:* This project applies King Rama IX's philosophy of sufficiency economy[1] to train people in prison to learn about farming so that they can rely on themselves and use the knowledge they obtain to help themselves and others. Thailand is an agricultural country, and many prisoners have experience working in agricultural occupations. Accordingly, there are programs in prison to assist people to develop skills to return to agricultural employment after being released from prison. This particular program aims to focus prisoners on adjusting their thoughts, developing discipline, and applying the program's principles to solve real-life problems. Participants who are in the pre-release phase of their sentence have been given a Royal Pardon. Since its commencement, 33,928 prisoners have received training; 19,962 (58.84%) have found employment following release, and only 2.2% have recidivated according to the Bureau of Rehabilitation, Department of Corrections (2022).

3 The *Library Project with Intelligence* is a project supported by Princess Maha Chakri Sirindhorn. It is the Princesses hope that all Thai people will have access to education, to be literate and to be interested in reading. People in prison are considered vulnerable and underprivileged and are included in this remit since many have not had educational opportunities in the community earlier in their lives. The aim of the project is to encourage people to read, and to have the opportunity to gain knowledge from reading. Libraries in participating prisons are required to have at least 3,000 books and the proportion of books by type is expected to be: "professional" books (30%), books on "religion or morality" (20%), entertainment books (20%), documentary or general academic books (15%) and books on the law and criminal justice system (15%).

4 The *Encouragement Project,* an idea of Princess Bajrakitiyaba Narendira Debyavati, is focused on improving the living conditions of females in prison with particular attention given to women who are pregnant and to prisoners' children. This initiative is designed to bring Thailand's prisons in line with the standards for the treatment of female prisoners under the Bangkok Rules and the United Nations Rules for the Treatment of Women Prisoners and Non-custodial Measures for Women Offenders. In addition to supporting females in prison to have satisfactory living conditions, the project also provides female prisoners with educational and vocational training programmes.

5 The *TO BE NUMBER ONE* Project of Princess Ubolratana Rakalanya applies the concept of peer support and cooperation with the Department of Corrections, Ministry of Justice and the Department of Mental Health, Ministry of Public Health in order to prevent prisoners from returning to drug use through various social activities and annual contests. Little information on these activities is publicly available and there has been no formal evaluation.

Religious Projects

1 The *Prisoners' Mind Improvement Project,* known as "the Sakkhasasamathi Course" is run according to the guidelines of Phra Phrommongkolyan (Luang Phor Wiriyang Sirintharo) (Nutchanart Plodhuang, 2017). According to Nutchanart Plodhuang (2017) this is a form of therapy involving a meditation course lasting 20 days. It is designed to "balance the prisoners' mental state", helping them to adjust their attitude as well as to help focus on working and living happily, ultimately leading to external behaviour change. Evaluations have revealed positive impacts for people who participate in this course, showing increased control over emotions and behaviours and in some cases, reducing the risk of recidivism. Phra Thamnu Chaiyasrisa and Jomdet Trimek (2021) reported that prisoners who had participated in the course thought the meditations were relevant and helpful and that following completion of the programme their mental state and life in general was improved.

2 The *Balinese Language Course* is a project supported by Princess Maha Chakri Sirindhorn. This programme provides opportunities for people in prison to study Buddha's teachings, which can be used to adjust their thoughts, behaviours and ways of living.

3 The *Phatcharatham Project* under the Encouragement Project of Princess Bajrakitiyaba Narendira Debyavati is a six-month course

offered in most prisons that seeks to "change prisoners" minds' by encouraging self-reliance through Buddha's teachings as well as adjusting the behaviours of people who have offended in order to prepare them for release. Speakers with knowledge and skills of Buddhism and Buddhist laws as well as the officers of the Phatcharatham Project are invited into the prisons to teach this course.

4 The *Trainings and Lectures about Religious Teachings Project* is led by Buddhist, Christian, Islamic, and other religious leaders. Although Buddhism is the national religion, the Department of Corrections coordinates the involvement of local religious leaders around the prisons to facilitate lectures about religious teachings to provide guidelines for living in a prosocial manner.

Educational and Occupational Development Projects

The aim of educational and occupational development projects is to develop knowledge and skills for people in prison. Certificates are provided for successful completion. The trainees' occupational skills inside and outside the prisons are developed by cooperating with the public and private sectors. In general, Thai society is supportive of the rehabilitation of people who have offended. These projects consider the potential of people in prison as well as their physical and mental impediments to determine expectations about working hours. The main purpose of these programmes is to provide occupation and to develop skills that can assist people in prison secure employment following release from custody. Occupational skills training in prisons involves cooperation between the Department of Corrections and private-sector employers. Programmes include work in industry, service centres, as well as offline and online shops.

Community Disposal

Thailand's penal code allows for alternatives to incarceration, including:

1 *Probation:* If the offence is punishable by imprisonment and the court imposes a term of imprisonment not to exceed five years and if the following conditions are met then the court may consider postponing or delaying the imposition of the sentence or punishment and substitute probationary measures. Requisite conditions include: the person has not been imprisoned before, or, a person has previously been imprisoned for an offense committed through negligence or a

petty offence, or for a term of imprisonment not exceeding six months, and, having served imprisonment before, but having been released from imprisonment more than five years previously, and then committing another crime. The latter offense is an offence committed through negligence or a misdemeanour.

The following conditions may be imposed during probation:

- Report to the probation officer periodically and arrange for community service.
- Participate in employment.
- Refrain from association with criminal peers, or engage in any other behaviour that may lead to the same misconduct again. Seek treatment for drug addiction, physical or mental impairment, or other mental health problems.
- Receive training at the place and time specified by the court.
- It is forbidden to leave the premises or enter any place during the time specified by the court. Electronic-monitoring devices may be used, or travel restrictions may be imposed.
- As agreed between the offender and the injured party, the offender must compensate the injured party and compensate for the damage done to damaged property and environment
- Other conditions deemed necessary by the court to rehabilitate, or prevent the offender from committing offences again.

2 *Entering drug rehabilitation in accordance with the law:* If the defendant has been charged with a drug-related crime and if they are not considered a drug dealer, he or she is eligible for drug treatment instead of being incarcerated. There is a subcommittee on drug addict rehabilitation responsible for recommending therapeutic interventions and reviewing treatment progress.

3 Receive mental health treatment if the offending was caused by mental illness and the offender cannot be held accountable or compelled to change, or if the reintegration of the person is regarded as too risky for release without treatment. The court may consider detaining the offender in a hospital for treatment until the patient does not pose a risk to himself/ herself and the public. A patient that is discharged from the hospital can resume living in the community. There will be additional follow-up care for patients to prevent the recurrence of mental health conditions.

Forensic Mental Health Processes in Thailand

Forensic mental health processes can be categorised into three phases:

Pre-Trial

If it is suspected by police officers or the courts that a person who has been charged with a criminal offence may have a mental illness, the person will be referred for assessment according to Section 14 (2478) of the Criminal Code, which states that "during investigations or considerations, if there are reasons to believe that suspects or defendants are psychotic and unable to defend themselves, the investigation officers or courts may order physicians to assess the individuals and give a medical opinion". In the case that the investigation officers or courts consider that the suspects or defendant is unable to contribute meaningfully to their defence, then the investigations will be halted until the person is treated and able to contribute meaningfully. The investigation officers or courts have the authority to refer the individuals to a psychiatric hospital for treatment. In cases when the courts halt the legal process, the courts may nullify the cases temporarily.

Trial

The Criminal code Section 65 (1956) states that "Whenever any person commits an offence at the time of not being able to appreciate the nature, or illegality of his act or not being able to control himself on account of defective mind, mental disease or mental infirmity" then the person should not be punished. However, if the person is considered "partially able to appreciate the nature or illegality of his act, or is still partially able to control himself, such person shall be punished for such offence, but the court may inflict less punishment to any extent than that provided by the law for such offence".

Offenders with mental illness are exempted from punishment because punishment does not offer any advantage in terms of behaviour modification (rehabilitation) or prevent other people from emulating their behaviour (general deterrence). However, it does not mean that the mentally ill person will always be exempt from punishment; this is determined by the severity of the mental health problems and the relationship between the illness and the person's criminal actions. If they suffer from a severe enough mental disorder leading to being unable to appreciate the nature of their acts or unable to control themselves, they will be exempted from punishment. Nevertheless, if they suffer from some degree of mental illness leading to being partially able to appreciate the nature of their acts or control themselves, they will still be punished, but the court may administer less punishment to any extent than that provided by the law. Similarly, if the person is able to appreciate the nature of their acts or control themselves, they will receive the same punishment as an individual without mental illness. Hence, the forensic psychiatric assessment aims to answer two questions: did the person suffer from mental illness at the time of committing the crime, and were they unable to appreciate the nature of their acts or control themselves?

Post-Trial

According to the Criminal Code, patients are not punished if they commit crimes because of mental illness. Section 48 of the Criminal Code (1956) authorises the courts to transfer patients for treatment: "if the courts consider that releasing the individuals with the psychotic or mental disorders being not punished or being punished less severely under the Section 65 will be dangerous for people, the courts can give orders to send them to hospitals at any time and the orders can be cancelled at any time". There is only one forensic psychiatric hospital in Thailand – the Galva Rajanagarindra Institute of Forensic Psychiatry. There are an additional 17 psychiatric hospitals across Thailand, which are overseen by the Department of Mental Health, Ministry of Public Health. The Galya Rajanagarindra Institute provides a forensic mental health service for those 17 hospitals when they admit forensic psychiatric patients, as well as general psychiatric patients with forensic issues.

Treating individuals with mental disorders is not only beneficial for the patient, but it may also prevent them from reoffending and ultimately, it protects people in the community. Forensic psychiatric patients are detained in hospital until they are no longer deemed to present a risk of harm to others. This is a clinical decision by a multi-disciplinary team; accordingly, the courts will be informed to nullify their detainment orders, so that they can return to their communities. These patients will continue to receive outpatient care and monitoring in the community.

Prisoners with mental disorders may be transferred to hospital for treatment according to Section 246 (1956) of the Civil Code, in view of the following circumstances:

1 The defendants are psychotic.
2 It is suspected that the defendants may die if they are imprisoned.
3 The defendants are pregnant.
4 It has been less than three years after the defendants have given birth, and the defendants have to raise the children. The court will specify the restrictions as well as the necessary monitoring and supervision by the officers.

The rehabilitation and placement plans must be appropriate to the circumstances of the defendants so that they can desist from engaging in further harmful criminal behaviour. For patients with a psychotic illness, imprisonment may be regarded as dangerous for the patient and other prisoners or if there are managemen issues within the prisons if these people are imprisoned. Hence, it is recommended that the patients be treated before they are imprisoned with the general prison population.

Opportunity for Growth and Development in Thailand's Forensic Mental Health Services

There are various areas within Thailand's correctional and forensic mental health services that can be improved. The following are ideas that may help build the capacity and working of the forensic mental health system.

1 Preventing criminal behaviour due to mental illness is essential. Experts and multidisciplinary teams are needed in mental health networks to ensure appropriate levels of professional care, supervision, and treatment.
2 Continuity of treatment is necessary so that patients receive uninterrupted care. Gaps in the transmission of information regarding treatment can result in inconsistent or incomplete treatment. As such, a connected information system is required for the continuity of health services, and ultimately, better outcomes for the patients.
3 Care for psychiatric patients does not end in hospitals or prisons. Forensic psychiatric patients eventually return to the community; they participate in community activities and return to their families. Increasing awareness of pertinent issues within the community, equipping the professional and supporting agencies with the relevant knowledge, as well as providing information for families who are caring for people with mental illness who have offended may assist in bridging the gap in patient care. This is important to create a good environment for the treatment and rehabilitation of patients when they return to their families and communities.
4 Because many forensic psychiatric patients have complex needs in multiple dimensions there is a need to provide care that may extend beyond their involvement within mental health and justice systems to education and employment-related support services.

Note

1 Sufficient Economy is a philosophy based on moderation, prudence, and social immunity, one that uses knowledge and virtue as guidelines in living. Significantly, there must be intelligence and perseverance which will lead to real happiness in leading one's life.

References

Chaiyasrisa, P. T., & Treemek, J. (2021). The Factors of Education and Meditation Trainings in the Sakkhasasamathi Course with the Guidelines of Phra Phrommo gkolyan Wi. (Luang Phot Wiriyang Sirinutro). Related to the Mental Qualities of the Prisoners in the Klong Prem Central Prison. [Paper Presentation], 16th Presentation of the Master Degree Research Results in the Academic Year of 2021, Pathum Thani, Thailand.

Narcotics Act (No. 8) B.E. 2564 (2021). Rett. Legal Affairs Bureau, Office of the Narcotics Control Board, Ministry of Justice. ISBN: 978-616-7777-40-5. Bangkok, Thailand.

Plodhuang, N. (2017). The Sakkhasasamathi Course in Prisons. *Journal of Philosophical Vision*, 22(2), 112–124.

The Act Promulgating the Criminal Procedure Code B.E. 2400. (1956). *Government Gazette*, Volume 73, Chapter 95, Special Issue, 1–123.

The Behavioral Development Division, Department of Corrections. (2022). *Annual Report in 2021.* https://drive.google.com/drive/folders/1EFqlBUl_Jy83WJiyTl0TrYOtxft6n8_r.

The Department of Corrections, Ministry of Justice. (2022). *The Annually Operational Reports of the Public Sector for the Public's in the Fiscal Year of 2021.* https://drive.google.com/file/d/1X_r5kWijxh3H68Ys_4rdKupcMZm2omTN/view

SOUTH ASIA

12

CORRECTIONAL AND FORENSIC MENTAL HEALTH SERVICES IN BANGLADESH

Al Aditya Khan[*]*, Howard Ryland*[*]*, Md. Amir Hussain, and Andrew Forrester*

Bangladesh

Mental Health in Bangladesh

Bangladesh is located in Southern Asia and has a population of 170 million people. It is the most densely populated country in the world, with an average of over 1,000 people per square kilometre. It is classified as a lower-middle income country, with a per capita gross domestic product (GDP) of USD1,855 (for comparison GDP is USD2,100 in India and USD1,285 in Pakistan) (World Bank, 2021). Mental disorders are common in Bangladesh, with an overall prevalence of 6.5% to 31.0% for adults and 13.4% to 22.9% for children (Hossain et al., 2014). The Bangladesh Mental Health Survey 2019 found an overall prevalence of mental disorder in adults of 18.7%, and 12.6% in children aged 7 to 17. Rates in men were 15.7%, in women 21.5%, and the elderly (60 years and over) 28.1%. Rates were similar in urban (18.9%) and rural (18.7%) populations. Mental health care is not prioritised by the government and negative social attitudes towards those with mental illness are commonplace (Hasan et al., 2021).

Bangladesh has an estimated 260 psychiatrists, or approximately 0.16 per 100,000 population, as well as 700 mental health nurses (0.4 per 100,000) and 565 psychologists (0.34 per 100,000). Almost all specialists are concentrated in major urban areas. General nurses trained in mental health are found only at the country's two mental hospitals (Bangladesh WHO Special Initiative for Mental Health Situational Assessment, 2020). There is approximately one physician per 2,000 population, but just one

DOI: 10.4324/9781003360919-16

mental health worker for every 200,000 people. Health expenditure in Bangladesh equates to 1% of GDP, from which only 0.44% is spent on mental health. Although people may have health insurance plans, they often do not cover mental illness (Alam et al., 2021; Hossain et al., 2014).

Bangladesh's new Mental Health Act was ratified in 2018, replacing the decades-old Lunacy Act. The new Act has yet to be fully implemented but has mostly been welcomed as a significant step forward. Some, however, believe that it does not go far enough to protect the human rights of people with mental illness (Karim & Shaikh, 2021). The new Act allows mentally disordered offenders to be involuntarily admitted to hospital for assessment and treatment under the direction of a magistrate, using a "reception order", although there is no specific provision for individuals at other stages of their criminal justice proceedings (e.g., on remand or pretrial, presentence, or post-sentence). Meanwhile, the Prison Act is being revised to increase the emphasis on rehabilitation (Khan et al., 2021), although full details have yet to be provided.

Crime and the Prison System in Bangladesh

Despite increasing urbanisation, about 60% of the Bangladeshi population lives in villages (The World Bank, 2020). The traditional Shalish system is the most used method of dealing with both civil and criminal dispute resolution; 60% to 70% of rural disputes are resolved through this system (Islam, 2009). Institutions implementing formal legal systems (e.g., court and police stations) are scarce in rural areas, and informal criminal justice systems such as the village Shalish often play a significant role in resolving disputes and addressing criminal behaviour. The village arbitration council or Shalish goes back to traditional forms of conflict resolution through mediation; it is not part of the judicial system which was given its present form during the colonial period (Amnesty International, 1993; Hoque & Zarif, 2019)). It has no legal standing but persists as a body that passes informal judgements like a council of elders seeking compromise solutions in local disputes (Hoque & Zarif, 2019). There are no uniform terms of reference for the Shalish, and there is no legislation governing it. Villages are usually close-knit communities, and this can result in a stronger sense of community responsibility and informal mechanisms to monitor and manage criminal behaviour. Local power structures, such as influential families, community leaders (political and non-political) and landlords may influence how crimes are addressed and potentially affect the fairness and transparency of the process. The Amnesty International Report of 1993 highlights several concerns with regard to human rights violations. We are of the view that there may also be a lack of awareness of legal rights and formal legal systems amongst villagers, with resultant reduced access to justice.

Although British rule in the subcontinent ended in 1947, Bangladesh maintains a legal system that was introduced by the British (i.e., Indian Penal Code of 1860). The idea of a fair trial, legal representation and offenders' rights are based on the justice system from that time. However, sentences such as capital punishment, established during colonial British rule, remain (Department of Law University of Dhaka, 2010).

Bangladesh is a democratic country that has faced various political upheavals since its liberation in 1971 and there were periods when the country was ruled by dictators. This has invariably had a significant impact upon the criminal justice system. Bangladesh is a signatory to several human rights treaties and conventions, and there are various international agreements with regard to matters related to the criminal justice system; the country has an obligation to uphold these (National Human Rights Commission, Bangladesh, n.d.). Bangladesh receives international aid and assistance from various governments and international organisations to strengthen its criminal justice system. For example, in Bangladesh, USAID aims to work with public institutions to support human rights, to reduce corruption, increase transparency of government and increase accountability (USAID, 2017). It may be considered that honouring the obligations is important in continuation of the aid and support.

According to Islam et al. (2022) the crimes most reported to police between 2010 and 2019 involved narcotics, while murder, narcotics, smuggling and *dacoity* (described as violent robbery by armed gangs) were identified as the most common offences. Most offences gradually reduced in number over the decade, with a sharp decline in the number of all offences recorded in 2019. The number of murders declined significantly from 3,988 in 2010 to 351 in 2019, with a peak of 4,514 in 2014; smuggling declined from 6,363 in 2010 to 361 in 2019, but peaked at 6,788 in 2014; while dacoity declined from 656 in 2010 to 32 to in 2019. Although Islam et al. (2022) do not offer an explanation for these marked changes in crime rate in 2019, it is possible that the figures represent variations in levels of reporting over the years, rather than an accurate reflection of underlying crime.

During this decade, the number of narcotics-related crimes increased in every region of the country except for Dhaka (the capital) and Chittagong (a South-Eastern division bordering with India and Myanmar and with port access through the Bay of Bengal) where more cases were recorded. The number of narcotics offences increased from 29,344 in 2010 to

112,549 in 2018, then declined to 9,069 in 2019. According to the Department of Prisons (2017), the most common offences amongst people in prison are: Drug carrying and trade (12%), Substance misuse (8%), Burglary and theft (7%), Homicide (6.5%), Offences against women (including those related to dowry and acid throwing) (5%), Arms and explosive related offences (5%), and Robbery (5%) (Department of Prisons, 2017).

As of 2016, Bangladesh had 13 central jails and 55 district jails, with a total of 73,177 prisoners (Department of Prisons, 2017). This is equivalent to 45 prisoners per 100,000 population, which is one of the lowest incarceration rates in the world, similar to Pakistan and India (Baranyi et al., 2019). Despite this, prison occupancy rates are more than double capacity, indicating considerable overcrowding. Around 4% of the prison population is female; there is only one female-only prison, near Dhaka, while other prisons provide separate accommodation for men and women. Most prisoners (approximately 75%) are on remand, which is one of the highest rates in the world. This presents a major problem because many people can wait for years before they are tried (Yesmen, 2022). Sentences can be severe, with 4,905 prisoners of those convicted serving a life sentence and 1,204 under a death sentence. There is under-recognition of mental illness, with only 385 prisoners recorded to be "mentally challenged" and a further 7,667 classified as "addicted" (Department of Prisons, 2017). No data exists regarding prisoners' requirements for transfer to a psychiatric hospital.

Bangladesh has three national Juvenile Development Centres with the capacity to take 300 children; 150 girls and 150 boys respectively. According to the country's Child Act 2013, children under 18 years old should be sent to one of these centres following criminal charges or conviction. Concerns have been raised regarding overcrowding of these Centres (at one point there was 941 boys in the institution with a capacity of 300) and ill-treatment of the children in the Juvenile Detention Centres (Mamun & Zaman, 2020). There have been also concerns about children being incarcerated with adult offenders, in contravention of the law.

In total, 173 prisoners are reported to have died in 2016, with a prison mortality rate that is similar to India. There were 15 deaths between 2002 and 2016 recorded as "unnatural". There were 4,596 prisoners whose illness was recorded as "drug-related", while no data were provided for mental illness. Regarding service provision, one clinical psychology post was funded for the prison estate across the whole country, but it remained vacant as of 2016 (Department of Prisons, 2017).

Legal Status of Rehabilitation in Bangladesh Including International Obligations

Prison conditions are generally poor and overcrowding is common. The need for prisons to act as an institution to rehabilitate offenders is not universally accepted and the public have been reported by some commentators to show little interest in the human rights of offenders (Chowdry, 2014; Yesmen, 2022). The combination of outdated legal frameworks and poor prison environments means that inadequate resources are available to ensure effective rehabilitation and reintegration of individuals back into society. Meanwhile, educational, skills development and income-generation programmes are seldom made available to prisoners. Former prisoners face many barriers when seeking employment in the community, and this is exacerbated by prevailing negative attitudes towards ex-offenders, as a result of which they may struggle to achieve community and family acceptance.

According to a report on the probation service in 2014 by Bangladesh Legal Aid and Service Trust (BLAST) and Penal Reform International (PRI), the Bangladeshi penal system is regulated by the Penal Code 1860, the Prison Act 1894, and the Prisoners Act 1900, all of which were enacted during the British colonial period. There are no sentencing guidelines in place. In practice, sentencing involves imprisonment of two kinds, either *rigorous* or *simple*. The Probation of Offenders Ordinance 1960, also enacted pre-Independence during the Pakistan period, is the principal law governing probation. Post-independence, this was supplemented by the Children Act 1974, recently replaced by the Children Act 2013, which focuses on child offenders, and by the Special Privileges for Convicted Women Act 2006. The report also indicates that Bangladesh has a legal framework for the full exercise of probation. Following independence, the Children Act 1974, and the Children Rules 1976, were enacted, addressing probation in the context of child offenders. This Act was repealed and replaced by the Children Act 2013. It allows the juvenile courts to grant probation to children in conflict with the law irrespective of the offence committed. The Special Privileges for Convicted Women Act 2006 has extended the scope to release women prisoners conditionally under the supervision of a Probation Officer. With respect to probation for adult men, the Probation of Offenders Ordinance 1960 is in effect.

As a member state, Bangladesh also has obligations to follow international instruments to promote alternatives to imprisonment including probation. In this respect, Rule 1.5 of United Nations Standard Minimum Rules for Non-custodial Measures states as follows:

"Member States shall develop non-custodial measures within their legal systems to provide other options, thus reducing the use of imprisonment, and to rationalise criminal justice policies, taking into account the observance of human rights, the requirements of social justice and the rehabilitation needs of the offender".

Although it is enshrined in law, there is no established probation service to oversee the rehabilitation and progress of prisoners after they are released from prison (Chowdry, 2014; Khan et al., 2021). The BLAST and PRI report states that Justice M. Imman Ali of the Appellate Division of the Supreme Court of Bangladesh had reported: "The use of [probation] by our trial Courts is very rare, possibly due to the punitive attitude of the learned Judges which appears to be prevalent across the country".

The report states that a Probation Officer is recruited by the Department of Social Services (DSS) under the Ministry of Social Welfare. It is reported that at that time there were 44 probation officer posts in 64 districts. Though Probation Officers may be appointed by the Government under different laws, in practice they are recruited primarily by the DSS. The presence of the concerned Probation Officer is mandated by the Children Act, 2013 during Children's Court trials.

It is reported that lawyers were generally neither aware of nor interested in the law concerning probation of adults. In this context, individuals who may otherwise be released on probation are sent to prison, with the result that very few convicted individuals are found in the probation system. There is also a lack of administrative and logistic capacity within the Department of Social Services to provide appropriate support to promote the probation system.

The concept of rehabilitation is not explicitly stated in the constitution of the People's Republic of Bangladesh. The Prisons Act specifies the separation of different types of prisoners, such as women, minors and those on remand, and guarantees the provision of clothing to remand prisoners, but contains nothing on rehabilitation. While a new Act governing prisons has been discussed by the government, it has yet to be enacted. A draft Jail Code was reportedly approved in 2008 by the Special Prison Committee, which provides some advancements such as the use of "open prisons" and provision of separate toilet facilities for prisoners. Recommendations of the Jail Reform Commission include alternatives to imprisonment (such as bail, conditional discharge, suspension of sentence, probation, binding-over, fines, community service order, compensation, restitution), and separate, exclusive institutions for juveniles (Yesmen, 2022). To help ensure some improvements within the wider system, the Department of Prisons published a five-year plan which aimed to "Ensure healthy and safe custody of the prisoners through providing rehabilitation training, counselling and after-release follow-up" between 2016 and 2020 (Department of Prisons, 2017).

The Universal Declaration of Human Rights (UDHR) (1948) sets out principles that are relevant for prisoners' rehabilitation under international law, despite not expressly using the term "rehabilitation". Article 10 of the International Covenant on Civil and Political Rights (ICCPR) of 1966 states that "the penitentiary system shall comprise treatment of prisoners, the essential aim of which shall be their reformation and social rehabilitation", creating a mandatory requirement to provide rehabilitation. Bangladesh is a signatory of the ICCPR but has made declarations limiting the application of Article 10 on the grounds of financial constraints and limited logistical support (Yesmen, 2022).

The convention on the Rights of the Children declares that incarcerated minors should be treated in a manner consistent with the promotion of the child's sense of dignity and worth, which reinforces the child's respect for the human rights and fundamental freedoms of others. These sentiments are echoed by the Convention against Torture (1984), Convention on the Rights of the Migrant Workers (1990), and Rome Statutes of International Criminal Court (2011). Bangladesh is a signatory of all of these international instruments and is therefore required to ensure proper rehabilitation of prisoners (Yesmen, 2022).

The "Standard Minimum Rules for the Treatment of Prisoners" are not legally binding, but are highly influential, especially given their promotion by the United Nations (United Nations, 2015). Rule 58 states that the purpose and justification of a sentence of imprisonment is ultimately to protect society against crime. This can only be achieved if the period of imprisonment is used to ensure that upon returning to society the offender is not only willing but able to lead a law-abiding and self-supporting life (Chowdry, 2014).

Recidivism and Rehabilitation in Bangladesh

A huge case backlog in the judicial system, estimated to amount to some two million cases, is seen as the primary contributory factor to the predominance of remand, or pre-trial, prisoners within the prison system in Bangladesh (approx. 50,000 prisoners, constituting around 70% of the prison population: Department of Prisons, 2017). The demand placed on the system by these unsentenced prisoners inevitably limits the resources that are available for rehabilitation. Poverty has been identified as a key causal factor in this backlog, because many remand prisoners do not have the funds to pay for legal representation to progress their cases.

Internationally funded efforts to allow Non-Governmental Organisation paralegals to operate within the system to help identify and assist relevant individuals have been piloted, with some success (Foreign Commonwealth and Development Office, 2022).

There is limited data on recidivism in Bangladesh, although it is considered an important issue, with a recent increase in the rate of return to prison (Yesmen & Mou, 2022). It has been suggested that approaches such as amendment of outdated laws and procedures, increasing family and community support for released prisoners, reducing stigma towards offenders, and improving opportunities for employment may be helpful. The low level of education and poor socio-economic situations of many prisoners and severe delays within the justice system have also been identified as major barriers to rehabilitation.

The primary focus of correctional programmes in Bangladesh has historically been to improve public safety by effectively detaining and supervising offenders. Little thought has been given to rehabilitation. The existing legal framework governing the treatment of prisoners is encapsulated by the Jail Code of 1920, which is now over a century old. The code is based on legislation enacted in the colonial era (Chowdry, 2014). Considerable stigma is attached to imprisonment, which can act as a barrier to reintegration. There is currently no mechanism for removing minor convictions from an individual's record, meaning that even a single night's imprisonment can have detrimental effects on a person's standing in society.

Rehabilitation Programmes within Bangladeshi Prisons

Several skill development programmes are provided inside the country's prisons, with an estimated 11,198 participants (out of 73,177 prisoners) taking part in activities designed to assist with their future reintegration and return to society in 2016 (Department of Prisons, 2017). It has been suggested that these schemes could support prisoners towards earning a living independently on release and being able to live with greater dignity. Activities included handicrafts, weaving, tailoring, ironworking, making paper bags, packets, and brooms, and repairing televisions, radio and watches (Yesmen, 2022).

While there does not appear to be a coordinated approach to rehabilitation, and there is a lack of adherence to internationally recognised rehabilitation models several initiatives have been introduced to support people in prison. The Ministries of Home Affairs, and Law, Justice and Parliamentary Affairs, and the prison directorate have been working for many years providing training, group counselling around drug addiction, and training on life skills through a partnership with German non-governmental organisation, *Gesellschaft für Internationale Zusammenarbeit* and local non-governmental organisations. The programme also aims to develop the knowledge and skills of prison staff on substance misuse and mental health issues. Gesellschaft für Internationale Zusammenarbeit also provides support and follow-up to prisoners after release, to help them find employment and remain abstinent from illicit substances. In response to the COVID-19 pandemic, Gesellschaft für Internationale Zusammenarbeit provided prison staff with basic mental health training, which included stress management, anger management and mindfulness (Khan et al., 2021).

Some institutions, including the Dhaka and Moulvibazar Central Jails, have reported the establishment of income generation, skill development and education programmes for prisoners, including the development of a garment factory, complete with 26 knitting machines in Dhaka. Initiatives to benefit minors in the prison system have focused on the need to keep such prisoners separated from their adult counterparts, to safeguard their educational needs. This has been facilitated by the Children Act 2013, which is meant to conform to the Convention of the Rights of Child (Chowdry, 2014).

Forensic Mental Health in Bangladesh

Bangladesh offers some services for people with mental illness who come in to contact with the criminal justice system. Courts, for example, can refer defendants to psychiatric institutions, and limited forensic mental health inpatient facilities are provided for the most unwell. However, limited psychiatric support is available for those who remain in the criminal justice system – for example, no psychiatrists are based in prisons. Meanwhile, psychosocial interventions in Bangladesh are often unavailable beyond the national psychiatric hospital and national medical teaching hospital (Khan et al., 2021).

Senior psychiatrists describe significant psychiatric morbidity in the prison population in Bangladesh, although no formal prison psychiatric services are provided to meet those needs (Khan et al., 2021). Training in mental health for the prison workforce is limited. There are prison medical officers who can assess and refer individuals with serious psychiatric symptoms, but they will usually have a general bachelor's level qualification in medicine, without specialist training in psychiatry. Essential psychotropic drugs – such as first-generation antipsychotics, lithium, valproic acid, benzodiazepines and amitriptyline – are usually available to prisoners free of charge, while other drugs may be available to purchase. There are medical assistants who are trained as paramedics, but no nurses with specific mental health qualifications work in prisons (Khan et al., 2021).

Currently there are no systematic processes in place to identify and refer those with mental illness to hospital from prison. Therefore, if a member of staff believes that a mental health opinion is required, the person is usually referred informally to a nearby psychiatric hospital for psychiatric assessment. However, this usually only occurs in cases of severe and acute illness when an individual's behaviour is actively disruptive. In Dhaka, prisons can refer inmates to the nearby National Institute of Mental Health Hospital. Elsewhere, similar arrangements for assessment and treatment may exist, as all teaching hospitals have a psychiatry department. In circumstances in which no local teaching hospital is available, mentally disordered prisoners may be transferred to a neighbouring district to access services. In Dhaka, the police can arrange for people with physical or mental health problems to be admitted to a general hospital (Khan et al., 2021). There are separately run hospitals for people with a history of substance misuse, and these hospitals can be asked to provide assessments for prisons or courts. Psychiatrists do not visit prisons to conduct assessments, so police officers will usually escort prisoners from prison to attend psychiatric reviews in hospitals.

Prisoners are evaluated by a medical board, including psychiatrists, who assess them to determine whether they have a major or minor psychiatric disorder (i.e., a secondary care level, or primary care level, mental disorder). In practice, hospital admissions are brief and only for acute cases, but treatment can then be provided within outpatient or inpatient contexts, and prisoners can be transferred to hospital at any point during the criminal justice pathway. Usually, prisoners are returned to prison from hospital as soon as they are established on medication and prescriptions are continued in prison; they may be referred to hospital or outpatient services on release. Male and female prisoners are handled in a similar way as regards the assessment and treatment of mental illness. Defendants may be directly referred by the courts to local psychiatric institutions; however, psychiatric reports are rarely obtained, and although there is usually hardly any gap between the verdict and sentencing, a judge may commute the death penalty for defendants who are severely psychiatrically ill (Khan et al., 2021).

Conclusion

There are significant challenges to offender rehabilitation in Bangladesh. These seem to stem from a lack of resources and logistics, and this results in difficulty meeting the needs of people in prison, particularly those with mental health issues, who are among the most stigmatised people in the population. Incarceration rates are relatively low however this does not necessarily signify a liberal approach towards offenders. There is a huge problem of overcrowding and delays within criminal justice processes. Although the law of the country allows for community sentences and supervision by probation services, in practice these are rarely used, and there is limited tailoring of sentencing options beyond "simple or rigorous" imprisonment.

Rehabilitation approaches are mostly focused on occupational and vocational training schemes that are established in some prisons. There has been no development of psychological approaches to offence-related work to support offenders' rehabilitation and reintegration. Discussions concerning reform of the Prison Act are occurring and this may lead to further development of rehabilitative activities.

There is little information available on the state of sub-populations within the justice system, including children and women and there is significant scope for research in these areas. There are significant gaps in information on general crime trends and recidivism rates, which makes the planning of rehabilitation approaches difficult. Mental health services within the criminal justice system (both in prison and in the community) is another area that is in much need for research and there is scope for significant development.

Note

* **Joint first authors.**

References

Alam, F., Hossain, R., Ahmed, H. U., Alam, M. T., Sakar, M., & Halbreich, U. (2021). Stressors and mental health in Bangladesh: current situation and future hopes. *British Journal of Psychiatry International*, *18*, 91–94.

Amnesty International. (1993). *Bangladesh: taking the law in their own hands: the village salish*.

Baranyi, G., Scholl, C., Fazel, S., Patel, V., Priebe, S., & Mundt, A. P. (2019). Severe mental illness and substance use disorders in prisoners in low-income and middle-income countries: a systematic review and meta-analysis of prevalence studies. *Lancet Global Health*, *7*, e461–e471.

Chowdry, M. (2014). Punishment fails, rehabilitation works. *Dhaka Tribune*.

Convention against Torture and Other Cruel, Inhuman or Degrading Treatment or Punishment (1984). Retrieved from: https://www.ohchr.org/en/instruments-mechanisms/instruments/convention-against-torture-and-other-cruel-inhuman-or-degrading

Department of Law; University of Dhaka (2010). Living under sentence of death.

Department of Prisons. (2017). Prison population statistics. *Dhaka, Bangladesh.*

Foreign Commonwealth and Development Office (2022). *Access to Justice through Paralegal and Restorative Justice Services in Bangladesh.* London, UK: Foreign, Commonwealth and Development Office, UK.

Hasan, M. T., Anwar, T., Christopher, E., Hossain, S., Hossain, M. M., Koly, K. N., Saif-Ur-Rahman, K. M., Ahmed, H. U., Arman, N., & Hossain, S.W., (2021). The current state of mental healthcare in Bangladesh: part 1 – an updated country profile. *British Journal of Psychiatry International, 18*(4), 78–82.

Hoque, M. R., & Zarif, M. M. M. (2019). Traditional Shalish system for rural dispute resolution in Bangladesh: An analytical study of its structure and operational mechanism. *Islamic University Chittagong Studies, 16,* 35–56

Hossain, M. (2012) Bangladesh jails children, report says. *BBC News, South Asia.*

Hossain, M. D., Ahmed, H. U., Choudry, W. A., Niessen, L. W., & Alam, D. S. (2014). Mental disorders in Bangladesh: a systematic review. *BMC Psychiatry, 14,* 216.

International Convention on the Protection of the Rights of All Migrant Workers and Members of Their Families (1990). Retrieved from: https://www.ohchr.org/en/instruments-mechanisms/instruments/international-convention-protection-rights-all-migrant-workers

Islam, Z. (2009). Strengthening state-led rural justice in Bangladesh: views from the bottom. *Dhaka: CCB Foundation.*

Islam, S. S., Haque, S., Miah, S. U., Sarwar, T.B., & Bhowmik, A. (2022). A trend analysis of crimes in Bangladesh. *Proceedings of the 2nd International Conference on Computing Advancements, 501–508.*

Karim, M. E., & Shaikh, S. (2021). Newly enacted mental health law in Bangladesh. *British Journal of Psychiatry International, 18,* 85–87.

Khan, A. A., Ryland, H., Pathan, T., Ahmed, H. U., Hussain, A., & Forrester, A. (2021). Mental health services in the prisons of Bangladesh. *British Journal of Psychiatry International, 18,* 88–91.

Mamun, S., & Zaman, T. (2020). Juvenile development centres or torture cells? *Dhaka Tribune.*

National Human Rights Commission, Bangladesh (n.d.). The International Covenant on Civil and Political Rights: A Study on Bangadesh Compliance.

Rome Statute of the International Criminal Court (2011). *International Criminal Court.* The Hague: The Netherlands.

United Nations. (2015). United Nations Standard Minimum Rules for the Treatment of Prisoners (the Nelson Mandela Rules).

USAID. (2017). Bangladesh: Democracy, Human Rights and Governance.

World bank. (2020). Rural Population (% of Total Population) – Bangladesh.

World Bank. (2021). The World Bank in Bangladesh. World Bank.

World Health Organisation. (2020). Bangladesh WHO special initiative for mental health situational assessment. World Health Organisation.

Yesmen, N. (2022). The state of prison in Bangladesh: disparities between law and practices. *Science, Technology & Public Policy*, 6, 23–38.

Yesmen, N., & Mou, R. (2022). Recidivism of prisoners in Bangladesh: trends and causes. *Scholars International Journal of Law, Crime and Justice*, 5, 80–86.

13

CARE, MANAGEMENT AND REHABILITATION OF OFFENDERS IN INDIA

Bhavika Vajawat, Guru S Gowda, Jaydip Sarkar, and Pratima Murthy

Introduction

Offender rehabilitation is a multidisciplinary field, drawing upon various areas of expertise to assist offenders in reintegrating into society and reducing the likelihood of reoffending (Robinson, 2009a). A range of philosophies and disciplines drive rehabilitation policies and practice in many jurisdictions, reflecting society's position in terms of its willingness and ability to care for and manage this population. Interdisciplinary involvement includes *criminology, sociology* and *social work, psychology* and *psychiatry*. Such interdisciplinary integration reflects the challenging nature of work in this area and the complexity of this population's needs and risks (Robinson, 2009b).

A criminological perspective of offender rehabilitation represents a shift from a punitive, penal-based approach of deterrence and retribution to a community-focused rehabilitative process. Named "restorative justice", this approach focuses on the reparation of harm to society caused by crime (Jeffery 1960; Robinson, 2009b). It contends that offenders can lead pro-social lives through agency, a sense of purpose and meaning in life, and by enhancing capacities for moral reasoning and encouraging offenders to take responsibility for their actions. The incorporation of spiritual and religious elements can contribute to this process (Holmes, 2016). Two notable theoretical frameworks, the risk-need-responsivity (RNR) model and the Good Lives Model (GLM), seemingly disparate in their conceptualisation, are widely regarded as the premier models for guiding offender assessment and treatment. The RNR model encourages the use of

DOI: 10.4324/9781003360919-17

psychometrically valid offender assessment instruments to gauge criminogenic needs and to determine the level of risk (Andrews et al., 1990). The GLM sets itself apart from RNR by its positive, strengths-based, and restorative rehabilitation approach. In addition, GLM hypothesises that enhancing personal fulfilment will lead naturally to reductions in criminogenic needs, whereas RNR posits that criminogenic needs have to be managed and/or treated (Andrews et al., 2011; Ward, 2002a). Some attempts have been made to highlight the overlap between these models, and some have argued that using a combined approach, whereby the RNR model helps identify and address potential risks of reoffending, and GLM helps build resilience and promote positive change, may help achieve optimal outcomes (Maruna, 2003). Much of the evidence gathered through the use of such models in informing offender management programs in prisons has been critical in converting the inherent pessimism of the 1970s, from the notion that "nothing works" in altering criminal thinking and behaviours in offender behaviour programs, to identify a range of intervention principles and practices that helps foster change – the "what works" literature (Cullen & Gendreau, 2001).

General Profile and Crime Trends in India

General Profile of India

India is located in South Asia with a large geographical distribution spread over 28 states and eight union territories. It is the world's largest democracy, with a parliamentary government system and the world's second-most populous country. The population is composed of various ethnic, linguistic, and religious groups. The median age of India's population is around the third decade, and about 65% is below 35, making it a relatively young population. Most of the population identifies as Hindu and other major religions include Islam, Christianity, and Sikhism. India is rapidly urbanising, with over 34% of people living in urban areas. The literacy rate in India is around 77%, and the country has a large and rapidly growing educated middle class. India is a developing country with a wide income gap; about 22% of the population lived below the poverty line in 2011–2012. However, the government has seen significant economic growth in recent years (India at a Glance, GOI).

Prisoner Profile and Crime Trend in India

India has one of the lowest incarceration rates in the world, with an estimated 40 prisoners per 100,000 population. Despite this, India still ranks fourth in the world for the total prisoner population, with

554,034 prisoners held in various prisons as of 2021. Moreover, India's prison population has almost doubled, while the overall population has only increased by about 30% over the last two decades. This suggests India's incarceration rate may be growing at a faster pace than its population.

Most prisons in India are designed to hold men and most prisoners are aged between 18 and 50 years of age. The majority were remand prisoners (77.1%), also called "under-trial" prisoners, followed by convicted prisoners (22.2%) and detenues (0.6%). Detenues are different from remand prisoners and are defined as any persons detained in prison on the orders of the competent authority under relevant preventive laws. Around 1% of the prisoners were citizens of other countries. Over two-thirds were poorly educated; a quarter of all prisoners had no formal education, and another 40.2% did not pass their school finals (Crime in India, 2021; NCRB, 2021). Around 4.1% of the prisoners were women. Notably, the percentage of women was slightly lower than in some Western jurisdictions, but not significantly so (Sarkar & Di Lustro, 2011). Although females are a minority in prison, their specific rehabilitative needs may not be catered to, and this becomes an important consideration while planning rehabilitative measures in prisons.

Prison System in India

India has 1,319 different types of prison institutions, including central, district, sub, women's, borstal, open, and special prisons. Central prisons have a larger capacity, with rehabilitation facilities, and they are used for prisoners sentenced to imprisonment for a long period (more than two years). District prisons serve as the main prisons in those states and union territories of India where no central prisons exist. There is little difference between district prisons and central prisons. Sub prisons are smaller prisons with a well-organised prison set-up, and they play the role of sub-divisional level prisons in India. Women's prisons are designed for women to ensure their safety and protection and to address their specific needs. Borstal schools are institutions designed for young offenders, with a focus on their welfare, care, and rehabilitation. Juveniles in borstal schools receive various kinds of education and vocational training. Open prisons in India are a form of correctional facility that allows inmates to live in a relatively open and unrestricted environment while still being under the supervision of prison authorities. Open prisons are typically located in rural areas, and inmates are expected to engage in farming and other agricultural activities to learn new skills and become self-sufficient.

Special prisons are high-security prisons made for people convicted of violent crimes, including terrorism and insurgency (Understanding Open Prisons in India, 2021). The overall median prison occupancy rate is 130%. Overcrowding in prisons appears to have resulted from various factors such as an increase in the crime rate, an increase in the proportion of remand prisoners awaiting judgement, and a disproportionate increase in the number of prisons compared to offenders. The central prisons hold the highest number of convicted prisoners (66.4%), followed by district prisons (27.8%) and sub prisons (2.0%) (NCRB, 2021).

Prisoner Mental Health

In India, the number of mentally disordered people in prisons increased from 1420 in 2001 to 9180 in 2021, a 646% increase over the last two decades. During this period, the prevalence of mental disorders increased from 0.11% to 1.65% of the prison population (NCRB, 2021). Compared to the overall increase in the prison population, the prevalence of mental illness has increased approximately eightfold. The higher rate of identification of mentally disordered people in prisons over the last decade may be due to the increased emphasis on mental and physical health issues among prisoners. Table 13.1 lists various prison-based studies conducted in India, which show variability in the rates of psychosis.

Prisoner Suicides

Suicide is a complex public health issue. In 2000, the rate of completed suicides in prisons was 6.62 per 100,000, which increased to 27.04 per 100,000 in 2021, an increase of 400% in the last 20 years and 2.5 times higher than in the general population. Between 2017 and 2021, suicides accounted for 7% of all deaths reported in Indian prisons. From 2015 to 2021, India's average prison suicide rate of 24 per 100,000 was comparable to the United States' rate (World Prison Brief, 2023). Lower suicide rates are likely due to open jails, dormitory barracks, and limited access to methods of suicide. Additionally, any deaths in custody are thoroughly investigated by the state (Fazel, 2016; Gowda, 2021).

Hanging is the most common method of suicide in Indian prisons, ranging from 82% to 94.3%, followed by poisoning. This pattern is consistent from 2016 to 2021 and is similar to previous studies in other parts of the world. It is also consistent with the general population's most common method of suicide in India. It is hypothesised that suicides by hanging are more likely when victims are in isolation or segregated cells or when staffing is minimal, such as at night or on weekends

TABLE 13.1 Prison-based Studies

Study	Sample Size	Sampling	Instrument	Total (%)	Substance Use Disorders (%)	SCZ (%)	Psychosis (%)	BPAD (%)	Major Depression (%)	Anxiety Disorder (%)
Math et al. (2011)	5024	Population sampling	MINI-Plus	79.6#	52.01	1.1	2.2	0.6	12.9	2
Goyal et al. (2011)	500	Random sampling	PSE	23.8*	56.4	0.4	2.6	1.2	18	1.2
Kumar and Daria (2013)	118	Random sampling	IPIS	33*	58.1	3.4	6.7	2.5	16.1	6
Ayirolimeethal et al. (2014)	255	Population sampling	MINI-Plus	68.6#	47.1	1.6	6.3	4.		1.6
Joshi et al. (2014)	50	Population sampling	N/A	82#	40	N/A	4	N/A	32	2

BPAD: bipolar affective disorder; IPIS: Indian psychiatric interview schedule; MINI: mini international neuropsychiatric; N/A: not available; PSE: present state examination; SCZ: schizophrenia.

*Prevalence of mental illness excluding substance use; #prevalence of mental illness, including substance use.

(Prison Statistics India, 2021). These risk factors are also consistent with evidence from the UK and Europe (Sarkar, 2011).

Death Row Prisoners in India

India is a capital jurisdiction and still retains the death penalty as a form of extreme punishment for the "rarest of rare" crimes (Bachan Singh vs State of Punjab, 1980). In 2015, there were 325 prisoners on death row, but by 2021, this number had increased to 472 prisoners facing death. The United National Secretary-General (UNSG), in their report on the state of the death penalty in the world, has acknowledged that socio-economically marginalised and vulnerable communities are disproportionately affected and are overrepresented among those sentenced to death. The UNSG also notes that the death penalty is discriminatorily applied against persons with mental or developmental and intellectual disabilities, a sentiment echoed by the UN Special Rapporteur on extreme poverty and human rights (United Nations Economic and Social Council, 2020).

Empirical evidence from India shows that 74.1% of the death row population is economically vulnerable, and more than 76% of the prisoners sentenced to death belong to marginalised communities, including religious minorities. In addition, death row prisoners have experienced significant childhood adversities and deprivation, consistent with the evidence that such adversities are substantial risk factors for a crime later in life. For example, a study found that 82% of prisoners on death row experienced three or more adverse childhood experiences, and 90% had been exposed to traumatic experiences (Surendranath et al., 2016; Misra et al., 2021). According to the Deathworthy report, out of 88 death row prisoners who were interviewed, 51 (62.2%) were diagnosed with at least one mental illness. Major Depressive Disorder, Generalised Anxiety Disorder, and Substance Use Disorder were found to be the most prevalent (Misra et al., 2021).

Interface of Religion, Culture and Crime

India's diverse cultural and religious practices can influence what constitutes an offence and its consequences. There continue to be reports of rare instances of honour killings, caste-based clashes, and unethical justice delivery, often through Khap panchayats. Khap is a group of 84 villages typically composed of influential individuals who settle disputes at the local level. Although deemed illegal by the Supreme Court, they remain popular due to their ability to resolve conflicts and maintain social order with fewer resources and less time than the legal system. Honour killing is the act of committing a crime against someone who is perceived to bring dishonour to the community or society. This is an extremely rare and very sensitive issue and a deep-rooted social problem in India. Some perpetrators involved in these acts have been identified with mental illnesses and psychopathologies surrounding religion. Offending by these people can incite public outrage, leading to harmful actions such as mob lynching.

Historical Aspects of Offender Rehabilitation in India

This section captures longitudinally a series of changes proposed in Indian prisons to meet the needs of the prisoners and uphold the rights of people detained in prison. Several committees have recommended reformative measures over the last century to ensure the welfare of prisoners. These include the Indian Jail Reform Committee (1919–20), Pakwasa Committee (1949), Mahajan Committee (1949), Mulla Committee (1980), Justice V.R. Krishna Iyer Committee (1987), and Under Trial Review Committee (2015). Recommendations made by these committees include improving the conditions of prisons, separating prisoners according to gender, age, and crime, providing education and vocational training to acquire new skills and monetary benefits, centralised prison administration, the use of alternatives to imprisonment, expanding the use of parole, having a separate juvenile justice system, allowing the press and public inside correctional settings to periodically have first-hand information about the prison, providing facilities for women and children, and treating prisoners humanely and with dignity. The Under Trial Review Committee was formed after the Supreme Court in 2015 ordered an improvement in the plight of remand prisoners. This committee evaluates the status of remanded prisoners. It is headed by the District & Sessions Judge with the District Magistrate, Superintendent of Police, Secretary DLSA and Prison Superintendent as members to discuss the clinical and legal details of the patients. Doctors involved in the care of the prisoners are also invited to these weekly meetings and are required to provide an update about the patient.

The Indian government published the Model Prison Manual in 1960, and again in 2016, which is based on recommendations of various committees and commissions. Although it is not mandatory to implement, it provides guidelines for improving prison services. It emphasises the rehabilitation and reintegration of prisoners into society as the primary goal of the prison system, rather than punishment alone. The Supreme Court of India has issued directives that all the prisons in India should comply with the guidelines, and various states have taken measures to implement some of the recommendations. Thus, they have only been partially implemented across different prisons in the country.

Management of Mentally Disordered Offenders

There is a high rate of psychiatric and substance use morbidity amongst the prisoner population in India. There are two settings in which this group is managed – prison services or secure psychiatric (forensic) units in hospitals.

Categories of Mentally Disordered Offenders

Four categories of mentally disordered offenders (prisoners with mental disorders) exist within prison services, three of which are pre-trial and one for people who have been convicted:

a Mentally disordered offenders on remand (under trial prisoner with mental illness)
b Mentally disordered offenders found unfit to plead and stand trial
c Mentally disordered offenders acquitted on the grounds of legal insanity (Section 84 Indian Penal Code) but detained in "safe custody", and
d Convicted Prisoners with mental disorders.

Protection for Prisoners with Mental Illnesses

The Indian Mental Health Care Act (MHCA, 2017), in Chapter IV, has outlined a set of minimum standards (Mental Healthcare (Rights of Persons with Mental Illness) Rules, 2018), for the management of prisoners with mental illnesses. These rules lay out several provisions for the safety and protection of prisoners with mental disorders (Section 100), seek to enhance resources within the prisons (Sections 31 and 103), call for both inspection of prisons by the Mental Health Review Board (MHRB) (Section 82), and for the existence of a medical wing in at least one prison in each state (under section 103). In addition, minimum standards of care now require psychiatric and substance use screening for all individuals on reception and ensure holistic care. This includes the provision of psychiatric medications, psychosocial interventions, rehabilitation and de-addiction services, formulation of aftercare plans, and protocols for dealing with difficult behaviours, including self-harm. It also calls for implementing the National Mental Health Programme and providing dedicated telemedicine services in all centrally administered prisons, availability of a medical doctor, two nurses, four counsellors, and a 20-bed psychiatric facility for every 500 prisoners. The District Mental Health Programme team now provides prison-based services in several districts across India.

Until a decade ago, a fifth category of mentally disordered offenders also existed within prisons: the "non-criminal lunatic". These were non-criminal psychiatric patients who were homeless, vagrant, and considered a public nuisance and perceived risk to the safety of others on account of their presentation and behaviours associated with untreated mental disorders. The previous two iterations of mental health legislation in India, the Mental Health Act 1987 and the Indian Lunacy Act 1912, appeared silent regarding the plight of this group of patients. They were allowed to be detained for no more than 24 hours before a court order authorising further detention and treatment in a place of safety, ideally a registered psychiatric facility. In reality, many such individuals ended up in prisons. Many remained there for long periods, including some who spent their entire lives there (Sarkar & Dutt, 2006).

Prison Psychiatric Service

The state government provides psychiatric services in Indian prisons through the Department of Health and Family Welfare. These services include treatment of mental illnesses and substance use disorders and referral to specialised psychiatric hospitals/forensic psychiatry units if necessary. Although the minimum standards of care in prison were laid down nearly four years ago, the implementation has been sporadic. Broadly, the central prisons, such as Tihar prison, generally have better resources in terms of having full-time psychiatrists, psychologists and social workers. On the other hand, state-administered prisons, especially those with low prisoner numbers, generally depend on visiting psychiatrists from district health services to provide periodic weekly or monthly consultations (under the District Mental Health Programme). Additionally, to bridge this gap and address resource constraints, the government has implemented telemedicine services in some prisons to improve access to psychiatric care for prisoners, and started training prison staff in identifying and managing mental health issues (Agarwal, 2019).

There is a prison referral system wherein mentally ill prisoners are transferred to psychiatric facilities in other prisons or forensic psychiatric unit facilities. They return to the referring prison once the assessment and initiation of treatment have been carried out, with written care plans for their management. The District Mental Health Programme team monitors their further care. Anecdotal evidence from staff working in prisons suggests that prisoners still have unmet needs. A high rate of suicide and suicidal behaviour among prisoners may be a proxy marker of these unmet needs. According to the Deathworthy report, out of 72 death row prisoners who volunteered for an interview about suicidality, 34 (47%) had lifetime suicidal thoughts, and 8 (11%) had lifetime suicidal attempts in prison (Misra et al., 2021). However, there is still a long way to go to ensure that all prisoners in India have access to quality psychiatric and medical services. Ongoing monitoring and evaluation of these services are crucial in meeting prisoners' health and well-being needs. Some of these efforts have led to the reduction of non-criminal mentally ill individuals in prison, mainly due to the advocacy for their rights by various NGOs and efforts of the National Human Rights Commission.

Prison Psychiatric Units in India

Most Indian prisons have a medical ward with a doctor to treat physical illnesses. Some larger prisons, such as Tihar Central and Bengaluru Central prisons, have specialised psychiatric beds. Whilst there is little data on the nature and quality of services delivered in most prisons, the Tihar Medical Services provide comprehensive care to mentally disordered offenders (160 beds), including drug and alcohol services. Additionally, psychiatric emergency services in the Central Prison Hospital are available round the clock in Tihar. Almost 98 medical doctors and 71 nursing staff provide care. As of 2020, 299,532 prisoners received outpatient care, 35,452 received emergency care, and 7,754 received inpatient care (Department of Tihar Prisons, 2020).

In Tihar Central Prison, all admitted prisoners are offered screening assessment upon reception. Those requiring intervention for substance use disorder are managed accordingly in the De-addiction Centre. Available services include detoxification and post-detoxification care such as counselling and rehabilitation. In addition, oral substitution therapy is available. This helps prevent the spread of HIV among injecting drug users. In addition, Non-government organisations provide rehabilitation services, especially "Aasra", "India Vision Foundation", "AIDS Awareness Group", and "Divyajyoti".

Forensic Psychiatric Units in India

Forensic psychiatric units are being established in India to provide care for individuals with mental illness under judicial or police custody. These units are generally attached to tertiary care hospitals in the country. These units are staffed by multidisciplinary teams, including psychiatrists, psychologists, nursing staff, and psychiatric social workers. One example of a large forensic psychiatric centre in India is the National Institute of Mental Health and Neurosciences (NIMHANS) in Bengaluru, an institute of national importance. In the forensic ward at NIMHANS, a specialised team is responsible for assessing, diagnosing, treating, and providing legal opinions to the court (Gowda, 2019). They use various assessment tools to document the ward behaviour of mentally disordered offenders and carry out legal tests such as fitness to stand trial, criminal responsibility concerning the insanity defence, and risk assessment. A number of tests are administered, including the NIMHANS Detailed Workup Proforma for Forensic Psychiatry Patients (NDPFPP), NIMHANS Behavioural Observation Report (to document daily ward observation, fitness to stand trial, risk assessment using the HCR-20 and other relevant assessments (Math, 2015; Gowda, 2019). In India, a single team caters to both treatment and legal aspects for prisoners with mental illness, leading to a "dual role" dilemma. NIMHANS also actively trains all the junior residents (psychiatry trainees) in forensic psychiatry through a compulsory one-month rotation and offers specialisation posts such as Doctorate in Medicine (which is equivalent to speciality training in the United Kingdom) and post-doctoral fellowships in forensic psychiatry.

Fitness to Stand Trial

Every individual is considered fit to stand trial unless proven otherwise in India. When a judge or lawyer believes that a prisoner with mental illness or intellectual disability is not able to understand the legal charges, the nature of the punishment, court proceedings, assist their defence attorney, or behave appropriately in court, they are referred to a psychiatrist for fitness to stand trial assessment. If the psychiatrist certifies that the individual is permanently unfit for trial, they are diverted to a psychiatric hospital to receive treatment or released to the care of their families. The course of action in such scenarios is described in sections 328–335 of the Criminal Procedure Code (Math, 2015; Malathesh, 2020).

The court generally considers various factors, such as the nature of the crime, associated risks of recidivism and availability of family to provide surety to decide whether the offender can safely live in the community or needs to be in safe custody. If deemed safe in the community and the family members are willing to provide surety, the prisoner is handed over to the family. In cases where the family does not provide surety or if the individual is deemed unsafe to live in the community by the court, they are detained in "safe custody". Unfortunately, no defined or dedicated facilities for "safe custody" exist. As a result, may continue to stay in prisons or forensic psychiatry units. Another barrier is that many prisoners with mental illness often commit crimes against their own families, and so their families may be hesitant to have them back. These instances and arrangements arguably violate the individual's autonomy in various ways because the state is not responsible for safeguarding their rights. Community services, such as Assisted Outpatient Treatment and Forensic Assertive Community Treatment, are not available in India. These services could provide crucial support for individuals with mental illness who come in contact with the criminal justice system, helping to reduce recidivism rates and improve the quality of life for those affected.

Criminal Responsibility and Unsoundness of Mind

The assessment of criminal responsibility in India is based on Section 84 of the Indian Penal Code, which states that "Nothing is an offence which is done by a person who, at the time of doing it, because of unsoundness of mind, is incapable of knowing the nature of the act, or that what he is doing is either wrong or contrary to law". The elements of McNaghten's rules are reflected in how the law is worded [M'Naghten's Case: 8 Eng. Rep. 718, 1843]. This section recognises that individuals with mental illness cannot be held responsible for their actions, as they lack rational thinking or guilty intent required for culpability. However, the presence of mental illness alone is insufficient under Section 84 IPC, and other factors must be considered. These include the circumstances surrounding the crime, the mental state of the accused, and their motive. The burden of proof for a defence of unsoundness of mind lies entirely on the accused, and expert evidence from a psychiatrist is required in court. It is worth noting that, unlike in other parts of the world, India does not recognise other mental state defences such as provocation, duress, and diminished responsibility (Sarkar, 2009).

Prisoners in India are generally referred to hospital for mental health evaluations several months or even years after the alleged crime. This delay can pose challenges for the review team due to the absence of reliable informants, and the unavailability of past treatment records and relevant legal documents. Additionally, there are no clear guidelines on how the team should engage with the family and legal counsel during the assessments (Murthy, 2016).

A review published in 2019 estimates that the rate of successful unsoundness of mind defence pleas in Indian high courts is around 18%, compared to the United States, where 25% of these pleas are successful. However, there are only so many instances where such requests are made., Approximately three-quarters of such cases involve homicide as the index offence. The verdict of the lower court, the psychiatrist's opinion, and the presence of documentary evidence of mental illness before the commission of the crime are the most significant factors associated with the success of the unsoundness of mind defence in Indian courts.

Prison Rehabilitation in India

In India, rehabilitation programs for offenders within the prison typically include vocational training, education, and counselling services, determined by the community's resources such as non-government organisations. Some state prisons also have open or community correctional centres allowing low-risk offenders to serve their sentences in a less restrictive environment. In addition, some state prisons offer programs such as drug and alcohol addiction treatment and life skills training. The contemporary strategies in the Indian prison system are discussed below.

Health Services

Prisoners in India are entitled to medical and psychiatric treatment and healthcare services, as per the Indian Constitution and the Prison Act of 1894. Most prison medical departments screen individuals for pre-existing medical and psychiatric conditions at admission. Those requiring higher-level care are treated in collaboration with the state-run Department of Health and Family Welfare.

Health Promotion Measures

Vipassana is a form of meditation first introduced in Tihar Prison in 1993 as part of the reform program. The course typically lasts ten days and is taught by trained Vipassana teachers. It aims to help inmates develop self-awareness, self-control and mental discipline. Inmates learn to observe their thoughts, emotions and physical sensations with an attitude of equanimity, which can help reduce stress and increase inner peace. The Vipassana course is voluntary and open to all inmates; however, the effectiveness of Vipassana intervention has not been tested in the prison population (Chandiramani, 2010).

Education Services

Tihar prisons and other central prisons are designed to provide formal and adult education with the help of government support and non-government organisations. Additionally, computer training is available for inmates through organisations such as the Indira Gandhi National Open University, and the National Institute of Open Schooling.

Additional education and computer training are available in Tihar Prison (Department of Tihar Prisons, 2020). Children of prisoners between three to six years of age are sent to Anganwadi (these are schools for children as part of a national program for all children in the country) near the prison campus. Children of prisoners over six years old are sent to a government school or admitted to residential schools/hostels in collaboration with the Child Welfare Committee and NGOs.

Livelihood and Vocational Rehabilitation

Indian prisons are designed to provide inmates with skills that can be used for employment after their release. Some vocational training programs in Indian prisons include tailoring, welding, carpentry, computer training, agriculture and handicrafts. Vocational training programs in Indian prisons typically partner with government agencies and non-government organisations. These programs are often provided free of charge to inmates and are considered a valuable resource for helping them reintegrate into society. Several prisons have also established manufacturing sites within the prison, such as steel and furniture units (Crime in India, 2021; NCRB, 2021).

Religious and Socio-cultural Rehabilitation in Indian Prisons

In India, religion is essential to many people's lives. Prisons often have facilities for religious worship and spiritual activities to help in their rehabilitation. Religious leaders and faith-based organisations commonly visit prisons to counsel and support prisoners. For example, the Hindu concept of "karma", which refers to the idea that our actions have consequences, both in this life and the next, can be relevant to prisoners. Encouraging prisoners to reflect on their past actions and the consequences of those actions, and to take positive steps in the present, can align with the principles of karma and may be helpful for their rehabilitation. Another relevant Hindu principle is the idea of "dharma", which refers to fulfilling one's duties and responsibilities in life. Encouraging prisoners to take on responsibilities within the prison, such as mentoring other prisoners or participating in vocational training programs, can align with the concept of dharma and provide a sense of purpose and meaning. In addition, Hindu traditions emphasise the importance of service to others and the value of forgiveness. Encouraging prisoners to participate in service projects and forgiveness can align with these principles. It may be helpful for their rehabilitation and reintegration into society. Similarly, religious leaders and faith-based organisations from Islam, Christianity and Jainism involved in spiritual teachings can also promote positive values such as forgiveness, compassion, and non-violence, which can help prisoners develop better attitudes and behaviours. Indian prisons promote creativity, social skills and self-expression. Inmates are involved in art and drama as part of the rehabilitation program.

Empowerment through E-Mulakat in Indian Prisons

To ensure regular contact with family and legal advisors, prison call and "E-Mulakat" (meaning virtual meeting) systems, which are video calling systems, are available in several Indian prisons. There are provisions for sending the wages earned by convicted prisoners to their family members by money order, bank or through visitors (Crime in India, 2021; NCRB, 2021).

Rehabilitation Measures for Special Populations in India

Women and Children

Indian prisons provide exceptional services and facilities for women and children. These include dedicated schools and vocational training centres for children in prison. Additionally, programs and services are provided to assist women with maternal health care and child-care issues. The care of children in conflict with the law is guided by the Juvenile Justice Act 2015 and various amendments to the Act after that. This Act is designed to ensure the psychological well-being, social reintegration and rehabilitation of children in a prison setting. When children between the ages of 16 and 18 stand accused of a heinous crime, mental health professionals are engaged to assess their physical and mental capacity to commit that crime (Snehil, 2020). Mental health services through the "Swatantra Clinic" are provided at NIMHANS for children referred from the juvenile justice system (Rajendra, 2021).

Transgender

The Transgender Persons (Protection of Rights) Act 2019 and its provisions advocate that transgender inmates should be treated with respect and dignity like other inmates and placed in a separate cell if they choose.

Foreign Nationals

Rehabilitation of foreign nationals in Indian prisons involves providing them with the necessary support and resources to help them adjust to their new surroundings, and prepare for their eventual release and return to their home country. Additionally, the Repatriation of Prisoners Act 2003 in India governs the transfer of prisoners between India and other countries. The Act provides a legal framework and enables foreign citizens imprisoned in India to return home. The Act is designed to facilitate the repatriation of prisoners in a timely and efficient manner and to ensure their rights are protected throughout the process (The Repatriation of Prisoner Act, 2003).

Non-governmental Organisations NGO Involved in Prisoner Rehabilitation in India

India's prison-based rehabilitation services rely heavily on Corporate Social Responsibility funds and NGOs. In 2021, 587 non-government organisations worked exclusively for prison reforms, and 202 worked exclusively for women's prison welfare. These non-government organisations provide a wide range of services, including legal aid, vocational training, counselling, and educational programs. Non-government organisations have been instrumental in filling the gaps in the prison system by providing services that the government does not offer. Non-government organisations also play an essential role in advocating for prisoners' rights and pushing for prison system reforms. They raise public awareness about prison conditions and the need for rehabilitation services. Non-government organisations also provide valuable feedback to policy makers and suggest reforms that can improve the effectiveness of rehabilitation programs. However, it is essential to note that non-government organisations can face challenges sustaining their services over time. They often rely on donations and grants, which can be unpredictable and may vary from year to year. As a result, non-government organisations continuity can be uncertain, and the quality of these services may vary across different regions.

Critical Observations and Ways Forward

India needs more standardisation and homogeneity in its prison-based interventions, including mental health interventions. Each state runs its programs, and there is considerable variability in the services offered. Rehabilitation programs are primarily offered to convicted prisoners rather than remand prisoners, who comprise the majority of the inmate population, meaning many people are deprived of the opportunity to participate in potentially helpful programs and services. Most incentives for good behaviour only apply to convicted prisoners, which can be detrimental to remand prisoners' rehabilitative progress. Although the facilities enumerated in this chapter reflect several progressive changes in prison care and rehabilitation, the specific interventions for mentally disordered offenders are minimal. Such interventions are essential not just within the prison but also in optimal aftercare for preventing relapse and recidivism. Mentally disordered offenders have more challenges in reintegration due to the dual experience of mental illness and incarceration.

Specific fundamental skills training should be made available across prisons. The model of training a small number inmates to deliver services to other prisoners could be further utilised to counter resource constraints. Liaising with companies and non-government organisations outside the prison and employing and supporting ex-prisoners could overcome stigma-related barriers. Providing support with employment opportunities and ensuring regular contact with family would facilitate re-socialisation and reintegration into the community.

References

Agarwal, P. P., Manjunatha, N., Gowda, G. S., Kumar, M. N. G., Shanthaveeranna, N., Kumar, C. N., & Math, S. B. (2019). Collaborative Tele-Neuropsychiatry Consultation Services for Patients in Central Prisons. *Journal of neurosciences in rural practice*, 10(1), 101–105. 10.4103/jnrp.jnrp_215_18

Andrews, D. A., Bonta, J., & Hoge, R. D. (1990). Classification for Effective Rehabilitation: Rediscovering Psychology. *Criminal Justice and Behavior*, 17(1), 19–52. 10.1177/0093854890017001004

Andrews, D. A., Bonta, J., & Wormith, J. S. (2011). The Risk-Need-Responsivity (RNR) Model: Does Adding the Good Lives Model Contribute to Effective Crime Prevention? *Criminal Justice and Behavior*, 38(7), 735–755. 10.1177/0093854811406356

Ayirolimeethal, A., Ragesh, G., Ramanujam, J. M., & George, B. (2014). Psychiatric Morbidity among Prisoners. *Indian Journal of Psychiatry*, 56(2), 150–153. 10.4103/0019-5545.130495

Bachan Singh vs State of Punjab. (1980). Available at https://indiankanoon.org/doc/307021/

Chandiramani, K., Verma, S. K., Khurana, A, & Pareek, U. (2010). Vipassana and Mental Health in Tihar Jail. Available at https://www.vridhamma.org/research/Vipassana-and-Mental-Health-in-Tihar-Jail.

Crime in India. (2021). National Crime Records Bureau, Govt of India. Available at https://ncrb.gov.in/sites/default/files/CII-2021/CII%202021%20SNAPSHOTS%20STATES.pdf

Cullen, F. T., & Gendreau, P. (2001). From Nothing Works to What Works: Changing Professional Ideology in the 21st Century. *The Prison Journal*, 81(3), 313–338. 10.1177/0032885501081003002

Department of Tihar Prisons. (2020). Available at http://health.delhigovt.nic.in/wps/wcm/connect/lib_centraljail/Central+Jail/Home/About+Us

Fazel, S., Hayes, A. J., & Bartellas, K., et al. (2016). Mental Health of Prisoners: Prevalence, Adverse Outcomes, and Interventions. *The Lancet Psychiatry*, 3, 871–881

Gowda, G. S., Komal, S., Sanjay, T. N., Mishra, S., Kumar, C. N., & Math, S. B. (2019). Sociodemographic, Legal, and Clinical Profiles of Female Forensic Inpatients in Karnataka: A Retrospective Study. *Indian Journal of Psychological Medicine*, 41(2), 138–143. 10.4103/IJPSYM.IJPSYM_152_18

Gowda, G. S., Shadakshari, D., Vajawat, B., Reddi, V. S. K., Math, S. B., & Murthy, P. (2021). Suicide in Indian Prisons. *The Lancet Psychiatry*, 8(8), e19. 10.1016/S2215-0366(21)00233-9

Goyal, S., Gargi, P., Garg, A., Singh, P., & Goyal, S. (2011). Psychiatric Morbidity in Prisoners. *Indian Journal of Psychiatry*, 53(3), 253.

Holmes, C., & Kim-Spoon, J. (2016 Mar). Why Are Religiousness and Spirituality Associated with Externalizing Psychopathology? A Literature Review. *Clinical Child and Family Psychology Review*, 9(1), 1–20. 10.1007/s10567-015-0199-1. PMID: 26662624; PMCID: PMC4755891.

India at a Glance. Available at https://knowindia.india.gov.in/profile/india-at-a-glance.php.

Jeffrey, C. R. (1959-1960) The Historical Development of Criminology. *Journal of Criminal Law and Criminology*, 50, 3. Available at https://scholarlycommons.law.northwestern.edu/cgi/viewcontent.cgi?article=4793&context=jclc.

Joshi, P., Kukreja, S., Desousa, A., Shah, N., & Shrivastava, A. (2014). Psychopathology and Other Contributing Stressful Factors in Female Offenders: An Exploratory Study. *Indian Journal of Forensic Medicine & Toxicology*, 8(2), 149–155.

Konrad, N., & Völlm, B. (2010). Forensic Psychiatry in Helmchen, Helmchen, H., & Sartorius, N. (eds.) *Ethical in Psychiatry–European Contributions* (pp. 363–381). Heidelberg, Germany: Springer Verlag.

Kumar, V., & Daria, U. (2013). Psychiatric Morbidity in Prisoners. *Indian Journal of Psychiatry*, 55(4), 366–370.

Malathesh, B. C., Gowda, G. S., Kumar, C. N., Moirangthem, S., Vinay, B., & Math, S. B. (2020). Fitness to Stand Trial in a Person with Intellectual Developmental Disorder – A Case Report. *Asian Journal of Psychiatry*, 50, 101964. 10.1016/j.ajp.2020.101964

Maruna, S., & LeBel, T. (2003). Welcome Home? Examining the Re-entry Court Concept from a Strengths-based Perspective. *Western Criminology Review*, 4(2) 91–107.

Math, S. B., Kumar, C. N., & Moirangthem, S. (2015). Insanity Defense: Past, Present, and Future. *Indian Journal of Psychological Medicine*, 37(4), 381–387. 10.4103/0253-7176.168559

editor (2011). Mental Health and Substance Use Problems in Prisons: *Local lessons for National Action*. Bangalore: NIMHANS.Math, S. Murthy, P. Parthasarathy, R. Kumar, C. M.

Misra, M., et al. (2021 October). *Deathworthy: A Mental Health Perspective of the Death Penalty, Project 39A [Internet]*. New Delhi: National Law

University, Delhi Press. 171 p. ISBN Number: 978-93-84272-31-9. Available from: https://www.project39a.com/deathworthy. ('Deathworthy').

Murthy, P., Malathesh, B. C., Kumar, C. N., & Math, S. B. (2016). Mental Health and the Law: An Overview and Need to Develop and Strengthen the Discipline of Forensic Psychiatry in India. *Indian Journal of Psychiatry, 58*(Suppl 2), S181–S186. 10.4103/0019-5545.196828

Prison Statistics India Chapters. (2021). National Crime Records Bureau, Govt of India. https://ncrb.gov.in/sites/default/files/PSI-2021/Chapters-2021.html

Rajendra, K. M., Jangam, K. V., Nambiar, P. P., Rehman, A. U., Shylla, D., Ramaswamy, S., & Seshadri, S. P. (2021). Swatantra Clinic: A Descriptive Study on the Specialized Child Mental Health Service for Children in Difficult Circumstances at a Tertiary Care Centre in India. *Asian Journal of Psychiatry, 66*, 102864. 10.1016/j.ajp.2021.102864

Ramamurthy, P., Chathoth, V., & Thilakan, P. (2019). How does India Decide Insanity Pleas? A Review of High Court Judgments in the Past Decade. *Indian Journal of Psychological Medicine, 41*(2), 150–154. 10.4103/IJPSYM.IJPSYM_373_18

Robinson, G., & Crow, I. (2009a). *Introducing Rehabilitation: The Theoretical Context*. SAGE Publications Ltd. 10.4135/9781446216460

Robinson, G., & Crow, I. (2009b). *Rehabilitation in a Historical Context*. SAGE Publications Ltd. 10.4135/9781446216460

Sarkar, J. (2009). Care and Treatment of Mentally Disordered Offenders in India. In Annie Bartlett & Gillian McGauley (eds.), *Forensic Mental Health: Concepts, Systems, and Practice*. Oxford University Press. p. 375.

Sarkar, J. (2011). Short-term Management of Repeated Self-harm in Secure Institutions. *Advances in Psychiatric Treatment, 17*(6), 435–446. 10.1192/apt.bp.110.008045

Sarkar, J., & Di Lustro, M. (2011). Evolution of Secure Services for Women in England. *Advances in Psychiatric Treatment, 17*(5), 323–331. 10.1192/apt.bp.109.007773

Sarkar, J., & Dutt, A. B. (2006). Forensic Psychiatry in India: Time to Wake Up. *The Journal of Forensic Psychiatry & Psychology, 17*(1), 121–130. 10.1080/14789940500445775

Snehil, G., & Sagar, R. (2020). Juvenile Justice System, Juvenile Mental Health, and the Role of MHPs: Challenges and Opportunities. *Indian Journal of Psychological Medicine, 42*(3), 304–310. 10.4103/IJPSYM.IJPSYM_82_20

Surendranath A, Rastogi S, et al. (2016 February) *Death Penalty India Report, Project 39A [Internet]*. New Delhi: National Law University, Delhi Press; 172 p. ISBN: 978-93-84272-06-7. Available from: https://static1.squarespace.com/static/5a843a9a9f07f5ccd61685f3/t/5b68a29a6d2a73cbec1ec89f/1533584200675/Vol.I_Death+Penalty+Report.pdf.

The Juvenile Justice (Care and Protection of Children) Act. (2015). Available From: Https://Cara.Nic.In/PDF/JJ%20act%202015.Pdf

The Mental Healthcare Act. (2017). Available from: https://www.indiacode.nic.in/bitstream/123456789/2249/1/A2017-10.pdf.

The Repatriation of Prisoners Act. (2003). Available at https://legislative.gov.in/sites/default/files/A2003-49.pdf

Understanding Open Prisons in India. Available at https://www.epw.in/engage/article/understanding-open-prisons-india. Last accessed on 1st January 2023.

United Nations Economic and Social Council. (2020 April 17). Capital Punishment and Implementation of the Safeguards Guaranteeing Protection of the Those Facing the Death Penalty [Internet]. 51 p. Report No. E/2020/53. Available from https://documents-dds-ny.un.org/doc/UNDOC/GEN/V20/022/02/PDF/V2002202.pdf?OpenElement

Ward, T. (2002a). Good Lives and the Rehabilitation of Offenders: Promises and Problems. *Aggression and Violent Behavior*, 7, 513–528.

World Prison Brief. Available at https://www.prisonstudies.org/highest-to-lowest/prison-population-total?field_region_taxonomy_tid=All

14

FORENSIC REHABILITATION IN SRI LANKA

Angelo de Alwis and Susitha Mendis

Introduction

Sri Lanka is an island-nation located near the Southern tip of the Indian subcontinent with a population of 22 million people. Close to three-quarters of the population live in rural areas and depend on agriculture for a living. Sri Lanka is a multi-ethnic nation, with Sinhalese, Tamils, and Muslims making up more than 99% of the population. The country's population is relatively young, with about one-fourth being under 15 years and around half of the population being under 30 (World Bank, 2022).

Sri Lanka is a democratic socialist republic governed by a semi-presidential system. The executive branch of the government is the President, the Prime Minister, and the cabinet. The national legislative body of the country is the parliament. Sri Lanka has an independent judiciary consisting of the Supreme Court of Sri Lanka (the highest court in the land), the Court of Appeal, high courts, district courts and magistrate courts. Criminal law and procedure are based on English common law, a legacy of the over 150 years of colonial rule by the British (Nadaraja, 1997).

The crime rate in Sri Lanka has been steadily decreasing since 2009 (World Bank, 2022); the crime index for the country is 41.39 – ranked 83rd in the world. Police statistics suggest the most common crimes are property offences, followed by assault, fraud, and drug-related offences. The Global Organised Crime Index ranks Sri Lanka as a country with low levels of organised crime with a lower criminality score when compared with its neighbouring countries (The Global Initiative Against

DOI: 10.4324/9781003360919-18

Transnational Organized Crime (GIATOC), 2021). In the year 2019, there were 3.48 intentional homicides per 100,000 population, lower than the global average of 6.1 (United Nations Office on Drugs and Crime (UNODC), 2019).

In recent years Sri Lanka has emerged as an important regional hub for international criminal activities such as transshipment of drugs (especially opiates), arms and human trafficking (Sutton & DeSilva-Ranasinghe, 2016). Drugs are smuggled into Sri Lanka for both domestic use and transshipment. Sri Lanka has also attracted some international attention as an origin point, as well as a hub for transit of asylum seekers and economic migrants. The severe economic crisis the country has been facing since 2021 is also suspected to have led to an increase in crime, with the total crimes reported to the police increasing in 2021 and 2022.

Health Services in Sri Lanka

The Government of Sri Lanka is the major provider of healthcare in the country. Sri Lanka spent 3.8% of its GDP in 2021 on health expenditure (both public and private). This is lower than what is spent by lower-middle-income countries but higher than South Asian counterparts. Only 1.5% of the GDP is used for public health spending (UNICEF, 2021).

The Ministry of Health in Sri Lanka provides primary, secondary, and tertiary healthcare that is free of charge to all citizens. The public health system is comprehensive, consisting of public hospitals, dispensaries, follow-up clinics and a community health service that focuses on maternal and child care, vaccination, communicable diseases, and disease prevention. Additionally, private health services are developing and are now available in most cities (Rajapaksa et al., 2021). Due to the COVID-19 pandemic and economic crisis, public health services have been under enormous stress, resulting in the public service experiencing a shortage of drugs, equipment and trained staff (George et al., 2022).

Sri Lanka spends 1.7% of the health budget (around USD 8.5 million) to provide mental health services. This amounts to only USD 0.44 per capita expenditure. Close to three-quarters of this expense is used to maintain large mental health hospitals. Only 0.4% of the health budget is available for mental health promotion. Despite relatively low resources allocated to mental health, Sri Lanka has managed to lower its suicide rate and grow the total number of mental health professionals. According to the World Health Organisation (WHO), in 2020, the burden of mental disorders in the country as measured by disability-adjusted life years is 1,379.4 (per 100,000 population), which is lower than other South Asian countries (WHO, 2022).

The Legal Framework of the Forensic Mental Health System in Sri Lanka

Involuntary treatment of mental illness is regulated by the Mental Diseases Ordinance of Sri Lanka. This ordinance dates to the Lunacy Ordinance of 1873 (De Alwis, 2017). The last amendments to this law were made in 1956. Mental Diseases Ordinance contains provisions related to the admission and treatment of civil as well as forensic patients to mental hospitals. In addition to the Mental Diseases Ordinance, two other statues, the Criminal Procedure Code and the Prison Ordinance contain provisions for the disposal and discharge of forensic patients.

There are three types of forensic patients identified in Sri Lankan law. They include those who have been found of unsound mind and not criminally responsible, those who have been found unable to make their defence at the time of the trial (unfit to stand trial) and mentally ill prisoners needing treatment. The insanity defence is codified in Section 77 of the Penal Code of Sri Lanka. The circumstances in which a person may be found unfit to stand trial is defined in case law and is not in statute (De Alwis, 2014). The Criminal Procedure Code stipulates how offenders acquitted due to insanity and those who have been found unable to make their defence should be disposed. The Mental Health Ordinance and the Prisons Ordinance provide the statutory framework for the transfer and treatment of mentally ill prisoners.

To receive an insanity defence, a defendant must prove on a balance of probabilities that at the time of the offence, by reason of unsoundness of mind, they were incapable of knowing the nature of the act, or that they were doing what is either wrong or contrary to law (Section 77 of the Penal Code). The defence is a modified and expanded version of the M'Naghten rules in English Law (De Alwis, 2019). Chapter 31 of the Criminal Procedure Code stipulates that those found to be not guilty due to reasons of insanity and those who are unfit to stand trial must not be released but be detained in safe custody. The place of safe custody could be in a prison or a secure mental health facility, such as the Forensic Psychiatry Unit in the National Institute of Mental Health. The period of detention is undefined and may easily exceed the amount of time they would have been imprisoned if found guilty (De Alwis, 2014). During detention these forensic patients are periodically reviewed by the Visitor's Board, which is a tribunal made up of representatives from the Ministry of Justice and Health. Additionally, a medical member (a psychiatrist) will provide independent medical opinions about the risks and rehabilitation needs of these forensic patients. The medical opinion is not based on any structured risk assessment but on clinical judgement through the perusal of clinical notes (which may be supplemented by a clinical assessment). The disposal laws in Sri Lanka are based on the first Indian Criminal Procedure Code which was passed over 150 years ago. Since its passage, the laws have remained unchained and are currently in breach of human rights treaties to which the Sri Lankan government is signatory (De Alwis, 2014).

Forensic Mental Health Service in Sri Lanka

Specialised forensic mental health services are relatively new in Sri Lanka. The first board-certified forensic psychiatrist qualified in 2014. Nevertheless, general psychiatrists and general mental health services have been providing forensic mental health services for over a century. Forensic mental health services are available in most districts of the country through general mental health services. These regional services are limited to providing treatment to mentally ill prisoners, providing expert opinions to the court on matters related to fitness to stand trial, and determinations on unsoundness of mind in relation to criminal responsibility. Over the last decade or so, local courts and judicial medical services have been seeking the assistance of mental health services for assessments of victims of torture and drug-dependant individuals. Moreover, parents who are involved in custody disputes are referred to local mental health services for parental capacity assessments. These additional pressures reflect the gradual recognition by judicial services of the value of expert psychiatric opinions. However, these additional demands are being placed on already over-stretched mental health services that are struggling to meet the treatment needs of people with serious mental illness without any extra allocation of resources. Almost all requests for opinions are diverted to medical doctors working in public hospitals with little use of private practitioners, including psychologists. This is likely due to the historical precedent where public health services have always provided reports to courts without a fee.

There is only one dedicated forensic mental health facility to accommodate forensic patients in the country, in Colombo – the Forensic Psychiatry Unit (FPU) of the National Institute of Mental Health (NIMH). Other locked general psychiatry inpatient units across the country may hold forensic patients for short periods of time for treatment or assessments. Additionally, the psychiatry ward in the Welikada Prison Hospital and the prisons accommodate forensic patients.

Forensic Psychiatry Unit (FPU)

The NIMH is the largest of the dedicated mental health hospitals recognised by the Mental Health Ordinance of Sri Lanka to involuntarily detain patients with mental illness. The FPU consists of two locked units, a 103-bed male unit and 24-bed female unit within the NIMH. Occupancy in the male unit is often close to 100% or higher, while the occupancy rate in the female unit is lower at 60–70%. The security levels present in these two units are similar to a medium secure unit in England. The male FPU is located in the upper two floors of a large building which was opened in the 1920s. The top floor is a dormitory-style ward with 100 beds and the lower floor is a dedicated forensic rehabilitation unit. The female FPU is located separately from the male FPU and consists of a ground-level unit comprising a secure section with beds and a lower security section for rehabilitation work.

The FPU is one unit of several general psychiatry units located within the NIMH. Mental health services in each of these units are provided by a multidisciplinary team consisting of a psychiatrist, medical officers of mental health, psychiatry trainees (registrars in psychiatry), psychiatric nurses, mental health attendants and allied health staff consisting of a social worker and an occupational therapist. None of the units employs a psychologist. In addition to the forensic psychiatrist, on average there would be between two and six doctors specialising in psychiatry (registrars and senior registrars as well as medical officers of mental health) providing care for close to 130 forensic patients.

Patient profile in the FPU

All patients in the FPU are forensic patients. Patients in the FPU are those sent by courts for either treatment or assessment. A large portion of the patients are sent through a magistrate's directive (outside of any existing mental health or disposal statute), for treatment prior to their matter being taken up at court. These individuals are placed on remand and transported via the prison's department to the FPU for treatment purposes with the expectation that upon completion of treatment, the person would be well enough to proceed with their legal matter. This group of patients is often unfit to stand trial and in need of acute psychiatric care. There is rapid turnover of this group with court matters being taken up every two weeks. This type of patient comprises close to 40–50% of the FPU population in both male and female units. Another group of patients sent for assessment and treatment is those found to be unfit to stand trial. These forensic patients require treatment to restore their capacity to be able to stand trial. Upon recovery of this capacity a report will inform the judiciary of this and the trial or inquiry will restart. Some patients on the unit are those who have been found NGRI and are being detained under the Criminal Procedure Code. A small portion of mentally unwell convicted prisoners are also transferred to the FPU for treatment.

Forensic rehabilitation at the FPU

The lower floor of the male FPU and the outer less secure area of the female FPU are used as rehabilitation units. The rehabilitation section of the male FPU was opened in 2010. It also coincided with the appointment of an occupational therapist dedicated to the FRU. Prior to that, no rehabilitation occurred other than biological treatment. Several years after the opening of the FRU, a piece of land next to the building in which the FPU is housed was provided for horticultural activities.

Ad hoc religious and supportive counselling measures are occasionally available when students of counselling programs or other religious organisations offer to talk to patients. In the opinion of the authors, while these interventions serve as important supports to forensic patients, they are unlikely to mitigate any of the risk factors that have led to offending. Between ten and 30 patients of the male FPU and almost all the female patients take part in rehabilitation activities daily. The rest of the patients sleep, play board games and engage in unstructured activities. On the male FPU, despite smoking being banned and tobacco products being prohibited, there is a high prevalence of smoking. In the opinion of the authors, there are no other drugs of abuse being used regularly on the male FPU. There is no substance use in the female FPU. This is most likely due to very low prevalence of alcohol, tobacco, and drug use among the female population in Sri Lanka (Randeniya & Weerasooriya, 1989).

Individual needs and functional assessments are performed by the occupational therapist on patients identified as having significant deficits, or those who are willing to participate in rehabilitation. However, it is rare for these functional assessments to be used to tailor a rehabilitation program for an individual patient. Most rehabilitation consists of group activities. Art and craft work groups, music, exercise, and horticulture are regular groups in the unit. Once a week there is a cooking group where the patients prepare themselves lunch. Depending on the availability of trained facilitators, drama groups, relaxation groups and yoga groups are conducted. The land that belongs to the FPU is used once or twice a week to engage in sports activities like cricket, football, and volleyball. The FPU has been running an organic vegetable cultivation over the last several years. Hand-sewn carpets, clothes, and handkerchiefs are sold to purchase equipment to conduct more rehabilitation activities on the unit. Similarly, the harvest of the horticulture project is sold and income reinvested in more rehabilitation activities. A few patients who have been on the unit for a long time have been given a daily wage to act as cleaners. Little to no structured risk assessment is done prior to selecting patients for rehabilitation activities other than to ensure that they are not acutely unwell.

Correctional Services in Sri Lanka

Sri Lanka had close to 22,000 people imprisoned in various correctional facilities at the end of 2021 (Department of Prisons Sri Lanka (DOPSL), 2021). Around 5% of the prison population is female and 0.1% are juveniles (under 18 years). Close to 60 secure locations around the country serve as prisons. All are centrally administered by the Ministry of Justice and Law Reform. There are four prisons for convicted offenders, 18 remand prisons, ten work camps, two open prison camps, three facilities for young offenders and 23 police lock-ups. The prison population in Sri Lanka has significantly increased over the last 20 years (DOPSL, 2021b). The incarceration rate in Sri Lanka is 102 per 100 000 population which is below the average compared to other countries in the Asia Pacific region (World Prison Brief, 2021).

Prisons have always been overcrowded in Sri Lanka (DOPSL, 2021a). At present the prisons in Sri Lanka have the capacity to house only 11,768 people. Thus, the occupancy rate sits close to double its capacity (186.9%). While the occupancy rate is increasing, the funding allocation for food, clothes and rehabilitation has fallen in recent years (DOPSL, 2018). The Sri Lankan government spends close to USD 5.4 million per year for the upkeep of prisoners. This is about USD1 per day per prisoner. Prison overcrowding leads to a neglect of rehabilitation activities (DOPSL, 2021a; HRCSL, 2019).

More than 50% of the prison population is on remand (DOPSL, 2021b). Due to a poorly resourced and overworked judicial system, there are long delays between remand and conviction or acquittal (Ministry of Justice, 2021). The annual performance report of the Ministry of Justice Sri Lanka states that there are 982,793 court cases pending as of June 2021; 90% are at the district and magistrate court level. This problem is further complicated by the fact that Sri Lanka only has 15 judges per one million population (Ministry of Justice, 2021). This has resulted in long delays before a matter can be resolved (Pinto, 2017). Consequently, many people spend long periods of time in remand prisons, with over 5% having spent more than two years on remand (DOPSL, 2021b). Remandees do not have as many opportunities to work or to engage in rehabilitation activities as a convicted prisoner.

Sri Lanka does not have a national sentencing policy or guideline that focuses on offender rehabilitation. In its absence, there is neither a central mechanism to monitor sentencing trends in the country nor a mechanism to ensure uniformity in sentencing. Some argue that this has led to a highly punitive form of sentencing that does not encourage rehabilitation (Wickramasekera, 2017). Close to 95% of those in custody have been sentenced for an imprisonment period of less than two years and close to 75% of receptions to Sri Lankan prisons in 2020 were due to the individual's inability to pay a fine (DOPSL, 2021b). While alternative sentencing strategies exist for such individuals there appears to be some reluctance among judges to use them. Consequently, correctional centres are overcrowded, and prisoners stay for a relatively short period of time (often not enough to engage in rehabilitation activities).

Forensic Rehabilitation in Custodial Environments

Rehabilitation comprises vocational and drug rehabilitation. In addition, opportunities for prisoners to complete formal educational qualifications are also offered in certain prisons. In certain sentences, there is an expectation that the prison will ensure prisoners engages in "hard labour" for a certain number of hours each day as punishment. Forensic patients detained in prisons have opportunities to engage in the various prison-based rehabilitation and work activities.

Like the situation in the FPU, prison-based rehabilitation programmes are not individualised. None of the prisons offer the services of occupational therapists or psychologists to perform needs assessments or functional assessments of prisoners to understand rehabilitation needs. Moreover, apart from the separation of those who are awaiting capital punishment, none of the prisons separate or classify prisoners according to risk. This makes it challenging to offer rehabilitation activities when these may allow access to potentially risky equipment or material.

In addition to correctional staff, prisons employ health staff (including doctors and nurses) as well as rehabilitation staff. However, the number of these staff is inadequate. According to prison statistics, for over 20,000 prisoners, the Department of Prisons has employed just over 150 rehabilitation officers, seven counsellors and about 170 technical-grade vocational instructors (DOPSL, 2021b). The prison study conducted by the Human Rights Commission of Sri Lanka (HRCSL) in 2019 revealed that staff struggled with prison overcrowding, lack of resources and lack of training (HRCSL, 2019). Most of the vocational training opportunities that were found in prison were low-level labouring jobs such as masonry, brick making, and agriculture-based activities that would not help prisoners escape the cycle of poverty. The HRCSL also noted that even these activities took place without any proper technical instructions, often using old and broken equipment.

In addition to rehabilitation opportunities, all prisons offer work opportunities. Work in prison helps prisoners engage in productive activities while incarcerated and to make a small income. The work opportunities in closed prisons are only available inside the prison. However, in open prison camps, prisoners have the option of leaving the prison to be employed in the community and to return to prison at the end of the day. This type of work release program is underutilised despite being popular among the prisoners (HRCSL, 2019). In a closed prison, the work available is diverse. It ranges from relatively light work (helping in an office), to hard labour (cleaning toilets or chopping wood for cooking). Prisoners have little choice in deciding which type of work they do. Depending on a prisoner's criminal history, conduct in prison and reliability, prison officers make the decision as to where a prisoner will work. In open prisons or in work camps the work is often manual, such as cultivation or brick-making. Work conditions are often harsh with little regard to work health and safety. Prisoners complain of having to use outdated and broken equipment that make the work difficult (HRCSL, 2019). Remuneration rates offered to prisoners have not been revised in close to 35 years. The highest a prisoner can make for a full day's work is less than 0.01 USD (2.50 rupees).

A study of 30 convicted prisoners in Welikada prison in 2019 revealed they spent 29.5% of the day engaged in work parties. Prisoners were unhappy due to not having a choice about the type of work they did. Moreover, they did not think prison work prepared them to make a living once released. The study also demonstrated that there was very little choice in recreation other than reading and listening to the radio. Participants only spent 17% of the day on rest and leisure. The study found that the prisoners were deprived of occupational choice and autonomy and that work was for merely passing the time (Gunarathne et al., 2020).

Treatment of Forensic Patients Inside Prison

There are close to 60 doctors and 90 dispensers (i.e., those who have a licence to dispense medication) employed by the Department of Prisons (DOPSL, 2021b). They are responsible for the day-to-day healthcare needs of prison inmates. Most prisons rely on external medical input from the

Ministry of Health, in the form of in-reach clinics, to support their staff to treat prisoners with serious mental illness. These clinics apply an outpatient model of care for serious mental illnesses such as depression, psychosis, and PTSD. When an inmate's conduct is too risky to be managed within a prison environment, they are either moved to FPU in the NIMH or moved to Welikada Prison psychiatry unit.

Welikada Prison Hospital – Psychiatry Ward

Welikada prison hospital is a large hospital in Colombo run by the Department of Prisons, within the Welikada prison complex. In addition to several medical wards, the hospital has a psychiatry ward with capacity for close to 30 patients, but it is often overcrowded. There are only a few beds, and most patients sleep on the floor on mats. There is one permanent medical officer appointed to care for these patients. All patients on this ward are prisoners either from the main Welikada prison or from other prisons. The forensic psychiatrist from the FPU visits this ward once a week. Due to the limited facilities available in this ward, acutely unwell patients are moved to the FPU at the NIMH. No formalised rehabilitation activity is available for this group of patients. For some prisoners, admission to this unit is short, until an acute mental illness settles. But for a significant group of other prisoners, especially for those who are unmanageable in the general prison population by prison authorities, this may be a long period.

Drug Rehabilitation in Forensic Patient Populations

WHO data suggests that Sri Lankan adults (over 15 years) consume 4.1 litres of pure alcohol per capita per year. The prevalence of alcohol use disorder and alcohol dependence is 3.1 and 2.6, respectively. These values are slightly better than the estimated values for the South-East Asia Region (WHO, 2018). Cannabis is the most used illicit drug in Sri Lanka with a prevalence of 1.9% (~300,000 users), and heroin is next, with a prevalence of 0.6% (~45,000 regular users). Nonmedical use of prescription drugs is increasing with 0.15% of total population reporting use. Stimulant use (e.g., methamphetamine and cocaine) has also become problematic over the last several years (National Dangerous Drug Control Board (NDDCB), 2019; Senanayake et al., 2021). This is a concern in prison populations; a study conducted in the Welikada Prison Complex revealed that close to 50% of the population have admitted to lifetime alcohol use disorder and close to 25% admitted to opioid use disorder (Hapangama et al., 2021).

Sri Lankan law allows courts to direct those who have been caught with smaller quantities of illicit drugs to drug treatment and rehabilitation services. This may be done either voluntarily or through a compulsory detention order to a residential rehabilitation facility run by the NDDCB and the Bureau of the Commissioner General of Rehabilitation. The NDDCB runs four treatment centres, in Colombo, Galle, Kandy, and Nittambuwa. These centres are designed to provide rehabilitation for heroin, cannabis and methamphetamine using a mix of pharmacological and psychological treatment. They accept voluntary as well as court-directed admissions. However, they do not provide rehabilitation services to sentenced prisoners. The Bureau of the Commissioner General of Rehabilitation runs one of the largest rehabilitation facilities in Sri Lanka in the North-Central province in Kandakadu. Kandakadu Drug Rehabilitation Centre, along with the Senapura Rehabilitation Centre, provides rehabilitation services for mostly heroin-dependent individuals who have been sent to these facilities by the court in lieu of a sentence to prison. In addition to these centres many prison facilities across the country offer drug rehabilitation services for prisoners. According to data from NDDCB, 1,649 individuals received drug rehabilitation services from these centres in 2020 (Senanayake et al., 2021). Out of this population, 45% have received treatment from the centres managed by the NDDCB and 30% from the Kandakadu Drug Rehabilitation Centre. The prison-based rehabilitation programmes provided services to only 226 individuals.

The 12-month treatment and rehabilitation programme managed by the NDDCB provides their services freely; these include assessment, detoxification treatment, and individual and group counselling. The first two months are residential, followed by a non-residential relapse prevention programme. The residential programme includes various structured and non-structured activities including art and music therapy, horticulture, and exercise. In addition, there is a strong emphasis on religious activities. Family involvement is very much encouraged.

The programme in the Kandakadu Rehabilitation Centre is also a 12-month residential programme with the first six months focussed on formal therapies to address drug use. After completion of the first six months of training, the prisoners are referred to a six-month vocational training programme. The vocational training provides an opportunity for the person to have formal training in carpentry, masonry, plumbing, house wiring amongst other tradecrafts that may be useful in obtaining employment upon leaving the centre.

The treatment programmes used in the above facilities do not fall into a strict treatment model but is a combined approach of the 12-step model, the therapeutic community, pharmacological and psychological treatment. Faith-based activities take centre stage in many of the programmes. Another characteristic feature appears to be the emphasis on the use of the family of the client to support them to access treatment as well as maintain abstinence.

Rehabilitation for Female Prisoners

Female prisoners have been overlooked when resources are being allocated for rehabilitation inside prisons (HRCSL, 2019). Females are detained in separate and segregated sections of the main prisons in Sri Lanka. Prison authorities allow female prisoners to bring infants up to five years of age into prison with them. This introduces unique challenges in the female prison environment. Female prisoners do not have the same opportunities for rehabilitation such as access to industries, education, and vocational rehabilitation as male prisoners. Female prisoners only have access to sewing and upkeep of the premises they live in as a form of rehabilitation activity.

Young Offenders

There are three correctional centres dedicated to young offenders (16–22 years) in Sri Lanka; Pallansena, Watareka, and Thaldena. There are about 300 young people in these centres at any given time. These centres conduct vocational training including instruction in agriculture, carpentry, welding, baking, weaving, etc. In addition, there are structured and unstructured activities that make up the daily routine of these centres including games, exercise and religious activities.

Children in Custody

Child victims, child suspects or child offenders below 16 years of age can be detained in state institutions following a court order. There are 14 remand centres across the various provinces in Sri Lanka for child suspects. Children over the age of 12 years can be detained at these facilities if charged with serious criminal offences. In addition, there are four safe homes (in the Northern and Eastern provinces) that act as transition housing for child victims, witnesses and suspects until the end of a court matter. Certified schools detain children who are convicted under the Children and Young Persons Ordinance for a maximum of three years. There are several certified schools in Sri Lanka; Western province

(Makaola and Ranmuthugala), Southern province (Hikkaduwa), Central province (Keppetipola) and Northern province (Jaffna). These schools are administered by the Department of Probation and Child Care Services. At a census conducted in 2019, there were 745 children between the ages of eight and 16 years in these institutions (Department of Census and Statistics [DCS], 2021). Only 325 of these children were being held as suspects or convicts. The others were child victims (victims of abuse, trafficked and exploited children) or witnesses who had no other place to go, thus had to be placed with offenders (Hettiarachchi et al., 2018).

Residents in remand homes and safe homes have very low educational attainment, with more than half of the children not engaged in any learning activities. This may be due to short turnover time, preventing children from properly engaging in available educational or vocational activities. In contrast, in certified schools where children stay for relatively longer periods, there are more opportunities for education and vocational training. Some programmes allow the participants to complete a vocational training qualification that is recognised nationally – National Vocational Qualifications (NVQ). Some programmes offered in these institutions include sewing and dressmaking, information technology, beauty culture, motor mechanics, electrical technology, carpentry, cookery, horticulture, baking, plumbing, landscaping, Juki machine operator training, metal cutting and welding. In addition to these training programmes many of these institutions have facilities for children to engage in sports, exercise and religious activities. All institutions have library facilities, with some subscribing to daily newspapers and magazines.

Role of Religion in Forensic Rehabilitation in Sri Lanka

In Sri Lanka, religion is an indispensable part of most citizens' lives. Sri Lankan national identity, its politics and social structures are inextricably blended with the state religion, Buddhism. Buddhists believe that everyone will have to suffer for any wrongdoings (including crimes) in their next life, even if they manage to escape justice in this life (Karma). This allows for a certain level of tolerance to those who are being punished by the law and branded as "criminals".

There are many drug rehabilitation centres in the country that are run by religious organisations. Their approach to rehabilitation is heavily informed by the principles of their religion. Every full-moon day of the month is declared a Buddhist Public Holiday by the Sri Lankan Government (Poya days) to commemorate influential events in Buddhism. On Poya days, it would be common for prisons to organise religious activities. These religious ceremonies involve Buddhist clergy chanting prayers (pirith) followed by a sermon about how to live a good life. These ceremonies often involve donations of food and equipment to prisoners from the public. Such acts are popular as they are considered to be of high merit in the afterlife of the donor (Dhanna). In many rehabilitation facilities, religious-based activities form the mainstay of rehabilitation outside their formal programme of rehabilitation. Rehabilitation programmes that are informed by religion include meditation, shramadhanna (voluntary free labour) and aesthetic activities (such as songs and dance) inspired by religion. Some prisoners are pardoned and released by the government on days of religious significance. In 2019, 762 prisoners were pardoned on the Vesak Poya Day in May. It would be quite common for religious figures such as Buddhist monks, priests, and imams to visit prisons to talk to prisoners and to conduct religious activities. These are well-received by most inmates and prison officials. Many participants (of which many are sentenced to life imprisonment) in a religious meditation programme said they participated every time it was offered. They reported that the programme helped them adjust to prison life and to let go of feelings of anger they had towards the prison authorities and society. They reported that they have taken up reading religious texts and have started to practise meditation on their own (Edirisinghe, 2002).

Effect of the COVID Pandemic and the Economic Crisis

The pandemic and the 2021–22 economic crisis have led to political instability as well as fuel and food shortages in Sri Lanka (Central Bank of Sri Lanka [CBSL], 2022; World Food Programme [WFP], 2022). GDP fell in 2022 and is expected to fall in 2023. This economic crisis has been described as the worst the country has faced since it gained independence from the British in 1948. With the government reserves shrinking, the government has put in place restrictions on imports. This will continue to hamper health services that depend on imported medicines. This will also impact the government's ability to invest in new infrastructure and programs for the forensic population.

Forensic Rehabilitation in Sri Lanka: Future Directions

It is the opinion of the authors that to improve forensic mental health services, there are certain problems that need to be resolved in the correctional system. One of the most critical would be to reduce overcrowding. Overcrowding in prison influences the number of admissions received by the FPU and the amount of work that specialised mental health teams can do. Overcrowding is a function of a poorly resourced judiciary, inadequate use of alternate sentencing options and an overloaded court system. Resolving the issue of overcrowding will require a multipronged approach involving increased funding, as well as investing in human resources and education.

We are pleased to note that all specialised psychiatrists have received at least three months of specialised training in forensic psychiatry and are therefore aware of the challenges and opportunities of working with forensic populations. While medical expertise has increased, there has been no increase in other disciplines such as psychology, occupational therapy, or social work. Employment in prisons with mentally unwell offenders continues to be unpopular. In addition, there is a need to invest in recruiting vocational skills training instructors and rehabilitations officers. There needs to be greater investment in infrastructure, equipment and human resources in vocational training opportunities made available to prisoners.

The current economic crisis is forcing many skilled citizens of the country to emigrate from Sri Lanka to find better economic opportunities. There is a risk that it may become difficult to encourage skilled professionals to work in forensic settings. Thus, the Government of Sri Lanka needs to implement short- and long-term measures to improve forensic rehabilitation.

References

Central Bank of Sri Lanka (CBSL). (2022). *CCPI based headline inflation recorded at 64.3% on year-on*. Central Bank of Sri Lanka. https://www.cbsl.gov.lk/en/news/inflation-in-august-2022-ccpi

Criminal Procedure Code Act 15. Chapter 31, Sect. 31 1979. (Sri Lanka). https://www.parliament.lk/uploads/bills/gbills/english/5997.pdf

Department of Census and Statistics (DCS). (2021). *Census of Children in Child Care Institutions 2019*. Department of census and statistics. http://www.statistics.gov.lk/Resource/refference/CensusofChildreninChildCareInstitutions 2019Final

De Alwis, A. (2014). Fitness to plead in Sri Lanka. *Sri Lanka Journal of Psychiatry*, 5(1), 3. 10.4038/sljpsyc.v5i1.6578

De Alwis, L. A. (2019). Historical origins of the insanity defense in Sri Lanka and India. *Sri Lanka Journal of Psychiatry*, 10(2), 4. 10.4038/sljpsyc.v10i2.8211

De Alwis, L. A. P. (2017). Development of civil commitment statutes (laws of involuntary detention and treatment) in Sri Lanka: A historical review. *Medico-Legal Journal of Sri Lanka*, 5(1), 22. 10.4038/mljsl.v5i1.7351

Department of Census and Statistics (DCS). (2021). *Census of children in child care institutions 2019*. Department of census and statistics. http://www. statistics.gov.lk/Resource/refference/CensusofChildreninChildCareInstitutions 2019Final

Department of Prisons Sri Lanka (DOPSL). (2021). *Prison statistics of Sri Lanka 2021*. Department of Prisons Sri Lanka. http://prisons.gov.lk/web/wp-content/ uploads/2021/05/prison-statistics-2021.pdf

DOPSL. (2018). *Performance report 2018*. Department of Prisons Sri Lanka. https://www.parliament.lk/uploads/documents/paperspresented/performance-report-department-of-prison-2018.pdf

DOPSL. (2021a). *Prison overcrowding – Short-mid-long term plan to overcome the challenge*. Department of Prisons Sri Lanka. http://prisons.gov.lk/web/wp-content/uploads/2021/11/prison-overcrowding-overcome-plan.pdf

DOPSL. (2021b). *Prison statistics of Sri Lanka 2021*. Department of Prisons Sri Lanka. http://prisons.gov.lk/web/wp-content/uploads/2021/05/prison-statistics-2021.pdf

Edirisinghe, M. E. (2002). Role of religion in the rehabilitation of offenders. *The International Association of Buddhist Universities (IABU)*.

George, A. S. H., George, A. S., & Baskar, T. (2022). Sri Lanka's economic crisis: A brief overview. *Zenodo*. 10.5281/zenodo.6726553

Gunarathne, G. P., Rodrigo, M. D., & Mendis, T. S. S. (2020). *Occupational engagement in prisons: An evaluation of time-use in Sri Lankan correctional settings*. 13th International Research Conference – General Sir John Kotelawala Defence University. http://192.248.104.6/bitstream/handle/345/2881/pdfresizer. com-pdf-split%2041-45.pdf?sequence=1&isAllowed=y

Hapangama, A., Dasanyake, D. G. B. M. S., Kuruppuarachchi, K. A. L. A., Pathmeswaran, A., & De Silva, H. J. (2021). Substance use disorders and their correlates among inmates in a Sri Lankan prison. *Journal of the Postgraduate Institute of Medicine*, 8(2), 157. 10.4038/jpgim.8334

Hettiarachchi, L. V., Kinner, S. A., Tibble, H., & Borschmann, R. (2018). Self-harm among young people detained in the youth justice system in Sri Lanka. *International Journal of Environmental Research and Public Health*, 15(2). 10.3390/ijerph15020209

HRCSL. (2019). *Prison study by the Human Rights Commission of Sri Lanka*. Human Rights Commission of Sri Lank. https://www.hrcsl.lk/wp-content/ uploads/2020/01/Prison-Report-Final-2.pdf

Mental Diseases Ordinance 1956 (Sri Lanka). http://www.health.gov.lk/moh_final/ english/public/elfinder/files/publications/publishpolicy/7_Mental%20Health.pdf.

Ministry of Justice. (2021). *Annual performance report of the year 2021*. Ministry of Justice Sri Lanka. https://www.moj.gov.lk/images/pdf/progress_report/2021/ English.pdf

Nadaraja, T. (1997). *The legal system of Ceylon in its historical setting (Asian studies)* (p. 311). Brill Academic Pub.

NDDCB. (2019). *National prevalence survey on drug use – 2019*. National Dangerous Drugs Control Board (NDDCB). http://www.nddcb.gov.lk/Docs/ research/National%20Prevalence%20Survey%20on%20Drugs%20Use %202019.pdf

Pinto, M. (2017). *Report of the Special Rapporteur on the Independence of Judges and Lawyers on her mission to Sri Lanka (Report of the Special Rapporteur on the Independence of Judges and Lawyers)*. United Nations. https://digitallibrary.un.org/record/1301719?ln=en

Prisons Ordinance 1980 (Sri Lanka).

Raja, S., Wood, S. K., de Menil, V., & Mannarath, S. C. (2010). Mapping mental health finances in Ghana, Uganda, Sri Lanka, India and Lao PDR. *International Journal of Mental Health Systems, 4*, 11. 10.1186/1752-4458-4-11

Rajapaksa, L., De Silva, P., Abeykoon, P., Somatunga, L., Sathasivam, S., Perera, S., Fernando, E., De Silva, D., Perera, A., Perera, U., & Weerasekara, Y. (2021). Sri Lanka health system review (Health Systems in Transition, Vol. 10, No. 1). *New Delhi: World Health Organization (on behalf of the Asia Pacific Observatory on Health Systems and Policies)*. https://apps.who.int/iris/handle/10665/342323

Randeniya, B., & Weerasooriya, W. A. (1989). Smoking patterns in Sri Lanka. *Colombo, Sri Lanka: National Cancer Control Program*.

Senanayake, B., Darshana, T., Wathsala, H., & Tissera, N. (Eds.). (2021). *Handbook of drug abuse information 2021*. National Dangerous Drugs Control Board (NDDCB). http://www.nddcb.gov.lk/Docs/research/Handbook_of_Drug_Abuse_Information_2021.pdf

Sutton, M., & DeSilva-Ranasinghe, S. (2016). *Transnational crime in Sri Lanka: Future considerations for international cooperation*. Australian Strategic Policy Institute. https://s3-ap-southeast-2.amazonaws.com/ad-aspi/import/SR94_Sri-Lanka.pdf?_uwZvpXxdXtxWaHS3FfIVy6Qnb6d9wBC

The Global Initiative Against Transnational Organized Crime (GIATOC). (2021). *Global organised crime index 2021*. The Global Initiative Against Transnational Organized Crime. https://ocindex.net/assets/downloads/global-ocindex-report.pdf

UNICEF. (2021). *Budget brief: Health sector – Sri Lanka 2021*. UNICEF Sri Lanka. https://www.unicef.org/srilanka/media/2716/file/BUDGET%20BRIEF:%20HEALTH%20SECTOR%202021.pdf

United Nations Office on Drugs and Crime (UNODC). (2019). *Global study on homicide 2019*. United Nations Office on Drugs and Crime.

WHO. (2018). *Global status report on alcohol and health 2018*. World Health Organisation. https://www.who.int/publications/i/item/9789241565639

WHO. (2022). *Mental health atlas 2020 country profile: Sri Lanka*. World Health Organisation (WHO). https://www.who.int/publications/m/item/mental-health-atlas-lka-2020-country-profile

Wickramasekera, N. (2017). *Alternative sentencing in Sri Lanka and its challenges from a rehabilitative perspective*. https://www.unafei.or.jp/publications/pdf/RS_No114/No114_11_PART_ONE_Participants_Papers_04.pdf

World Bank. (2022). *Sri Lanka. World Bank Data*. https://data.worldbank.org/country/LK

World Food Programme (WFP). (2022). *Sri Lanka: Rising prices reduce access to food for millions*. World Food Programme (WFP). https://www.wfp.org/stories/sri-lanka-rising-prices-reduce-access-food-millions

World Prison Brief. (2021). *Sri Lanka*. World Prison Brief. https://www.prisonstudies.org/country/sri-lanka

CONCLUSION

15

CULTURALLY RESPONSIVE OFFENDER REHABILITATION

Future Directions

Brandon Burgess and Alicia Nijdam-Jones

Introduction

Most existing models of rehabilitation, such as the Risk-Reed-Responsivity framework (RNR; Bonta & Andrews, 2017) and Good Lives Model (GLM; Ward, 2002), utilise a universal (etic) approach to rehabilitation. However, there is growing recognition of the need to incorporate cultural considerations and safety into rehabilitation services using culturally specific (emic) perspectives. An emic approach emphasises culture as a critical context for human behaviour. As cultural influences may play an essential role in individuals' cognitions, assumptions, and behaviours, it is vital to understand how cultural factors may impact rehabilitation services and how culturally adapted treatments may improve outcomes for individuals involved in the criminal legal system. This chapter aims to identify future directions for developing and implementing culturally-specific rehabilitation models for those involved in legal systems in Asian contexts.

Challenges to Culturally Informed Practice in Asia

A fundamental challenge to providing recommendations for developing culturally safe rehabilitation services in Asia is the diverse array of unique cultural and sociopolitical contexts found across this region. As highlighted in other chapters of this text, the correctional systems of some Asian countries may not have well-developed correctional mental health services or programming regimes. Other countries may face additional

DOI: 10.4324/9781003360919-20

challenges, such as overpopulated penal systems, geographical challenges, and resource limitations. This means that implementing culturally informed rehabilitation services and the respective challenges will vary from country to country. For example, practical barriers such as political climate, policy, and institutional structure can significantly challenge the development and successful implementation of culturally informed programmes. The countries highlighted in this chapter (i.e., New Zealand, Canada, and Australia) were chosen because they have taken significant steps to address cultural safety in corrections. While progress in this process of working towards culturally safe correctional practice is ongoing, part of the success in these endeavours has been due to specific cultural climate, systemic changes, and external pressures allowing these efforts to proceed (Nielsen, 2003).

In Canada, for instance, longstanding agreements between the government of Canada and Indigenous peoples have resulted in initiatives for culturally informed corrections, such as Section 81 of the *Corrections and Conditional Release Act* (1992; discussed further below) being codified in law. Between 2007 and 2015, the Canadian government invested approximately 72 million dollars in the Truth and Reconciliation Commission of Canada (TRC) to highlight the impact of systemic traumas caused by the residential school system (Government of Canada, 2022). The TRC produced a comprehensive list of calls to action to address historical and ongoing harms to the Indigenous peoples of Canada, including specific recommendations for changes in law and corrections to provide more culturally adapted and safe services (Truth and Reconciliation Commission of Canada, 2015).

Another example from New Zealand is the Treaty of Waitangi Act (1975) and subsequent Waitangi Tribunal created to address breaches of treaties between the Māori people and the New Zealand Government (Waitangi Tribunal, 2014). Increased attention to Māori issues culminated in initiatives beginning in the late 80s to modify the New Zealand correctional system (Ara Poutama) to better address identified issues (Hamer et al., 2021). The most recent of these attempts is the Hōkai Rangi strategy, an overarching initiative to improve outcomes of Māori involved in the legal system. Many countries in Asia may not have the existing foundations in place nor the political climate necessary to proceed with such initiatives without significant advocacy efforts to start the process (Nielsen, 2003).

It is important to note that political climate also has a drastic influence in countries which have already taken steps to include cultural safety in correctional programming. For example, in Canada, the Harper administration (2006–2015) was marked by increased support for more punitive correctional practices (Nielsen, 2016). Under this government, existing programmes experienced an extended period of stagnation (Nielsen, 2016). These ebbs and flows can significantly impact resources such as support, funding, and the ability to staff such programmes. Developing, implementing, and maintaining these programmes is complex and requires cooperation and buy-in at all levels of government, corrections, and the public.

With the previously identified challenges in mind, the following sections will provide an overview of commonly used rehabilitation models, describe the concept of cultural safety, and highlight specific examples. The goal of this chapter is to offer potential guidance on how existing Western rehabilitation models could be tailored for the specific needs, preferences, and cultural context of Asian countries.

Risk, Needs, Responsivity and the Good Lives Model

Two prominently used frameworks for rehabilitation services and crime prevention are the RNR (Bonta & Andrews, 2017) and GLM (Ward, 2002) frameworks. The RNR and GLM models have been adopted for practice in Canada, the United States, Britain, Europe, New Zealand, and Australia (Ward et al., 2007; Zeccola et al., 2021). Briefly, the RNR model focuses on three core principles which are used to guide incarceration and treatment parameters (i.e., risk, need, and responsivity) as well as eight central risk factors which predict criminal involvement (Bonta & Andrews, 2017). Despite its wide acceptance and the significant body of meta-analytical research supporting the effectiveness of the RNR model for reducing recidivism (Bonta & Andrews, 2017; Bonta et al., 2014; Gutierrez et al., 2013; Hanson et al., 2009; Smith et al., 2009), the model is not without criticism.

Of relevance to this book, the RNR model has been criticised because of its shallow consideration of the influence of cultural factors in offending and rehabilitation (Strauss-Hughes et al., 2022). Although culture is ostensibly captured by the "responsivity" factor of the RNR model, a common criticism is that "responsivity" is often neglected in actual practice, leading to a "one size fits all" application of the framework (Gannon & Ward, 2014; Ward et al., 2007). In addition, many authors have highlighted that the RNR model's focus on criminogenic factors and risk mitigation has rendered the model incompatible with many Indigenous group's traditional values and beliefs (Cunneen & Tauri, 2016; Leaming & Willis, 2016; Strauss-Hughes et al., 2019).

In response to criticisms of the RNR model, the GLM of rehabilitation was developed as a strengths-based approach focused on improving the individual's overall well-being to promote prosocial behaviour (Ward, 2002). Core to the GLM framework is the idea of "primary goods," phenomena that are fundamentally beneficial to humans and contribute to living a "good life" (Prescott & Willis, 2022; Ward, 2002; Ward & Stewart, 2003). Those working under the GLM approach focus on developing an individual's skills and capabilities in obtaining these primary goods, thus increasing the likelihood of desistance from antisocial behaviour (Ward, 2002; Ward & Stewart, 2003). Although the GLM model has been incorporated into clinical and correctional practice in multiple countries, empirical support for reducing recidivism using the GLM approach is limited (Netto et al., 2014; Zeccola et al., 2021).

The substantial body of empirical research and three decades of momentum behind the RNR model means it remains the dominant framework for rehabilitation services and treatment (Bourgon et al., 2018). The influence of the model can be seen in risk assessment and treatment interventions in Canada, Britain, the United States, Australia, and New Zealand (Ward et al., 2007; Zeccola et al., 2021) and has been touched on to varying degrees in research and practice throughout many countries in Europe and Asia including Singapore (Chua et al., 2014), Pakistan (Gul et al., 2021), the Philippines (Spruit et al., 2016), Indonesia (Arham & Runturambi, 2020), and Turkey (Tuncer et al., 2020). The focus on targeting risk and criminogenic factors has become a fundamental feature of rehabilitation efforts. Although the RNR model remains the most prevalent rehabilitation framework, the need for culturally informed practice in corrections and rehabilitation services grows increasingly evident. Service providers looking to adapt these models to audiences in Asia should consider the criticisms and limitations of these approaches.

Etic and Emic Approaches

To some extent, the GLM and RNR models focus on universal factors contributing to the etiology, maintenance, or prevention of criminal offending. This "universal" foundation places both models as etic approaches to rehabilitation when used cross-culturally. The etic perspective is based on the assumption of universality. Scholars and clinicians who utilise this approach emphasise similarities and differences across cultures by studying similar objects (e.g., aggression) and comparison standards (e.g., measurable levels of aggression using specific tools) rather than culturally specific norms, values, practices, or beliefs that could influence the object of study (Helfrich, 1999; Triandis, 1992).

Concerning rehabilitation programmes, etic approaches rely on universal factors and commonalities between groups and assume that theories and practices can be equally applied across cultural groups (Helfrich, 1999). Research and intervention practices based on an etic approach treat culture as an external influence that can highlight similarities and differences between cultures by focusing on a particular factor (e.g., response to offending) rather than considering how cultural factors and influence can affect those factors. For example, a fundamental assumption of the RNR framework is that the "big eight" criminogenic factors equally represent the risk of offending across all groups (Bonta & Andrews, 2017). Similarly, the GLM approach takes for granted that its outlined primary goods are intrinsic aspects of human nature and that the values con- tributing to "a good life" are equally valued across different cultures. This is particularly evident in the model's emphasis on autonomy and personal agency, which more collectivist cultures may not value (Prescott & Willis, 2022; Ward, 2002). Although the GLM has been adapted for use with diverse cultural populations (e.g., Māori groups: Leaming & Willis, 2016; Strauss-Hughes et al., 2022), its etic underpinnings necessitate a practi- tioner's understanding of the importance of cultural influences, a motiva- tion for incorporating these factors into the GLM framework, as well as an understanding of the limitations of the model (Prescott & Willis, 2022).

Practices which proceed and centre themselves around cultural consid- erations and perspectives in mind are known as emic approaches. Unlike etic approaches, which are intended to be implemented universally across groups, emic approaches are meant to incorporate culturally relevant considerations into practice (Helfrich, 1999). Emic approaches consider culture to fundamentally influence human behaviour (Helfrich, 1999). An individual's culture influences their values, decision-making processes, assumptions, and behaviours, including how or when they engage in violence or respond to aggression (Krug et al., 2002). In research and practice, etic and emic approaches are often integrated as both approaches have individual pros and cons that may be balanced when used in tandem.

Cultural Competency, Safety, and Responsiveness

When working with justice-involved individuals with diverse social, cultural, and linguistic needs, it is critical to adapt etic approaches to rehabilitation to be more culturally centred and responsive. Beginning in the late 1980s, clinical health professionals have become aware of the need to integrate cultural considerations in the design and delivery of services with the development of the construct of cultural competency (Cross et al., 1989). Cultural competency emphasises the need for individual providers and organisations to be aware of the behaviours, attitudes and policies that impact cross-cultural care and acknowledge and incorporate cultural knowledge in adapting services to respond to individuals' culturally unique needs (Cross et al., 1989). Often used interchangeably with other terms, such as cultural awareness, cultural sensitivity, cultural humility, cultural security, cultural respect, cultural adaptation, and transcultural competence or effectiveness (Curtis et al., 2019), cultural competency focuses on the development of knowledge, skills, and attitudes to improve services. Cultural competency is often critiqued because some believe it is something that can be achieved rather than something that should be continually developed and improved.

As our understanding of the impacts of structural racism and power differentials in health settings has grown, the emphasis has increasingly been placed on the importance of cultural safety and responsiveness in intervention and treatment practices. Cultural safety originated in the New Zealand healthcare context, specifically in working with Indigenous peoples, to address the limitations of cultural competency frameworks. It differs from cultural competency in that it moves the onus of responsibility onto the clinician and health setting to examine how interpersonal power dynamics and bias can impact the care the client receives rather than merely focusing on the client's context and their unique cultural, social, or linguistic characteristics. Developing cultural safety involves creating healthcare environments built on models of social justice and the need for equitable care and respect across cultural groups (McGough et al., 2018). To develop culturally safe services and spaces, service providers must reflect and challenge power differentials such as "repression, social domination, and structural variables such as class and power" (Doutrich et al., 2012, p. 144) and return power to the client. This is even more critical in the correctional and forensic context, where justice-involved individuals working toward recovery and rehabilitation are often stigmatised and disempowered across many contexts. Cultural competency and cultural safety are essential frameworks for forensic mental health and correctional contexts. Cultural competency necessitates professionals to continually develop their knowledge, skills, and understanding while working with diverse clients. On the other hand, cultural safety requires challenging historical power dynamics and oppression to foster equitable services.

Importance of Cultural Safety in Corrections

The consequences of systemic disempowerment in the legal system can be seen in the consistent overrepresentation of particular cultural and ethnic groups. This pattern is demonstrated across jurisdictions around the world. For example, Indigenous peoples comprise only 4% of the

Canadian population but a disproportionately large portion (29%) of the criminal legal system (Malakieh, 2019; Perreault, 2009). A similar pattern of overincarcerations can be seen in both Australia (Australian Bureau of Statistics, 2015; Durey et al., 2014) and New Zealand (Florencio et al., 2022; Nakhid & Shorter, 2014).

In Canada, a recent court case has highlighted concerns about using risk assessment measures with members of Indigenous groups or other groups not represented in the original development samples (*Ewert v. Canada*, 2018). With *Ewert*, the Supreme Court of Canada ruled that the Correctional Service of Canada must respect and be responsive to the cultural differences of those in its custody. The ruling also resulted in the court highlighting the need for researchers to demonstrate that a measure is unbiased before being used with Indigenous individuals. Similarly, Canadian courts must consider the individual circumstances and factors related to Indigenous identity when determining sentencing for Indigenous individuals (Criminal Code of Canada, 1985; *R. v. Gladue*, 1999).

Despite an increasing focus on the necessity of culturally safe practices in the world's legal systems, research on these practices is still quite limited. There is limited quantitative research evaluating the effectiveness of culturally responsive rehabilitation programmes for the reduction of recidivism. One meta-analytic review of correctional programmes offered by Correctional Services Canada (CSC) found a significant reduction in rates of recidivism in Indigenous service users who took part in correctional programming over those who did not (Usher & Stewart, 2014); however, this study did not specifically examine those who completed culturally safe programmes. A more recent meta-analysis of seven studies (*N* = 1731) examining correctional programmes which incorporated things such as traditional Indigenous practices and medicines, facilitation by community Elders, and Indigenous language found a decrease in recidivism for Indigenous individuals who took part in generic correctional programming (Gutierrez et al., 2018). Although the effect of culturally informed treatment was positive, the researchers highlighted the need for additional high-quality evaluations of culturally informed correctional programming.

Evaluating Culturally Responsive Rehabilitation Programmes

Research on culturally informed correctional practices often relies on qualitative methods such as narrative reviews and analyses of interviews with relevant stakeholders (e.g., past or present service users, staff, appropriate community members). Researchers emphasise the importance of conducting qualitative research with Indigenous communities to centre inquiry around their unique cultural perspectives by promoting their voices in programme development (e.g., Peltier, 2018). Additionally, Indigenous groups may be reluctant to engage in research suspected to be exploitative, especially in the context of corrections (Cunneen & Tauri, 2016). Participatory action research and community-based participatory research are essential and relevant approaches for conducting research with Indigenous communities and members of other cultural groups. Participatory action research seeks to include relevant community members and stakeholders throughout the research process to bridge the gap between research and practice (Munro et al., 2017), whereas community-based participatory research aims to develop equitable partnerships and co-learning between researchers and the community. Participatory research embodies an emic perspective to developing or evaluating services and seeks to promote respectful, reciprocal, and responsible research with Indigenous communities (Peltier, 2018).

As the goals of qualitative studies which use participatory research methods are grounded in the perspectives and values of those with lived experiences, much of the current research on culturally informed practice in legal settings does not include recidivism as an outcome measure. Researchers have highlighted issues with relying solely on recidivism as the definitive indicator of programme success due to its complex determinants; as such it may be unreasonable to expect a single programme or initiative to directly impact recidivism rates (e.g., Putt et al., 2005). Studies on culturally safe correctional programming emphasise factors such as greater motivation to participate in programming, higher programme completion rates, and service user outcomes such as increased well-being and connection to community and culture (Gutierrez et al., 2018). Although reducing recidivism rates is an important outcome of correctional programming, increases in user outcomes, such as increased willingness to participate in programming, correspond to an improvement in the "responsivity" of a programme, leading to more effective intervention overall, as per the RNR model. It is also important to note that in developing culturally safe rehabilitation programmes, service users may have many unique needs that must be addressed to ensure meaningful participation and treatment involvement.

Examples of Culturally Informed and Safe Practices

Correctional Institution-based Programmes/Practices

The earliest attempts to incorporate culturally informed practice into rehabilitation services occurred in correctional institutions. It gradually became understood that involving cultural practices in corrections led to improved outcomes and well-being for people belonging to Indigenous groups and increased Indigenous participation in correctional programming (Cox et al., 2009; Thakker, 2013; Zellerer, 2003). For example, in the early 1980s, Correctional Services Canada began allowing Indigenous people to participate in sweat lodges within prison walls, a common cultural practice amongst some Canadian Indigenous groups (Waldram, 1997). Since this time, cultural practices in correctional facilities have expanded to include things such as access to Elder-guided ceremonies, smudging, pow-wows, traditional art and music, carving, engagement with the community, sacred circles, and sacred medicines (Nielsen, 2003; Thakker, 2013; Trevethan et al., 2007). These inclusions aimed to address historical and ongoing trauma faced by Indigenous groups by reconnecting them with cultural practices, potentially enhancing responsiveness to rehabilitation programmes.

Over time, many countries and jurisdictions have developed correctional programmes which attempt to merge cultural practices with standard correctional programming. For example, one of North America's first culturally informed correctional programmes was a family violence programme implemented at Stony Mountain Institution in Manitoba, Canada (Zellerer, 2003). The programme was developed by the Ma Mawi Wi Chi Itata Centre (a community-based Indigenous services agency) and modified in conjunction with Correctional Services Canada (CSC) for delivery within the institution (Zellerer, 2003). The programme activities took place over four months and included group discussions, cultural ceremonies, and participating in sweat lodges. Although recidivism was not an explored outcome of the programme, evaluators identified high satisfaction with the programme from both staff and inmates. Many of those who participated in the programme gained benefits such as developing a better understanding of their violence, developing skills such as communication, and having an opportunity to learn about and engage with their cultural heritage.

Another notable example of a culturally informed correctional programme is the Tu Tahanga violence programme in Aotearoa/New Zealand (Florencio et al., 2022). The programme was adapted from the United States-based ManAlive programme (Gilligan & Lee, 2004) by a Māori cultural expert to be delivered to Māori adults in prison who had engaged in violent crime. The programme encapsulated a Māori approach to mental health (Te Whare Tapa Whā) and conflict resolution (Hohou Rongo) and provided service users with a culturally safe meeting place. A narrative review which interviewed both service users and providers highlighted several benefits of the programme, including being able to share their experiences and difficulties with others, increased emotional awareness, developing a better understanding of their pathway to violence, the development of coping skills, and a greater connection to their community. Service users also highlighted the importance of having Māori people involved in the delivery and facilitation of the programme.

Community-based Programmes and Alternatives to Traditional Correctional Institutions

Several jurisdictions have attempted to incorporate cultural safety into a more fundamental aspect of corrections than simply informing institutional programming. For example, a unique feature of the Canadian legal system is special correctional facilities known as healing lodges. These facilities are mandated by Section 81 of the *Corrections and Conditional Release Act* (1992) and represent an effort to bridge the gap between colonial correctional systems and traditional Indigenous practices (Nielsen, 2003, 2016; Trevethan et al., 2007) and to provide Indigenous communities increased latitude to provide care to their community members (Correctional Service of Canada, 2021). In this context, "healing" refers to improving an individual's physical, mental, and spiritual health and transitioning towards a prosocial lifestyle. This healing takes place through engagement with Elders, taking part in traditional knowledge and practices, and may incorporate Western counselling or therapy approaches depending on the facility.

In addition to programmes situated in correctional institutions, community-based programmes and community groups also play an essential role in the rehabilitative process. Community-based efforts can play several roles, including reducing the likelihood of recidivism through primary maintenance services (i.e., substance use programs; Ashdown et al., 2019; Munro et al., 2017), fostering and maintaining connections with the community (Nakhid & Shorter, 2014), providing recreation opportunities (English et al., 2022), and engaging in advocacy efforts. Community-based groups and communities can serve to gather and strengthen individual voices and inform the development and trajectory of programmes that will impact members of their community (Ashdown et al., 2019; Munro et al., 2017; Murdocca, 2020; Nakhid & Shorter, 2014; Wharewera-Mika et al., 2020).

Recommendations for Service Providers in Asia

To this point, the present chapter has given an overview of the frameworks for correctional rehabilitation commonly employed in Western countries. The chapter has also discussed how these approaches relate to the goals of providing culturally safe correctional programming and the potential benefits of these modifications, and highlighted several examples from research and practice. The following section offers recommendations for institutions and service providers in Asian countries to adapt these practices to their context and cultural considerations.

Actionable Steps/Recommendations

Prior to identifying several specific, actionable recommendations for service providers, it is crucial to recognise that there is a need for system-level changes to other areas of the criminal legal system. This need is especially important for countries with still-developing legal systems. While the content of this chapter has focused primarily on rehabilitation within the context of the correctional system and community resources, many aspects of the legal process may be modified to allow for culturally safe practices. As researchers have highlighted, a single programme alone is unlikely to change recidivism rates radically (Trevethan et al., 2007), just as modifying only one aspect of the interconnected web of the criminal legal system would likely have limited effect. Changes can be brought about in the courts, such as considering cultural factors in sentencing (Dickson & Smith, 2021), as well as by creating focused diversion courts (Maurutto & Hannah-Moffat, 2016) which seek to consider an individual within the unique social, cultural, and historical context which they reside, and providing individualised and culturally appropriate sentencing. This may be particularly relevant to those countries that inherited former colonial power laws. Cultural safety can also be incorporated into risk assessment practices (Muir et al., 2023; Shepherd & Anthony, 2018; Shepherd & Lewis-Fernandez, 2016; Wharewera-Mika et al., 2020) and treatment considerations (Danto & Zangeneh, 2022; Day, 2013; Durey et al., 2014; Strauss-Hughes et al., 2022). It is important to remember that the rehabilitation process does not begin or end with the correctional system.

Countries transitioning to a more rehabilitative approach in their legal and correctional systems can initiate the process by conducting research and implementing established correctional frameworks like the GLM or RNR models, tailoring them to their own nascent systems. This undertaking is no small task and may require time and effort to garner governmental and public support. It is advised that this process be done through collaboration with experts from similar countries or programmes that have already implemented the models. It is important to note that Western-developed models may not be directly translatable to Asian contexts, and so these frameworks should be adopted critically with the intent of modification to better address the cultural values of the country in question. Practice examples covered in this chapter may provide direction for how Western rehabilitation models may be tailored for Asian countries.

For countries amenable to developing culturally safe programming for their communities, service user buy-in may still pose a challenge. A fundamental hurdle of such aspirations is the process of merging culturally informed practices with a correctional system which has often played a central role in the historical and continued oppression of cultural minorities (Boyce, 2017; Murdocca, 2020). Specific concerns have arisen around correctional institutions and governments wielding a banner of cultural safety as a shield while promoting colonial hegemony (Boyce, 2017; Martel et al., 2011; Nielsen, 2016).

A commonly highlighted practical issue is that the inherent conflict between cultural practice and the correctional environment may prevent important cultural practices from occurring (Hyatt, 2020; Waldram, 1997). For example, some practices may require access to natural environments or sacred sites, which may not be feasible for incarcerated individuals (Ontario Human Rights Commission, 2015). Other factors, such as institutional requirements to search or screen sacred objects, have resulted in some Canadian Indigenous Elders refusing to conduct ceremonies within prisons (Waldram, 1997). Lack of suitability or buy-in from the targeted group may delegitimise a culturally safe programme and compromise potential benefits.

To address the issue of service user buy-in and successful incorporation of cultural safety into practice, it is crucial for service providers to approach this endeavour earnestly and collaboratively, respecting the autonomy and practices of those they are working with. A commonly highlighted issue is that individuals may be reluctant or unwilling to participate in programmes or research that appear exploitative, culturally inappropriate, or shallowly representative of their beliefs and values (Boyce, 2017). Thus, research and programme development in this area necessitates skilful and culturally informed researchers and substantial collaboration with relevant communities in developing and maintaining correctional programming (Nakhid & Shorter, 2014).

To ensure the meaningful inclusion of service users, it is essential to prioritise their voices throughout the development, staffing, implementation, and evaluation of programmes that will impact them (English et al., 2022). Successful collaboration empowers marginalised populations by giving them a voice in programmes that affect them and ensuring that programmes are relevant and valuable to the intended participants. The principles of participatory research should be integrated into programme development, while implementation should involve a continuous evaluation and improvement process. It is also important to involve cultural group members in programme delivery or guidance. For example, a common feature of culturally safe programmes for Indigenous populations is to provide access to Elders, figures of great importance in Indigenous cultures (Marchetti et al., 2022). A useful way of facilitating effective collaboration may be to connect with existing community-based organisations for guidance and support (Murdocca, 2020; Nielsen, 2003; Zellerer, 2003).

Another recommendation commonly identified through narrative reviews of Indigenous service users' experiences in corrections is that members of the relevant cultural group should be well-represented amongst programme facilitators (Durey et al., 2014; Murdocca, 2020). This both legitimises and facilitates a safe environment within the programme. Related to this, programme staff should ideally come from outside the correctional institution (Zellerer, 2003). The dynamics between an incarcerated person and a correctional officer are far too complex to facilitate a safe and trust-based environment present in many culturally adapted programmes.

A final recommendation is to maintain a willingness to step outside of the culturally dominant paradigms and values of the country in which you are operating from. Researchers and clinicians should actively embrace cultural humility and recognise that they are not experts on what is "right" for culturally or linguistically diverse groups. For instance, many Indigenous groups favour a more holistic approach to understanding mental health and may not recognise or respond to colonially-influenced approaches (e.g., Durey et al., 2014; Florencio et al., 2022). For example, when working with Indigenous populations in Western contexts, it is important to be prepared to set aside the Western biomedical model paradigm for conceptualising mental health and the treatment of mental illnesses (Day, 2013; Durey et al., 2014). This underscores the importance of modifying existing practices such as the RNR or GLM frameworks when adapting them to an Asian context. The degree of cultural diversity in Asian countries may present additional obstacles to creating meaningful culturally safe programmes. Terms such as "Indigenous" are often used to encompass diverse peoples, cultures, languages, and traditions (Martel et al., 2011). A one-size-fits-all approach to such heterogeneity can delegitimise a programme, exclude certain groups, and undermine programme effectiveness (Hyatt, 2020; Nakhid & Shorter, 2014). It is therefore essential to consider and address within-group diversity in programme design and implementation.

References

Arham, L., & Runturambi, A. J. S. (2020). Kebijakan Perlakuan Narapidana Teroris Menggunakan Risk Need Responsivity (RNR) di Lembaga Pemasyarakatan Kelas I Cipinang. *Deviance: Jurnal Kriminologi, 4*(1), 45–66.

Ashdown, J. D., Treharne, G. J., Neha, T., Dixon, B., & Aitken, C. (2019). Māori men's experiences of rehabilitation in the Moana House Therapeutic Community in Aotearoa/New Zealand: A qualitative enquiry. *International Journal of Offender Therapy and Comparative Criminology, 63*(5), 734–751. 10.1177/0306624X18808675

Australian Bureau of Statistics. (2015). *Prisoners in Australia, 2015. Catalogue 4517.0.* https://www.abs.gov.au/AUSSTATS/abs@.nsf/Lookup/4517.0Main +Features100002015?OpenDocument

Bonta, J., & Andrews, D. A. (2017). *The psychology of criminal conduct* (6th ed.). Routledge.

Bonta, J., Blais, J., & Wilson, H. A. (2014). A theoretically informed meta-analysis of the risk for general and violent recidivism for mentally disordered offenders. *Aggression and Violent Behavior, 19*(3), 278–287. 10.1016/j.avb.2014.04.014

Bourgon, G., Mugford, R., Hanson, R. K., & Coligado, M. (2018). Offender risk assessment practices vary across Canada. *Canadian Journal of Criminology and Criminal Justice, 60*(2), 167–205. 10.3138/cjccj.2016-0024

Boyce, M. R. (2017). Carceral Recognition and the Colonial Present at the Okimaw Ohci Healing Lodge. *Sites: A Journal of Social Anthropology and Cultural Studies, 14*(1), Article 1. 10.11157/sites-vol14iss1id345

Chua, J. R., Chu, C. M., Yim, G., Chong, D., & Teoh, J. (2014). Implementation of the Risk–Need–Responsivity framework across the juvenile justice agencies in Singapore. *Psychiatry, Psychology and Law, 21*(6), 877–889. 10.1080/ 13218719.2014.918076

Correctional Service of Canada. (2021). *Indigenous healing lodges.* Correctional Service Canada. https://www.csc-scc.gc.ca/002/003/002003-2000-en.shtml

Corrections and conditional release act, C.20 § 81 (1992).

Cox, D., Young, M., & Bairnsfather-Scott, A. (2009). No justice without healing: Australian Aboriginal people and family violence. *Australian Feminist Law Journal, 30*(1), 151–161. 10.1080/13200968.2009.10854421

Criminal Code of Canada, RSC, (1985), c C-46.

Cross, T., Bazron, B., & Isaacs, M. (1989). *Towards a culturally competent system of care: A monograph on effective services for minority children who are severely emotionally disturbed.* CASSP Technical Assistance Centre. Georgetown University Child Development Centre.

Cunneen, C., & Tauri, J. (2016). *Indigenous criminology.* Policy Press.

Curtis, E., Jones, R., Tipene-Leach, D., Walker, C., Loring, B., Paine, S.-J., & Reid, P. (2019). Why cultural safety rather than cultural competency is required to achieve health equity: A literature review and recommended definition. *International Journal for Equity in Health, 18*(174). 10.1186/s12939-019-1 082-3

Danto, D., & Zangeneh, M. (Eds.). (2022). *Indigenous knowledge and mental health: A global perspective.* Springer International Publishing. 10.1007/978-3-030-71346-1

Day, A. (2013). Chapter 18. Culturally responsive CBT in forensic settings. In *Forensic CBT*. John Wiley & Sons, Ltd. 10.1002/9781118589878.ch18

Dickson, J., & Smith, K. (2021). Exploring the Canadian judiciary's experiences with and perceptions of Gladue. *Canadian Journal of Criminology and Criminal Justice*, 63(3–4), 23–46. 10.3138/cjccj.2021-0031

Doutrich, D., Arcus, K., Dekker, L., Spuck, J., & Pollock-Robinson, C. (2012). Cultural safety in New Zealand and the United States: Looking at a way forward together. *Journal of Transcultural Nursing*, 23(2), 143–150. 10.1177/1043659611433873

Durey, A., Wynaden, D., & O'Kane, M. (2014). Improving forensic mental health care to Indigenous Australians: Theorizing the intercultural space. *Journal of Psychiatric and Mental Health Nursing*, 21(4), 296–302. 10.1111/jpm.12105

English, M., Wallace, L., Evans, J., Diamond, S., & Caperchione, C. M. (2022). The impact of sport and physical activity programs on the mental health and social and emotional wellbeing of young Aboriginal and Torres Strait Islander Australians: A systematic review. *Preventive Medicine Reports*, 25, 101676. 10.1016/j.pmedr.2021.101676

Ewert v. Canada, (S.C.C. 30 2018).

Florencio, F., Healee, D., Ratahi, T., Wiki, N., & McKenna, B. (2022). Tū Tahanga: A qualitative descriptive study of a culturally adapted violence prevention programme in a forensic mental health service. *International Journal of Forensic Mental Health*, 21(2), 185–193. 10.1080/14999013.2021.1953194

Gannon, T. A., & Ward, T. (2014). Where has all the psychology gone? *Aggression and Violent Behavior*, 19(4), 435–446. 10.1016/j.avb.2014.06.006

Gilligan, J., & Lee, B. (2004). Beyond the prison paradigm: From provoking violence to preventing it by creating 'anti-prisons' (residential colleges and therapeutic communities) *Annals of the New York Academy of Sciences*, 1036, 300–324. 10.1196/annals.1330.030

Government of Canada. (2022). *Truth and Reconciliation Commission of Canada*. https://www.rcaanc-cirnac.gc.ca/eng/1450124405592/1529106060525

Gul, R., Muhammad, B., & Hussain, R. (2021). An analysis of Risk-Need-Responsivity Model to reform Pakistan's prisons. *Pakistan Journal of Criminology*, 13(3), 64–73.

Gutierrez, L., Chadwick, N., & Wanamaker, K. A. (2018). Culturally relevant programming versus the status quo: A meta-analytic review of the effectiveness of treatment of Indigenous offenders. *Canadian Journal of Criminology and Criminal Justice*, 60(3), 321–353. 10.3138/cjccj.2017-0020.r2

Gutierrez, L., Wilson, H. A., Rugge, T., & Bonta, J. (2013). The prediction of recidivism with Aboriginal offenders: A theoretically informed meta-analysis. *Canadian Journal of Criminology and Criminal Justice*, 55(1), 55–99. 10.3138/cjccj.2011.E.51

Hamer, P., Paul, J., & Hunia, M. (2021). Hōkai Rangi: Context and background to the development of Ara Poutama Aotearoa Strategy 2019-2024. *Practice: The New Zealand Correction Journal*, 8(1), 18–22.

Hanson, R. K., Bourgon, G., Helmus, L., & Hodgson, S. (2009). The principles of effective correctional treatment also apply to sexual offenders: A meta-analysis. *Criminal Justice and Behavior*, 36(9), 865–891. 10.1177/0093854809338545

Helfrich, H. (1999). Beyond the dilemma of cross-cultural psychology: Resolving the tension between etic and emic approaches. *Culture & Psychology, 5*(2), 131–153. 10.1177/1354067X9952002

Hyatt, A. (2020). Healing through culture for incarcerated Aboriginal people. *First Peoples Child & Family Review, 14*(1), 182–195. 10.7202/1071295ar

Krug, E., Dahlberg, L., Mercy, J., Zwi, A., & Lozano, R. (2002). *World report on violence and health*. World Health Organization.

Leaming, N., & Willis, G. M. (2016). The Good Lives Model: New avenues for Māori rehabilitation? *Sexual Abuse in Australia & New Zealand, 7*(1), 59–69.

Malakieh, J. (2019). Adult and youth correctional statistics in Canada, 2017/2018. *Juristat, 85-002-X*, 1–26.

Marchetti, E., Woodland, S., Saunders, V., Barclay, L., & Beetson, B. (2022). Listening to country: A prison pilot project that connects Aboriginal and Torres Strait Islander women on remand to Country. *Current Issues in Criminal Justice, 34*(2), 155–170. 10.1080/10345329.2021.2018813

Martel, J., Brassard, R., & Jaccoud, M. (2011). When two worlds collide: Aboriginal risk management in Canadian corrections. *The British Journal of Criminology, 51*(2), 235–255. 10.1093/bjc/azr003

Maurutto, P., & Hannah-Moffat, K. (2016). Aboriginal knowledges in specialized courts: Emerging practices in Gladue Courts. *Canadian Journal of Law and Society, 31*(3), 451–471.

McGough, S., Wynaden, D., & Wright, M. (2018). Experience of providing cultural safety in mental health to Aboriginal patients: A grounded theory study. *International Journal of Mental Health Nursing, 27*(1), 204–213. 10.1111/inm.12310

Muir, N. M., Viljoen, J. L., & Shepherd, S. M. (2023). Violence risk assessment tools and Indigenous peoples: Colonialism as an underlying cause of risk ratings on the SAVRY. *International Journal of Forensic Mental Health*, 1–13. 10.1 080/14999013.2023.2178554

Munro, A., Shakeshaft, A., & Clifford, A. (2017). The development of a healing model of care for an Indigenous drug and alcohol residential rehabilitation service: A community-based participatory research approach. *Health & Justice, 5*(1), 1–12. 10.1186/s40352-017-0056-z

Murdocca, C. (2020). Re-imagining 'serving time' in Indigenous communities. *Canadian Journal of Women & the Law, 32*(1), 31–60. 10.3138/cjwl.32.1.02

Nakhid, C., & Shorter, L. T. (2014). Narratives of four Māori ex-inmates about their experiences and perspectives of rehabilitation programmes. *International Journal of Offender Therapy and Comparative Criminology, 58*(6), 697–717. 10.1177/0306624X13476939

Netto, N. R., Carter, J. M., & Bonell, C. (2014). A systematic review of interventions that adopt the "Good Lives" approach to offender rehabilitation. *Journal of Offender Rehabilitation, 53*(6), 403–432. 10.1080/10509674.2014.931746

Nielsen, M. O. (2003). Canadian aboriginal healing lodges: A model for the United States? *The Prison Journal, 83*(1), 67–89. 10.1177/0032885502250394

Nielsen, M. O. (2016). Aboriginal healing lodges in Canada: Still going strong? Still worth implementing in the USA? *The Journal of Legal Pluralism and Unofficial Law, 48*(2), 322–345. 10.1080/07329113.2016.1157377

Ontario Human Rights Commission. (2015). *Policy on preventing discrimination based on creed.* https://www.ohrc.on.ca/en/policy-preventing-discrimination-based-creed/11-indigenous-spiritual-practices

Peltier, C. (2018). An application of Two-Eyed Seeing: Indigenous research methods with participatory action research. *International Journal of Qualitative Methods, 17*(1), 160940691881234. 10.1177/1609406918812346

Perreault, S. (2009). *The incarceration of Aboriginal people in adult correctional services.* Statistics Canada. http://www.statcan.gc.ca/pub/85-002-x/2009003/article/10903-eng.htm

Prescott, D. S., & Willis, G. M. (2022). Using the good lives model (GLM) in clinical practice: Lessons learned from international implementation projects. *Aggression and Violent Behavior, 63,* 101717. 10.1016/j.avb.2021.101717

Putt, J., Payne, J., & Milner, L. (2005). Indigenous male offending and substance abuse. Trends & Issues in crime and criminology. *Trends & Issues in Crime and Criminal Justice, 293.* https://www.aic.gov.au/publications/tandi/tandi293

R. v. Gladue, (1 SCR 688 1999).

Shepherd, S. M., & Anthony, T. (2018). Popping the cultural bubble of violence risk assessment tools. *The Journal of Forensic Psychiatry & Psychology, 29*(2), 211–220. 10.1080/14789949.2017.1354055

Shepherd, S. M., & Lewis-Fernandez, R. (2016). Forensic risk assessment and cultural diversity: Contemporary challenges and future directions. *Psychology, Public Policy, and Law, 22*(4), 427–438. 10.1037/law0000102

Smith, P., Gendreau, P., & Swartz, K. (2009). Validating the principles of effective intervention: A systematic review of the contributions of meta-analysis in the field of corrections. *Victims & Offenders, 4*(2), 148–169. 10.1080/15564880802612581

Spruit, A., Wissink, I. B., & Stams, G. J. J. M. (2016). The care of Filipino juvenile offenders in residential facilities evaluated using the risk-need-responsivity model. *International Journal of Law and Psychiatry, 47,* 181–188. 10.1016/j.ijlp.2016.04.005

Strauss-Hughes, A., Heffernan, R., & Ward, T. (2019). A cultural–ecological perspective on agency and offending behaviour. *Psychiatry, Psychology & Law, 26*(6), 938–958. 10.1080/13218719.2019.1644250

Strauss-Hughes, A., Ward, T., & Neha, T. (2022). Considering practice frameworks for culturally diverse populations in the correctional domain. *Aggression and Violent Behavior, 63,* 101673. 10.1016/j.avb.2021.101673

Thakker, J. (2013). The role of cultural factors in treatment. In *What Works in Offender Rehabilitation* (pp. 387–407). John Wiley & Sons, Ltd. 10.1002/9781118320655.ch21

Treaty of Waitangi Act 1975, No. 114.

Trevethan, S., Crutcher, N., Moore, J.-P., & Mileto, J. (2007). *Pê Sâkâstêw Centre: An in-depth examination of a healing lodge for federally incarcerated offenders (Research Reports).* Research Branch Correctional Service of Canada. https://www.csc-scc.gc.ca/research/r170-eng.shtml

Triandis, H. C. (1992). Cross-cultural research in social psychology. In *Social judgement and intergroup relations: Essays in honour of Muzafer Sherif* (pp. 229–243). Springer.

Truth and Reconciliation Commission of Canada. (2015). *Truth and Reconciliation Commission of Canada: Calls to action.* https://nctr.ca/records/reports/

Tuncer, A. E., Erdem, G., & de Ruiter, C. (2020). The impact of a brief RNR-based training on Turkish juvenile probation officers' punitive and rehabilitative attitudes and recidivism risk perceptions. *Journal of Community Psychology, 48*(3), 921–931. 10.1002/jcop.22310

Usher, A. M., & Stewart, L. A. (2014). Effectiveness of correctional programs with ethnically diverse offenders: A meta-analytic study. *International Journal of Offender Therapy and Comparative Criminology, 58*(2), 209–230. 10.1177/03 06624X12469507

Waitangi Tribunal. (2014). *Strategic direction 2014–2025.* https://www. waitangitribunal.govt.nz/assets/Strategic-Direction-2014-2025.pdf

Waldram, J. (1997). *The way of the pipe: Aboriginal spirituality and symbolic healing in Canadian prisons.* Broadview Press.

Ward, T. (2002). The management of risk and the design of good lives. *Australian Psychologist, 37*(3), 172–179. 10.1080/00050060210001706846

Ward, T., Melser, J., & Yates, P. M. (2007). Reconstructing the Risk–Need–Responsivity model: A theoretical elaboration and evaluation. *Aggression and Violent Behavior, 12*(2), 208–228. 10.1016/j.avb.2006.07.001

Ward, T., & Stewart, C. A. (2003). The treatment of sex offenders: Risk management and good lives. *Professional Psychology: Research and Practice, 34*(4), 353–360. 10.1037/0735-7028.34.4.353

Wharewera-Mika, J., Cooper, E., Wiki, N., Prentice, K., Field, T., Cavney, J., Kaire, D., & McKenna, B. (2020). The appropriateness of DUNDRUM-3 and DUNDRUM-4 for Māori in forensic mental health services in New Zealand: Participatory action research. *BMC Psychiatry, 20*(1), 61. 10.1186/s12888-020-2468-x

Zeccola, J., Kelty, S. F., & Boer, D. (2021). Does the good lives model work? A systematic review of the recidivism evidence. *The Journal of Forensic Practice, 23*(3), 285–300. 10.1108/JFP-03-2021-0010

Zellerer, E. (2003). Culturally competent programs: The first family violence program for Aboriginal men in prison. *The Prison Journal, 83*(2), 171–190. 10.1177/0032885503083002004

INDEX

9 781032 418674